Handbook of
Psychology and Health

Volume III

Cardiovascular
Disorders
and
Behavior

Handbook of
Psychology and Health

Volume III

Cardiovascular
Disorders
and
Behavior

edited by

DAVID S. KRANTZ
ANDREW BAUM
JEROME E. SINGER
Uniformed Services University of the Health Sciences

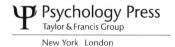

Psychology Press
Taylor & Francis Group

New York London

First Published by
Lawrence Erlbaum Associates, Inc., Publishers
365 Broadway
Hillsdale, New Jersey 07642

Transferred to Digital Printing 2009 by Psychology Press
270 Madison Ave, New York NY 10016
27 Church Road, Hove, East Sussex, BN3 2FA

Library of Congress Cataloging in Publication Data
Main entry under title:

Cardiovascular disorders and behavior.

   (Handbook of psychology and health ; v. 3)
   Bibliography: p.
   Includes index.
   1. Heart—Diseases—Psychological aspects—Addresses,
essays, lectures.   2. Cardiovascular system—Diseases
—Psychological aspects—Addresses, essays, lectures.
I. Krantz, David S.   II. Baum, Andrew.   III. Singer,
Jerome E.   IV. Series.
RC454.H353   vol. 3   610'.1'9s [616.1'001'9]   83-1562
[RC682]
ISBN 0-89859-185-6

Publisher's Note
The publisher has gone to great lengths to ensure the quality of this reprint
but points out that some imperfections in the original may be apparent.

Table of Contents

Preface

Cardiovascular diseases are arguably the largest cause of death in the United States. This statement attests to the importance of understanding these disorders, in order to be able to prevent, ameliorate, and reduce the devastation which this set of diseases can cause. Cardiovascular disorders have also been the most intensely studied of those health hazards that have come to the attention of behavioral scientists. The many ways in which these problems are influenced by environmental, social, and behavioral factors have provided a fertile ground for study by investigators of many disciplines and persuasions. For these two reasons, it is appropriate that a volume in this series be directed toward the study of cardiovascular disease.

The domains of health psychology and behavioral medicine constitute rapidly growing behavioral science fields. The area is not well organized in terms of taxonomy or characterization, and many ways of arranging or classifying the field have been offered. Some do so by type of disease—cardiovascular, cancer, metabolic, and so on. Other classify the field of health psychology/behavioral medicine according to the point at which behavioral interventions impact (e.g., prevention, treatment, or rehabilitation). Still others classify the field in terms of characteristics of the patient population such as age, and create sub-fields such as pediatric or gerontological health psychology. And finally, others will classify the field in terms of the nature of the disciplinary or sub-disciplinary contribution to the study of behavior and health and thus talk about social psychology and health psychology, clinical psychology and health psychology, and so forth. In this series, we have used several of these classifications of each of the volumes: Volume I—*Clinical Psychology and Behavioral Medicine: Overlapping Disciplines*—classified the field in terms of the nature of the psychological contribution. Volume II—*Issues in Child Health and Adolescent Health*—classified the field by the nature of a characteristic of the patient population. And this volume, Volume III in the series, defines its scope according to the type of disease being studied.

This volume also reflects the fact that the study of behavioral and psychological factors should complement rather than supplant other aspects of the study of cardiovascular diseases. Obviously, cardiology, physiology, pharmacology, and a variety of other biological and medical disciplines also come into play in a total understanding of the interplay of pathological processes involved in these disorders. This volume reflects the diversity of disciplinary interests in cardiovascular disease, and attempts to show the relationship of psychological and behavioral approaches to the physiological and biomedical ones. Consequently, the contributors are drawn from several disciplines, including psychology, physiology, medicine, and medical sociology. While the picture presented by the sum of all the chapters by no means gives a complete account of cardiovascular pathology, nevertheless, the interplay between behavioral and medical issues is clearly highlighted.

We have used the plural term "cardiovascular disorders" because in this volume we have tried to make distinctions among several of the major forms of cardiovascular pathology and not treat them as if they were identical. Whatever their biomedical similarities may be, there are at least three separable research streams—ischemic coronary heart disease, hypertension, and arrhythmia/sudden death. This tri-partite division has been used both to select material for inclusion and to arrange it within the volume itself. Where possible within each of the disease classifications, we have also attempted to examine animal models, human studies, and for human studies, to examine etiology, pathogenesis, treatment, and rehabilitation. The large matrix generated by all these cross classifications has, of course, not been completely filled. Such a volume would be a massive undertaking in itself and beyond the scope of the present series.

As with all such volumes much of the work in preparing the book has been done by people whose names otherwise will not appear. Direct material contributions have been made to this volume by Martha Gisriel who has been primarily responsible for shepherding the administrative aspects of the volume and who performed near heroic labors in the construction of the massive subject index. Along the way she had assistance from India Fleming, T. Kevin Blanc and Mary Janson. No less important, but less direct, were the contributions made by our families—particularly our wives, Marsha Douma, Carrie Baum, and Linda Singer. Although not as visible to the reader as a subject index or a chapter, their support and encouragement are invaluable to us. It is for these and a host of other reasons that we dedicate this volume to our wives.

David S. Krantz
Andrew Baum
Jerome E. Singer

Handbook of
Psychology and Health

Volume I
Clinical Psychology and Behavioral Medicine:
Overlapping Disciplines
Robert J. Gatchel, Andrew Baum, and Jerome E. Singer

Volume II
Issues in Child Health and Adolescent Health
Andrew Baum and Jerome E. Singer

Volume III
Cardiovascular Disorders and Behavior
David S. Krantz, Andrew Baum, and Jerome E. Singer

Volume IV
Social Aspects of Health
Andrew Baum, Jerome E. Singer, and Shelley E. Taylor

Volume V
Coping and Stress
Andrew Baum and Jerome E. Singer

Handbook of Psychology and Health

Volume III

Cardiovascular Disorders and Behavior

1 Behavior and Cardiovascular Disease: Issues and Overview

David S. Krantz, Andrew Baum, Jerome E. Singer
Uniformed Services University of the Health Sciences

Despite the fact that there has been a real decline in cardiovascular mortality in recent years (USDHEW, 1979a), the major cardiovascular disorders, including coronary heart disease (CHD), hypertension, and sudden death, still account for one in two deaths in the United States. Because of a confluence of factors, research on cardiovascular disorders is one of the most developed areas of inquiry in the study of behavioral influences on health. First, epidemiologic studies reveal that these diseases are not an inevitable consequence of aging and genetic make-up (Kannel, 1979). Numerous environmental and behavioral variables are involved in their etiology and pathogenesis. Second, considerable progress has been made in moving beyond the establishing of correlations between psychological variables and cardiovascular disorders, to explore basic *mechanisms* linking behavioral processes to particular manifestations of disease.

This book provides an intensive review and evaluation of the progress of biobehavioral research on the etiology, treatment, rehabilitation, and prevention of the major cardiovascular disorders (coronary heart disease, essential hypertension, and cardiac arrhythmia/sudden death). The aim has been to assemble scholarly reviews pertaining to all three disorders in a single location where they can be easily accessed by researchers and practitioners. As is generally recognized, for each of these disorders an understanding of pathogenesis, and the implementation of effective preventive and treatment strategies requires consideration of the *interplay* of hereditary factors, metabolic alterations, and the individual's lifestyle. Such an interdisciplinary perspective is reflected by the fact that the contributors to this volume span a range of disciplines, including the basic biomedical sciences; physiology; experimental, physiological, social and clinical psychology; psychiatry; social epidemiology, and medical sociology. This introductory chapter provides an overview of major research directions in behavior and cardiovascular diseases, and a foreshadowing of the themes considered in greater depth in the following chapters.

Scope of the Book

As noted, the chapters in this volume will focus primarily on the following major cardiovascular disorders: coronary heart disease and coronary atherosclerosis; sudden cardiac death; and essential hypertension. A brief description of these disorders is in order here. More detailed descriptions are, of course, provided in the following chapters.

Coronary atherosclerosis is a symptomless condition characterized by narrowing and deterioration of the coronary arteries, the blood vessels that nourish the heart. An excess accumulation of cholesterol and related lipids forms a mound of tissue, or atherosclerotic plaque, on the inner wall of one or more of the coronary arteries (Hurst, Logue, Schlant, & Wenger, 1978). The formation of atherosclerotic plaques may proceed undetected for years, affecting cardiac functioning only when they cause a degree of obstruction sufficient to diminish blood supply to the heart. Once this occurs, coronary atherosclerosis has evolved into coronary heart disease (CHD), also known as ischemic heart disease.

In one form of CHD, angina pectoris, occasional instances of inadequate blood supply (ischemia) cause the individual to experience attacks of chest pain. Although ischemia *per se* does not cause permanent tissue damage, angina is a painful condition that can lead to more serious complications. A more severe and frequently fatal consequence of CHD is myocardial infarction (MI), or heart attack, in which a prolonged state of ischemia results in death of a portion of the heart tissue. Many cases of MI are associated with the presence of thrombosis (or clotting), suggesting that clot formation with an already occluded artery may precipitate the clinical incident. The issue of whether coronary thrombosis plays a precipitating or a secondary role in MI has been the subject of much debate in recent years. Indeed, there is no evidence of occlusive thrombosis in many cases of sudden cardiac death (SCD) (Chapters 2 and 5; Eliot, 1979; Haerem, 1974). This observation has led some investigators to argue that MI and SCD are two forms of heart tissue death with distinct pathophysiological mechanisms (Eliot, 1979). Chapters 2 and 5 provide more in-depth discussions of these issues.

The cardiac arrhythmias, disturbances of the conductive or beat-regulating portions of the heart, constitute another clinical manifestation of coronary disease to be discussed in this volume. In some cases, certain types of ventricular arrhythmias are harbingers of sudden cardiac death. These arrhythmias are often sporadic and emerge without a readily identifiable physiological basis. While the presence of ischemia may predispose to cardiac arrhythmias, young and otherwise healthy subjects without demonstrable heart disease can be subject to such rhythm irregularities. (See Chapter 5).

Essential hypertension, another major cardiovascular disorder considered in depth in this volume, is a condition of unclear etiology in which blood pressure shows chronic elevations. When the disorder becomes developed fully, increased pressure is usually due to a constriction or contraction of blood vessels throughout the body (Page & McCubbin, 1966). Although high blood pressure (HBP) is a symptomless disorder, there is epidemiologic evidence that even mild blood pressure elevations are associated with a shortening of life expectancy (Kannel & Dawber, 1971) and the increased risk of coronary heart disease and stroke.

The importance of modifiable environmental and behavioral variables in the development and/or maintenance of cardiovascular disease is suggested by studies demonstrating variations in incidence of illness associated with components of individual lifestyle or the social milieu (Kannel, 1979). Exercise, smoking, obesity, diet, and stress have all been shown to account for some variation in disease incidence, as have social factors such as occupational status, income, education, and the like (Bruhn, Wolf, Lynn, Bird, & Chandler, 1968; Henry & Stephens, 1977; House, 1975; Kannel, 1979). Despite these demonstrations, however, the degree to which we can accurately predict who will develop cardiovascular disease is far from adequate. Moreover, the predictive value of many of the risk factors for clinical coronary heart disease is far from being a settled issue. For example, the role of diet in the etiology of ischemic heart disease is quite controversial (e.g., Mann, 1977). Identifiable biologic risk factors by themselves are also poor predictors of sudden death. (See Chapter 5.)

Physical Risk Factors.   The risk-enhancing effects of so-called "standard" or physical risk factors had been initially viewed in terms of their physiological influence (e.g., toxic effects of tars and nicotine in the pathogenesis of CHD; the role of salt intake in regulating blood pressure levels; the relationship between diet and serum cholesterol). However, *behavioral* research on cardiovascular disease was stimulated by these epidemiologic associations because many of the standard risk factors are determined, at least partially, by behavioral factors. For example, cigarette smoking is a preventable behavior undoubtedly brought about by psychosocial forces (Leventhal & Cleary, 1980). Enhanced risk due to sex and age may also derive from non-biological correlates of these variables, such as occupational pressure, stressful life events, and behavior patterns (Eisdorfer & Wilkie, 1977; Riley & Hamburg, 1981).

The list of behaviorally-related influences on standard biologic risk factors can be extended even further. Resting blood pressure levels differ between racial groups, socioeconomic strata, and cultures (Weiner, 1977) for reasons presumed to relate to styles of living. Family history of coronary disease, while in some cases linked to a specific genetic mechanism (e.g., Goldstein & Brown, 1974) may also lead to enhanced risk of CHD or high blood pressure through psychosocial channels such as family patterns of cigarette smoking, diet, and socioeconomic condition. There is even preliminary data that family patterns of social interaction may contribute to the aggregation (similarity) of blood pressure among family members previously regarded as solely genetic in origin (cf. Baer, Vincent, Williams, Bourianoff, & Bartlett, 1980).

As is the case for coronary heart disease, studies of both humans and animals have identified environmental factors related to behavior which might play a role in the initiation of high blood pressure (HBP). These factors and their possible pathogenic mechanisms are discussed in detail in Chapters 6, 7, and 9 and therefore will only be briefly described here. These factors include dietary intake of salt, obesity, and psychological stress.

Much has been written about the role of salt in essential hypertension, largely because excessive intake of sodium is thought to increase the volume of blood. However, as Campbell and Henry (Chapter 6) and Shapiro (Chapter 9) indicate, studies reveal that high salt intake may be associated with high blood pressure levels only in some cultures and population groups. The relationship between salt intake and HBP appears to be complex, and salt intake may result in sustained blood pressure levels only in genetically predisposed individuals (cf. Dahl, Heine, & Tassinari, 1962). Obesity is another cultural and behavioral phenomenon that plays an important role in hypertension, although the precise reasons for the higher prevalence of HBP in obese patients have not been determined. Nevertheless, recent studies have determined that weight loss can result in significant decreases in blood pressure (Chapter 9).

Psychosocial Risk Factors. Biobehavioral research on the etiology and pathogenesis of cardiovascular disease received further impetus from limitations in the ability of the standard biologic risk factors for coronary disease and hypertension to identify most new cases of the disorders (Jenkins, 1971; 1976). Some variable or set of variables appear to be missing from the predictive equations. A broadened search for mechanisms and influences contributing to risk of cardiovascular disorders now includes social indicators such as socioeconomic status and social mobility, and psychological factors such as anxiety and neuroticism, psychological stress, and overt patterns of behavior. These results have been encouraging, though not uniformly so. The two most promising psychosocial risk factors for CHD and hypertension to emerge in recent years are psychological stress, and the Type A "coronary-prone" behavior pattern in the case of coronary heart disease. Although the concept of "stress" is widely used and often imprecisely defined, we use the term here in a psychophysiological sense to refer to an internal state resulting from the perception of threat and/or physical harm (Lazarus, 1966; Mason, 1971). This use of the term places emphasis on the organism's perception and evaluation of potentially harmful stimuli, and considers the perception of threat to arise from a comparison between the demands imposed upon the individual and his/her felt ability to cope with these demands. A perceived imbalance in this mechanism gives rise to the experience of stress and to a "whole body" stress response simultaneously physiological and behavioral in nature.

Early stress research (Cannon, 1932; Selye, 1956) emphasized the generality or non-specificity of responses to a wide variety of stimuli. Subsequent work has recognized certain general physiological responses to stress centering on the sympathetic nervous system and the pituitary-adrenal cortical axis, but has also emphasized the finding that the link between stress and disease is not simple (e.g., Baum, Singer, & Baum, 1981; Mason, 1971). Stress and illness relationships depend upon the context in which the stressful agent occurs, how individuals appraise it, and the social supports and personal resources available (Lazarus, 1966; Cohen, Horowitz, Lazarus, Moos, Robins, Rose, & Rutter, 1981; Mason, 1971). There are wide individual differences in physiological responses to stressors, which depend on biological predispositions (Levi, 1979), but also on the individual's felt ability to cope with or master conditions of harm, threat, or challenge. For example, stressful events (e.g., unemployment, loss of loved ones, divorce, etc.) are inevitable throughout the life cycle, yet only a minority of individuals suffer lasting adverse effects. Research has shown that a variety of social and psychological factors (e.g., styles of coping, social supports provided by others) act to modify or buffer the impact of stressful events on illness (F. Cohen et al., 1981).

Several indices of psychological stress have been studied in relation to the development of coronary heart disease. For example, there is an increasing body of research which suggests that excessive workload and job responsibility and dissatisfactions may enhance coronary risk (Jenkins, 1971; 1976; Haynes, Feinleib, & Kannel, 1980; House, 1975). Other research, in which information regarding life events prior to sudden cardiac death was obtained from a survivor of the deceased (usually the spouse), reveals an accumulation in the intensity of life events in the 6 months prior to death (cf. Garrity & Marx, 1979). Research on stressful events as an antecedent of sudden death receives detailed consideration in Chapter 5.

Stress deriving from psychosocial causes is also a factor which has been implicated in the etiology and maintenance of high blood pressure. The notion here is that psychological stimuli that threaten the organism result in cardiovascular and endocrine responses that can play an important role in the development of hypertension (Julius & Esler, 1975). The brain and central nervous system, which are involved in determining whether situations are harmful or threatening, thus play a role in physiological mechanisms mediating the impact of noxious stimuli. On a societal level, there is some evidence that blood pressure elevations occur under conditions of rapid cultural changes and socioeconomic mobility. There are several studies, for example, in which "primitive" populations living in small cohesive societies were found to have low blood pressure that did *not* increase with age. When members of such societies migrated to areas where they were suddenly exposed to Western culture, they were found to have high levels of blood pressure that increased with age. This suggested some cumulative effect of the new living conditions that became evident over the course of the life span (Henry & Cassel, 1969).

We should note that several recent critical reviews of the epidemiologic literature on stress and hypertension have noted that there are a sizeable number of studies which fail to confirm an association between cultural change or social stress and the incidence or prevalence of hypertension in population groups (e.g., Ostfeld & Shekelle, 1967; Syme & Torfs, 1978). Well-designed epidemiologic studies can attempt to rule out confounding factors (e.g., diet, sanitation, etc.) by using carefully matched control groups and by employing statistical control techniques, but there are inherent limits to conclusions that can be reached from correlational research. It is here that experimental techniques for inducing HBP in animals, and experimental studies of behavioral-cardiac interactions in humans have contributed to our understanding of the role of behavioral variables in the development of essential hypertension.

A second psychological factor which has important implications for coronary heart disease is the Type A or "coronary-prone" behavior pattern, a complex set of behaviors described by Friedman and Rosenman (1959). Type A behavior, perhaps the most widely researched psychosocial risk factor for CHD, is characterized by excessive competitive drive, impatience and hostility, and accelerated speech and motor movements. A contrasting Type B pattern is defined as the relative absence of these characteristics. As described in Chapter 3, no sharp division exists between the two behavior patterns; instead, the Type B person is a generally more relaxed and easy-going person who exhibits little aggressive drive and who is relatively devoid of time urgent characteristics. It has been observed that the Type A pattern emerges in the presence of certain environmental challenges or stresses (Chapter 3; Glass, 1977; Krantz, Glass, Schaeffer, & Davia, 1982). Encouraged by the development of the field of behavioral medicine and also by a considerable body of data (including two large scale prospective studies) documenting an association between Type A and coronary disease, research in this area has become increasingly popular among biomedical and behavioral researchers alike (see Cooper, Detre, & Weiss, 1981; Dembroski, Weiss, Shields, Haynes, & Feinleib, 1978b). Research on the Type A pattern is considered in detail in this volume in Chapters 3, 4, and 8.

Mechanisms Linking Stress to Cardiovascular Disorders

As we indicated at the beginning of this chapter, behavioral research on cardiovascular disease has taken a leading role in exploring physiological processes which mediate the relationship between risk factors—whether physical or psychosocial in nature—and the occurrence of disease. As these mechanisms are the subject of considerable attention in this volume (cf. Chapters 2 through 7), they will be only briefly outlined here.

Atherosclerosis, Clinical Coronary Heart Disease, Sudden Death. Although the pathogenesis of coronary disease is not completely understood, several factors are believed to play a major contributing role. These include a variety of physiological and biochemical states which may enhance coronary risk by influencing the initiation and progression of atherosclerosis and/or by precipitating clinical CHD (Herd, 1978; Ross & Glomset, 1976; Chapter 2). Many of these physiological states have been observed in experimental studies of psychological stress. For example, hemodynamic effects such as elevated heart rate and blood pressure, and biochemical changes such as increased levels of serum cholesterol, are produced in animals under prolonged or severe stress (Chapter 2). It has been observed, in addition, that a reduction in blood clotting time occurs under conditions of stress and, in some cases, degeneration of heart tissue has been reported as well. Other animal research has linked laboratory stressors to a lowered threshold for ventricular arrhythmia and for ventricular fibrillation (e.g., Chapter 5), a state which leads to sudden cardiac death unless immmediate treatment is given. Schneiderman (Chapter 2) pursues this evidence further by discussing the role of catecholamines in stress-induced pathology, and a mechanism involving the neural innervation of the heart which might account for these effects.

Potentially pathogenic states have been observed in studies of psychological stress in healthy humans. For example, life stressors such as occupational pressure have been shown to produce biochemical changes such as elevated levels of serum cholesterol (Friedman et al., 1958). Other research has demonstrated an association of increased heart rate and blood pressure with stressors such as the performance of mental arithmetic, harassment, and threat of electric shock. Still other studies report that the stresses of automobile driving, public speaking, and discussion of emotionally-charged topics provoke ventricular arrhythmias (see Chapter 5). Chapter 5 also alludes to recent studies of so-called "trigger" patients who seem to be particularly susceptible to stress-induced arrhythmias.

A notable feature of the foregoing research is the measurement of physiological *reactivity* in response to stress, as distinct from the observation of basal or resting levels of physiological variables. These changes in functioning, which are not detected by basal risk-factor measurement, are believed to yield a better index of the pathogenic processes involved in coronary disease. In addition, by observing such changes in response to both real-life and laboratory-induced stressors, pathogenic states may be detected within the context of their psychosocial antecedents.

The physiological concomitants of psychological stress are believed to result from activation of the sympathetic-adrenal medullary system (SAM) and the pituitary-adrenocortical axis (PAC). Interest in the impact of SAM activation on bodily reactions to emergency situations may be traced to Walter Cannon's work on the fight-or-flight response. This neuroendocrine response appears to be elicited in situations requiring coping with threatening stimuli (Frankenhaeuser, 1971). The hormonal responses of the PAC axis were emphasized by Selye in his notion of a generalized physiological response to aversive stimulation. The PAC secretions include a number of hormones that influence bodily systems of relevance to the development of coronary disease. The corticosteroids, which include cortisol, regulate the metabolism of cholesterol and other lipids involved in the atherosclerotic process. Activation of the SAM system also may have a special significance in mediating stress-related pathophysiological changes. Particularly culpable in this regard is secretion of the catecholamines, epinephrine and norepinephrine, which are believed to induce many of the pathogenic states associated with psychological stress. These include increased blood pressure and heart rate, elevation of blood lipids, acceleration of the rate of damage to the inner layers of the coronary arteries over time, and provocation of ventricular arrhythmias, believed to lead to sudden death (See chapters 2 and 5).

Jennings (Chapter 4) discusses evidence suggesting that chronic processes relating to the physiological and psychological correlates of information processing and attention also may play a role in the development of coronary heart disease. This notion is based on earlier work by the Laceys (e.g., Lacey & Lacey, 1970), epidemiological research on work overload and coronary heart disease, and psychophysiological research on the attentional style of Type A individuals. First, it is proposed that chronic allocation of full attentional capacity for immediate use produces a pattern of cardiovascular and neuroendocrine responses which cause "wear and tear" on the vasculature which may be involved in the pathogenesis of coronary artery disease. It is further suggested by Jennings that cardiac decelerative responses linked to anticipatory attention states may be involved in cardiac arrhythmias. Third, Jennings proposes that purely psychological aspects of attention (e.g., ignoring potentially important symptoms, insensitivity to protective or disease-buffering social cues such as social support) may also be health-impairing.

Essential Hypertension.   As described in Chapters 6 and 7, essential hypertension is not a single, homogeneous disease. In the development of the disorder, blood pressure is thought to progress over a period of years from moderately elevated or "borderline" levels to more appreciably elevated levels, called "established" hypertension. Several pathogenic mechanisms may bring about blood pressure elevations, and different physiological and/or behavioral mechanisms are implicated at various stages of the disorder. For example, individuals with borderline hypertension are commonly observed to have an elevated cardiac output (i.e., amount of blood pumped by the heart), but little evidence of increased resistance to the flow of blood in the body's vasculature (Julius & Esler, 1975). As noted earlier, the physiological pattern observed in borderline hypertension is consistent with increased activation of the sympathetic nervous system, which is the body's initial reaction to psychological stress. However, in older individuals with more "established" high blood pressure, a different physiologic pattern is observed. Cardiac output is either normal or depressed, while the vascular resistance is elevated. Psychological stimuli such as emotionally stressful events have been shown to correlate highly with the exacerbation of hypertensive episodes in diagnosed patients (cf. Weiner, 1977) with established hypertension. However, recent research on behavioral influences has focused increasingly on earlier stages, rather than on the later stages of the disease.

In addition to cardiovascular adjustments and changes, the physiological mechanisms of high blood pressure probably involve the interaction of the central and autonomic nervous systems, the endocrine-hormonal system, and the kidneys. Accordingly, behavioral factors (in particular, psychological stress) might play a role in the etiology of HBP via a number of physiological pathways (Kaplan, 1980; Chapter 7). Recall that stress leads to discharge of the sympathetic nervous system and to increases in catecholamines. High levels of blood and tissue catecholamines have been found in some hypertensive humans and animals (Julius & Esler, 1975). Such elevations could lead to increased blood pressure via increased heart rate and force of heart action, constriction of peripheral blood vessels, and/or activation of a hormonal mechanism in the kidney that constricts the vasculature (Kaplan, 1980) and regulates the volume of blood.

It is likely that in humans, sustained elevations are produced by an interaction of a variety of genetic and environmental factors. Consider, for example, that family history of HBP is a significant, albeit imperfect predictor of whether a young individual will later develop high blood pressure (Julius & Schork, 1978). In addition, epidemiological studies reveal a difference in the prevalence of HBP among various social and cultural groups—a difference which cannot be accounted for by genetic factors alone (Henry & Cassel, 1969). For example, in the United States, hypertension is more common among blacks than among whites, but the prevalence of high blood pressure is greater in poor than in middle class black Americans (Harburg, Erfurt, Hauenstein, Chape, Schull, & Schork, 1973). Animal research described by Campbell & Henry (Chapter 6) similarly reveals examples where environmental factors such as dietary salt intake or environmental stress lead to sustained blood pressure elevations only in certain genetic strains. Closely related to this observation is the finding that family members tend to have similar blood pressures. As we have noted, the prevalent view attributes this solely to a genetic source, but there is emerging evidence suggesting joint genetic and environmental effects. A possible environmentally-determined behavioral factor, family social interaction, is illustrated by a recent study which observed more negative nonverbal behavior (e.g., grimacing, gaze aversion) among families with a hypertensive father, compared to families with a normotensive father (Baer et al., 1980).

Experimental work has sought to identify individuals who are at risk of developing HBP, and the types of situations that might activate genetic predispositions to high blood pressure. Since the aim is to understand mechanisms in the *cause* of the disorder, this research has focused increasingly on the beginning stage, rather than the culmination, of the disease.

Given that borderline high blood pressure is characterized by heightened responsiveness of the cardiovascular and sympathetic nervous systems to psychological stimuli such as mental stress (Julius & Esler, 1975), recent research has examined the tendency toward large episodic or acute increases in heart rate, blood pressure, and sympathetic nervous system hormonal (catecholamine) activity as possible mechanisms involved in etiology. Several groups of investigators including Manuck, and Obrist and colleagues (Manuck & Schaefer, 1978; Chapter 7) have found that cardiovascular responsiveness is a stable and persistently evoked response that can be measured reliably in a laboratory situation. Cardiovascular responsiveness to certain psychological stimuli has also been related consistently to family history of high blood pressure (a hypertension risk factor), even among individuals who have normal resting blood pressure levels and display no overt signs of the disorder (Chapter 7; Falkner, Onesti, Angelakos, Fernandes, & Langman, 1979). Obrist and his co-workers further report that cardiovascular responsiveness above the level that is efficient for the body's metabolic needs occurs uniquely in situations where *active coping* or behavioral adjustments are required, as opposed to stressful situations where the individual remains passive and does not take direct action to control the situation. Experimental evidence is also presented regarding possible cardiovascular and renal mechanisms which may link sympathetic responses to active coping with particular physiological changes of relevance to the etiology of HBP.

The Contribution of Animal Behavior Models.   Four chapters in this volume (Chapters 2, 5, 6, and 7) are devoted wholly or in substantial part to a discussion of the contribution of animal behavior models toward understanding the mechanisms involved in the major cardiovascular disorders. As Campbell and Henry (Chapter 6) note, the advantages of animal models include the ability to manipulate relevant variables, the ability to follow the course of disease over the animal's compressed life span, and the ability to control both genetic and environmental variables.

In the case of hypertension, Campbell and Henry outline a variety of animal models which have proven useful in the study of behavioral influences on this disorder. They further review the extensive research involving the controlled breeding of infrahuman species that has facilitated the study of genetic/behavioral interplay. For example, several strains of rats susceptible to stress- and salt-induced HBP have been produced through selective breeding. Campbell and Henry also discuss some of the more highly promising behavioral research involving the spontaneously hypertensive strain of rats.

Schneiderman's chapter on animal behavior models of CHD discusses in detail the catecholamine hypotheses of cardiovascular pathology, and the possible role of these hormones in the pathogenesis of atherosclerosis, stress-induced myocardial damage, and arrhythmias. An important direction taken by this review is a focus on "specificity", or the notion that distinctions can be made among specific types of pathology in terms of their associations with particular behavioral or psychological stimuli, and their mediation by differing physiological events. Scientific understanding of these disorders in humans is greatly furthered to the extent that separate identifiable psychophysiological processes are linked to specific types of pathology.

Verrier, De Silva & Lown (Chapter 5) review the literature on sudden death and on psychological influences on "ventricular vulnerability" (i.e., susceptibility to ventricular fibrillation). Both animal behavior models and recent human clinical research on arrhythmia/sudden death are discussed, and they evaluate the status of experimental research employing biofeedback and meditation on the treatment of arrhythmias. Other recent research on patients susceptible to psychologically-induced arrhythmias is also considered. This chapter is particularly notable for its review of research involving the interplay of animal models and human experimental and epidemiological work. The potential for future use of animal models is discussed in Chapters 2, 5, and 6.

Behavior and Prevention, Treatment, and Rehabilitation

It has also become clear to both researchers and practitioners that an understanding of behavioral issues is crucial in the implementation of effective prevention, treatment, and rehabilitation strategies for the major cardiovascular disorders (Krantz, Glass, Contrada, & Miller, 1981; Weiss, Herd, & Fox, 1981; USDHEW, 1979b). Among the more salient of such issues are motivating and sustaining compliance with antihypertensive medications, facilitating resumption of normal activities after heart attack, and prevention or modification of coronary risk behaviors, e.g., smoking, dietary habits, stress in young adults and high risk middle-aged subjects (Croog & Levine, 1977; USDHEW, 1979b).

Prevention.   Associations between the major cardiovascular disorders and seemingly modifiable behavioral variables have spurred intense interest in relating behavioral knowledge to the prevention of various stages of cardiovascular disease (see for example the Surgeon General's recent report on Health Promotion and Disease Prevention). The chapters in this volume by Roskies and Shapiro provide a comprehensive review and assessment of the state of research in this area. Primary prevention (i.e., before disease develops) of health impairing habits is a cost-effective approach to health. Encouraging prevention efforts have, for example, employed social-psychological techniques to deter smoking in adolescents (Evans, Rozelle, Maxwell, Raines, Dill, & Guthrie, 1981), and preliminary efforts are underway to alter patterns of dietary fat intake (e.g., Foreyt, Scott, Mitchell, & Gotto, 1979; Matarazzo, Connor, Fey, Carmody,

Pierce, Brischetto, Baker, Connor, & Sexton, in press) and Type A behavior (Roskies, Chapter 8). The current status of employing non-pharmacologic techniques in the prevention and control of borderline or early hypertension is assessed in Shapiro's chapter in this volume.

The terms "secondary prevention" and "tertiary prevention" refer, respectively, to interventions taken to arrest the progress of illness already in early asymptomatic stages, and interventions taken to stop the progression of a clinically manifest disease (Institute of Medicine, 1978). The life-style modification studies reviewed by Roskies (Chapter 8) might suggest that secondary and tertiary prevention activities may be more feasible than primary prevention from a policy point of view, given the present state of knowledge. Advantages of such interventions are that appropriate target groups can be more easily recognized and more motivated to change their behavior (Institute of Medicine, 1978).

In the case of essential hypertension, Shapiro's chapter reviews evidence relating to the effect of diet (i.e., sodium) modification, weight control, and physical exercise in the treatment of HBP. In addition, a variety of behavioral stress-reduction techniques have been employed in relatively small scale clinical trials. Shapiro reviews evidence regarding their comparative efficacy. At present, given the apparently greater efficacy of pharmacologic therapy, these behavioral techniques are best employed as supplements or adjuncts to other therapies. However, there have been some promising findings that behavioral techniques may be particularly effective means of reducing the effective dose of antihypertensive medications (Fahrion, 1980). It may therefore be possible to "wean" patients off medications by effective combinations of pharmacologic and behavioral techniques. In addition, as is the case with all non-pharmacologic approaches involving lifestyle alterations, effective treatment outcomes depend not only on producing transitory changes in behavior but also on the maintenance of these changes and sustained compliance with prescribed regimens.

The question of whether altering habits and behavior patterns such as dietary fat intake, smoking, and Type A behavior will reduce morbidity and mortality from cardiovascular diseases has become the major focus of numerous clinical trials, and a central area of research and controversy in the study of behavior and health (e.g.,Kasl, 1980; Krantz et al., 1981; Leventhal, Safer, Cleary, & Gutmann, 1980; Meyer, Nash, McAlister, Maccoby, & Farquher, 1980). The current status of research on modification of coronary-risk behaviors is reviewed and assessed in the chapter by Roskies. Approaches examined in her review include both single-factor and multiple risk factor intervention trials, employing techniques such as community-wide media-based attitude change techniques (e.g., the Stanford and North Karelia Projects); clinic-based health service delivery (e.g., the MRFIT project); social learning and modeling techniques to deter smoking in adolescents (e.g., the Houston project); as well as face-to-face psychotherapy and behavior therapy approaches (e.g., research on the modification of Type A behavior). The more ambitious of these studies measure disease endpoints of morbidity and/or mortality, often devoting lesser attention to, and occasionally neglecting, mediating processes of behavior change. Other studies focus more intensively on whether risk behaviors are altered, without necessarily being directly concerned with disease outcomes.

Several important challenges and questions are raised by efforts to modify cardiovascular risk factors. First, there are encouraging indications that established patterns of behavior can be changed in the short-term. However, a major difficulty has been maintaining these changes in substantial numbers of individuals over sustained periods of time (Bernstein & Glasgow, 1979; Hunt, Matarazzo, Weiss, & Gentry, 1979). This problem is illustrated by the remarkably similar relapse rates among subjects treated in programs aimed at weight reduction, smoking cessation, and reduction of alcohol consumption (Hunt et al., 1979). Two-thirds of such patients abandon the regimen and backslide by the end of three months, and only about one-quarter of the individuals maintain changed behavior at the end of a 1-year period. There is also a high early drop-out rate in various treatment programs (cf. Leventhal & Cleary, 1980) which may spuriously inflate success rates.

Moreover, the assumption that effective alteration of health-impairing habits, if achieved, will reduce cardiovascular morbidity and mortality, cannot be fully evaluated until data from pending clinical trials are available. For example, in the case of cigarette smoking, epidemiological data reveal that former cigarette smokers experience declining overall mortality rates as the years of discontinuance of the habit increase (USDHEW, 1964). Data on morbidity are more complex, and indicate that the benefits of being an ex-smoker are not as high as the benefits of never having smoked. Similarly, the data on the effects of reduced blood lipids on CHD are not conclusive (Kasl, 1980). Indeed, they suggest that factors such as the age at which reductions occur and the underlying mechanism for lipid elevations make a difference in the benefits that accrue. The clinical trials of lifestyle interventions reviewed by Roskies face the problems of behavioral measurement and of maintaining continued adherence to regimens (Kasl, 1980; Syme, 1978). Despite these advantages, such studies are major field trials of therapeutic and preventive measures which are relevant to the formation of public policy regarding behavior and cardiovascular health.

Rehabilitation. Substantial evidence is accumulating that behavioral and psychosocial characteristics of patients and their family environments are in many cases as important as physiologic processes in determining successful rehabilitation of cardiac patients (see Chapter 10; also Croog & Levine, 1977; Doehrman, 1977; Garrity, 1981). As Croog describes in Chapter 10, a large number of predictor variables have been implicated and studied as possible determinants of coping and adjustment after a heart attack (cf. Doehrman, 1977; Garrity, McGill, Becker, Blanchard et al., 1976). These include physical variables (e.g., severity of disease, symptom intensity, physical activity); psychological processes (e.g., perceptions of health, beliefs about the controllability of illness, coping styles); sociological and family characteristics (e.g., occupational, socio-economic and marital status); and characteristics of the health care system (e.g., communication with physicians). The patient's morale during recovery and the ability to return to work are the most frequently studied outcome variables. Several theories and conceptualizations of the recovery process have been proposed (see Krantz, 1980), but most of these apply to the acute (in-hospital) phase of recovery. However, it appears that medical and behavioral variables show differing patterns of relationships to recovery variables at various points in the time course of illness (i.e., the acute or in-hospital phase versus the convalescent post-hospital phase). Croog's chapter provides a conceptual overview and critique of research on psychosocial aspects of long-term recovery and rehabilitation of the heart patient. The focus of the review is on a number of inter-related life areas which are related to or directly affected by coronary heart disease as a chronic illness (e.g., family, work, doctor-patient relationship, individual coping and adjustment, etc.). Gaps and needs in the research literature are also discussed by Croog, and particular research, conceptual, and methodological issues are outlined. Hundreds of thousands of individuals survive acute myocardial infarction each year and the cardiac rehabilitation is clearly an important area for the study of behavior and health.

Conclusion

An important priority for further research on cardiovascular disorders is the continued integration of behavioral and biomedical knowledge in a way that elucidates the mechanisms underlying relationships between behavior and pathophysiological processes. Other priorities are the development and evaluation of techniques to produce sustained changes in behavioral risk factors and to develop effective psychosocial interventions in the treatment and rehabilitation of the cardiac patient.

Research on cardiovascular disorders has proven to be among the more promising areas for the study of behavioral influences on health. The body of research reviewed in this volume serves to highlight many of the important challenges and questions which remain.

REFERENCES

Baer, P. E., Vincent, J. P., Williams, B. I., Bourianoff, G. G., & Bartlett, P. C. Behavioral response to induced conflict in families with a hypertensive father. *Hypertension*, 1980, Supp. I, 2, I–70–77.

Baum, A., Singer, J. E., & Baum, C. Stress and the environment. *Journal of Social Issues*, 1981, 37, 4–35.

Bernstein, D. A., & Glasgow, R. E. Smoking. In O. F. Pomerleau & J. P. Brady (Eds.), *Behavioral medicine: Theory and practice*. Baltimore: Williams and Wilkins, 1979.

Bruhn, J. C., Wolf, W., Lynn, T., Bird, H., & Chandler, B. Social aspects of coronary-heart disease in a Pennsylvania German community. *Social Science and Medicine*, 1968, *2*, 201–212.

Cannon, W. B. *The wisdom of the body*. New York: Norton, 1932.

Cohen, F., Horowitz, M. J., Lazarus, R. S., Moos, R. H., Robins, L. N., Rose, P. M., & Rutter, M. Report of the subpanel on psychosocial assets and modifiers. Committee to Study Research on Stress in Health and Disease, Institute of Medicine, National Academy of Sciences, 1981.

Cooper, T., Detre, T., & Weiss, S. M. Coronary-prone behavior and coronary heart disease: A critical review. *Circulation*, 1981, *63*, 1199–1215.

Croog, S. H., & Levine, S. *The heart patient recovers*. New York: Human Sciences Press, 1977.

Dahl, L. K., Heine, M., & Tassinari, L. Role of genetic-factors in susceptibility to experimental hypertension due to chronic excess salt ingestion. *Nature*, 1962, *194*, 480–482.

Dembroski, T. M., Weiss, S. M., Shields, J. L., Haynes, S. G., & Feinleib, M. *Coronary-prone behavior*. New York: Springer-Verlag, 1978.

Doehrman, S. R. Psycho-social aspects of recovery from coronary heart disease: A review. *Social Science and Medicine*, 1977, *11*, 199–218.

Eisdorfer, C., & Wilkie, F. Stress, disease, aging, and behavior. In J. E. Birren & K. W. Schaie, (Eds.), *Handbook of the psychology of aging*. New York: Van Nostrand Reinhold, 1977.

Eliot, R. S. *Stress and the major cardiovascular disorders*. New York: Futura Publishing Company, 1979.

Evans, R. I., Rozelle, R. M., Maxwell, S. E., Raines, B. E., Dill, C. A., & Guthrie, T. J. Social modeling films to deter smoking in adolescents: Results of a three year field investigation. *Journal of Applied Psychology*, 1981, *66*, 399–414.

Fahrion, S. L. *Etiology and intervention in essential hypertension: A biobehavioral approach*. Unpublished manuscript, The Menninger Foundation, 1980.

Falkner, B., Onesti, G., Angelakos, E. T., Fernandes, M., & Langman C. Cardiovascular response to mental stress in normal adolescents with hypertensive parents. *Hypertension*, 1979, *1*, 23–30.

Foreyt, J. P., Scott, L. W., Mitchell, R. E., & Gotto, A. M. Plasma lipid changes in the normal population following behavioral treatment. *Journal of Consulting and Clinical Psychology*, 1979, *47*, 440–452.

Frankenhaeuser, M. Behavior and circulating catecholamines. *Brain Research*, 1971, *31*, 241–262.

Friedman, M., Rosenman, R. H., & Carroll, V. Changes in the serum cholesterol and blood-clotting time in men subjected to cyclic variation of occupational stress. *Circulation*, 1958, *17*, 852–861.

Friedman, M., & Rosenman, R. H. Association of specific overt behavior pattern with blood and cardiovascular findings. *Journal of the American Medical Association*, 1959, 169, 1286–1296.

Garrity, T. F., & Marx, M. B. Critical life events and coronary disease. In W. D. Gentry & R. B. Williams, Jr., (Eds.). *Psychological aspects of myocardial infarction and coronary care*, (2nd ed.) Saint Louis: C. V. Mosby, 1979.

Garrity, T. F. Behavioral adjustment after myocardial infarction: A selective review of recent descriptive, correlational and intervention research. In S. M. Weiss, J. A. Herd, & B. H. Fox (Eds.), *Perspectives on behavioral medicine*. New York, Academic Press, 1981.

Garrity, T. F., McGill, A., Becker, M., Blanchard, E., et al. Report of the task group on cardiac rehabilitation. In S. M. Weiss (Ed.), *Proceedings of the National Heart and Lung Institute working conference on health behavior*. DHEW Publication No. 76-868. Washington, DC: U.S. Government Printing Office, 1976.

Glass, D. C. *Behavior patterns, stress, and coronary disease*. Hillsdale, NJ: Lawrence Erlbaum Associates, 1977.

Goldstein, J. L., & Brown, M. S. Binding and degradation of low density lipoproteins by cultured human fibroblasts. *The Journal of Biological Chemistry*, 1974, *249*, 5153–5162.

Haerem, J. W. Mural platelet microthrombi and major acute lesions of main epicardial arteries in sudden coronary death. *Atherosclerosis*, 1974, *19*, 529.

Harburg, E., Erfurt, J. D., Hauenstein, L. S., Chape, C., Schull, W. J., & Schork, M. A. Socio-ecological stress, supressed hostility, skin color, and black-white male blood pressure. *Psychosomatic Medicine*, 1973, *35*, 276–296.

Haynes, S. G., Feinleib, M., & Kannel, W. B. The relationship of psychosocial factors to coronary heart disease. *American Journal of Epidemiology*, 1980, *111*, 37–58.

Henry, J. P., & Cassel, J. C. Psychosocial factors in essential hypertension: Recent epidemiologic and animal experimental data. *American Journal of Epidemiology*, 1969, *90*, 171–200.

Henry, J. P., & Stephens, J. P. *Stress, health, and the social environment*. New York: Springer-Verlag, 1977.

Herd, A. J. Physiological correlates of coronary-prone behavior. In T. M. Dembroski, S. M. Weiss, J. L. Shields, S. G. Haynes, & M. Feinleib, (Eds.), *Coronary-prone behavior*. New York: Springer-Verlag, 1978.

House, J. S. Occupational stress is a precursor to coronary disease. In W. D. Gentry and R. B. Williams, Jr., (Eds.), *Psychological aspects of myocardial infarction and coronary care*. Saint Louis: C. V. Mosby, 1975.

Hunt, W. A., Matarazzo, J. D., Weiss, S. M., & Gentry, W. D. Associative learning, habit and health behavior. *Journal of Behavioral Medicine*, 1979, *2*, 111–124.

Hurst, J. W., Logue, R. B., Schlant, R. C., & Wenger, N. K. (Eds.), *The heart*. New York: McGraw Hill, 1978.

Institute of Medicine, National Academy of Sciences. *Perspectives on health promotion and disease prevention in the United States*. Report to National Academy of Sciences, 1978.

Jenkins, C. D. Psychological and social percursors of coronary disease. *New England Journal of Medicine*, 1971, *284*, 244–255; 307–317.

Jenkins, C. D. Recent evidence supporting psychologic and social risk factors for coronary disease. *New England Journal of Medicine*, 1976, *294*, 987–94, 1033–38.

Julius, S., & Esler, M. Autonomic nervous cardiovascular regulation in borderline hypertension. *The American Journal of Cardiology*, 1975, *36*, 685–696.

Julius, S., & Schork, M. A. Predictors of hypertension. *Annals of the New York Academy of Sciences*, 1978, 38–52.

Kannel, W. B. Cardiovascular disease: A multifactorial problem (insights from the Framingham study). In M. L. Pollock & D. H. Schmidt (Eds.), *Heart disease and rehabilitation*. New York: John Wiley & Sons, Inc., 1979.

Kannel, W. B., & Dawber, T. R. Hypertensive cardiovascular disease. In G. Onesti, K. E. Kin, & J. Hayer, (Eds.), *The Framingham Study, hypertension: Mechanisms and management*. New York: Grune and Stratton, 1971.

Kaplan, N. M. The control of hypertension: A therapeutic breakthrough. *American Scientist*, 1980, *68*, 537–545.

Kasl, S. V. Cardiovascular risk reduction in a community setting: Some comments. *Journal of Consulting and Clinical Psychology*, 1980, *48*, 143–149.

Krantz, D. S. Cognitive processes and recovery from heart attack: A review and theoretical analysis. *Journal of Human Stress*, 1980, *6*(3), 27–38.

Krantz, D. S., Glass, D. C., Contrada, R., & Miller, N. E. Behavior and health. In the National Science Foundation's *Five Year Outlook on Science and Technology: 1981*. (Source materials, volume 2). Washington, D.C.: U.S. Government Printing Office, 1981.

Krantz, D. S., Glass, D. C., Schaeffer, M. A., & Davia, J. E. Behavior patterns and coronary disease: A critical evaluation. In J. F. Cacioppo & R. E. Petty (Eds.), *Perspectives on cardiovascular psycho-physiology*. New York: Guilford Press, 1982.

Lacey, J. I., & Lacey, B. C. Some autonomic-central nervous system interrelationships. In H. Black (Ed.), *Physiological correlates* of emotion. New York: Academic Press, 1970.

Lazarus, A. S. *Psychological stress and the coping process*. New York: McGraw-Hill, 1966.

Leventhal, H., & Cleary, P. D. The smoking problem: A review of research and theory in behavioral risk modification. *Psychological Bulletin, 1980, 88,* 370–405.

Leventhal, H., Safer, M. A., Cleary, P. D., & Gutmann, M. Cardiovascular risk modification by community-based programs for life-style change: Comments on the Stanford study. *Journal of Consulting and Clinical Psychology, 1980, 48,* 150–158.

Levi, L. Psychosocial factors in preventive medicine. In *Surgeion general's background papers for healthy people report*. U.S. Department of Health, Education and Welfare. USPHS Publication No. 79-55011A. Washington, DC: U. S. Government Printing Office, 1979.

Mann, G. V. Diet-heart: End of an era. *New England Journal of Medicine, 1977, 294,* 644–650.

Manuck, S. B., & Schaefer, D. C. Stability of individual differences in cardiovascular reactivity. *Physiology and Behavior, 1978, 21,* 675–678.

Mason, J. W. A re-evaluation of the concept of "non-specificity" in stress theory. *Journal of Psychiatric Research, 1971, 8,* 323–333.

Matarazzo, J. D., Connor, W. E., Fey, S. G., Carmody, T. P., Pierce, D. K., Brischetto, C. S., Baker, C. H., Connor, S. L., & Sexton, G. Behavioral cardiology with emphasis on the family heart study: Fertile ground for psychological and biomedical research. In T. Millon, C. J. Green, & R. B. Meagher, (Eds.), *Handbook of health care psychology*. New York: Plenum Press, 1982.

Meyer, A. J., Nash, J. D., McAlister, A. L., Maccoby, N., & Farquhar, J. W. Skills training in a cardiovascular education campaign. *Journal of Consulting and Clinical Psychology, 1980, 48,* 129–142.

Ostfeld, A. M., & Shekelle, R. B. Psychosocial variables and blood pressure. In J. Stamler, R. Stamler, & T. N. Pullman, (Eds.), *The epidemiology of hypertension*. New York: Grune & Stratton, 1967.

Page, I. H., & McCubbin, J. S. The physiology of arterial hypertension. In W. F. Hamilton & P. Dow (Eds.), *Handbook of physiology: Circulation*. Section 2, Volume 1, Washington, D.C.: American Physiological Society, 1966.

Riley, M. W., & Hamburg, B. A. Report of the Subpanel on Stress, Health, and the Life Course. Committee to Study Research on Stress in Health and Disease, Institute of Medicine, National Academy of Sciences, 1981.

Ross, R., & Glomset, J. A. The pathogenesis of atherosclerosis. *New England Journal of Medicine, 1976, 295,* 369–377, 420–425.

Selye, H. *The stress of life*. New York: McGraw-Hill, 1956.

Syme, S. L. Life style intervention in clinic-based trials. *American Journal of Epidemiology, 1978, 108,* 87–91.

Syme, S. L., & Torfs, C. P. Epidemiologic research in hypertension: A critical appraisal. *Journal of Human Stress, 1978, 4(1),* 43–48.

U.S. Department of Health, Education and Welfare. *Proceedings of the conference on the decline of coronary heart disease mortality*. NIH Publication No. 79-1610. Washington, DC: U. S. Government Printing Office, 1979a.

U.S. Department of Health, Education and Welfare. *Healthy people: A report of the surgeon general on health promotion and disease prevention*. USPHS Publication No. 79-55071. Washington, DC: U. S. Government Printing Office, 1979b.

U.S. Department of Health, Education and Welfare. *Smoking and health: A report of the surgeon general*. USPHS Publication No. 1103. Washington, DC: U. S. Government Printing Office, 1964.

Weiner, H. *Psychobiology and human disease*. New York, NY: Elsevier North-Holland, Inc., 1977.

Weiss, S. M., Herd, J. A., & Fox, B. H. *Perspectives on behavioral medicine*. New York: Academic Press, 1981.

2 Animal Behavior Models of Coronary Heart Disease

Neil Schneiderman
University of Miami

> *In modern society wrath,*
> *reinforced by sloth and*
> *gluttony, is the deadliest*
> *of the seven sins.*
> —M. E. Carruthers (1969)

INTRODUCTION

The Framingham study established cigarette smoking, elevated serum cholesterol, high systolic blood pressure and advancing age as risk factors for coronary heart disease (Dawber, Meadors, & Moore, 1951). Knowledge about these risk factors alone or in combination, however, still does not predict most new cases of coronary heart disease (CHD) in the United States (Jenkins, 1976). Search for additional risk factors, however, has led to identification by the Western Collaborative Group Study (WCGS) of the Type A coronary-prone behavior pattern as a potential risk factor for CHD (Rosenman, Brand, Jenkins, Friedman, Strauss, & Wurm, 1975). Although the Framingham study and the WCGS demonstrated associations between particular risk factors and CHD, the exact pathophysiologic mechanisms mediating the relationship between any risk factor and CHD are presently unknown.

In attempting to study some of the psychophysiologic factors that might be involved in the relationship between the Type A behavior pattern and CHD, several investigators have examined experimentally the physiologic reactivity of Type A and B individuals in various behavioral situations (e.g., Dembroski,

MacDougall, Herd, & Shields, 1979; Glass, Krakoff, Contrada, Hilton, Kehoe, Mannucci, Collins, Snow, & Elting, 1980). The outcome of such studies suggest that the person classified as Type A is an individual who shows a high degree of defensive sympathetic nervous system activation while struggling to cope with the social and work related challenges of everyday life.

The catecholamine and/or cardiovascular changes elicited by Dembroski et al. (1979) and by Glass et al. (1980) were short-term in nature, but they represent the kind of catecholamine-induced responses that pathophysiologic studies suggest could lead to atherosclerosis—and ultimately to CHD if elicited repeatedly over a prolonged period of time. This view is reinforced by the results of coronary angiography studies linking the Type A behavior pattern to the severity and progression of coronary atherosclerosis (Blumenthal, Williams, Kong, Schanberg, & Thompson, 1978; Krantz, Sanmarco, Selvester, & Matthews, 1979).

Although it is reasonable to examine physiologic reactivity in experiments conducted upon humans, and it is important to correlate behavior patterns with atherosclerosis in retrospective and prospective studies, it would be unethical deliberately to induce atherosclerosis or CHD by experimental means in humans. It is possible, however, to establish cause-effect relationships between emotional behavior and cardiovascular pathology by resorting to animal experimentation. At present the experimental study of how presumed pathophysiological mechanisms mediate relationships between behavior and cardiovascular pathology is still embryonic. Experimental evidence does exist, however, that behavioral variables can induce cardiovascular pathology, and testable hypotheses have been presented concerning the specific circumstances under which particular forms of pathology are likely to occur. In this chapter we first describe the presumed role of the catecholamines in the development of atherosclerosis and CHD, and then discuss the various animal models that have been used to study the biobehavioral bases of these disorders. We conclude with a discussion of relations among behavioral processes, physiologic responses and the specificity of cardiovascular pathology as well as directions for new research.

CATECHOLAMINE HYPOTHESES OF CARDIOVASCULAR PATHOLOGY

The major secretions of the sympathoadrenomedullary axis are the catecholamines, norepinephrine, epinephrine and dopamine. Since Walter B. Cannon (1911) established the association between emotional displays and the release of adrenomedullary secretions, the sympathetic nervous system and its secretions have played a central role in conceptions of emotional reactions to stressful situations. Typically, aggressive behaviors such as fighting have been found to elicit increases in blood pressure, heart rate, cardiac output, and a redistribution of blood flow from the splanchnic beds to skeletal muscles, the brain, and myocardium (e.g., Adams, Bacelli, Mancia, & Zanchetti, 1968; Caraffa-Braga, Granata, & Pinotti, 1973). Anticipation of fighting has also been associated with an increase in blood pressure, but in this case may occur concomitantly with bradycardia, decreased cardiac output, and hind-limb muscle and mesenteric vasoconstriction (e.g., Adams, et al., 1968). Such differences emphasize that the sympathetic nervous system is capable of more specificity than was once believed.

The sympathoadrenomedullary axis plays an important role in mediating relationships between emotional behavior and cardiovascular reactivity, but other factors such as neuroendocrine changes, metabolic adjustments and the parasympathetic nervous system also must be taken into account (Mason, Mangan, Brady, Conrad, & Rioch, 1961; Levy, 1977; Selye, 1961). Chronic physical or emotional stress, for instance, can cause an elevation in corticosteroid production. This, in turn, can augment the toxic effects of catecholamines and/or lead to increased water and sodium retention, thereby adversely influencing cardiovascular functions (Raab, 1966; Selye, 1961).

There are many ways in which the secretions of the sympathetic nervous system might mediate relationships between emotional behavior and cardiovascular pathology. These include (a) precipitation of life-threatening arrythmias, (b) alterations in the metabolism of myocardial cells, (c) induction of cardiac ischemia due to an increased need for myocardial oxygenation in conjunction with atherosclerotic stenosis of the coronary arteries, (d) deposition and incorportaion into coronary artery plaques of thromboembolitic components of the blood, and (e) facilitation of necrosis, calcification and rupture of plaques, which in turn could produce thrombosis and myocardial infarction. Emotional factors have actually been implicated in arrhythmias (Lown, Verrier, & Corbalan, (1973), atherosclerosis (Lang, 1967), hypertension (Graham, 1945), myocardial ischemia and infarction (Raab, 1966; Russek, 1973), sudden cardiac death (Lown, 1979), and thrombosis (Haft & Fani, 1973). Moreover, injections of even modest quantities of catecholamines have been shown to produce atherosclerosis (Friedman, Oester, & Davis, 1955), arrhythmias (Guideri, Barletta, Chav, Green, & Lehr, 1975), and myocardial ischemia and necrosis (Eliot, Todd, Clayton, & Pieper, 1978; Rona, Chappel, Balasy, & Caudry, 1959). In the face of this surfeit of dysfunctions and putative pathophysiologic mediators it might seem reasonable to ask whether (a) particular behavior patterns are linked by specific mediating variables to discriminably different cardiovascular pathologies, or (b) a wide range of emotional stressors can precipitate CHD nonspecifically in individuals previously made susceptible by factors possibly unrelated to behavior. The available evidence suggests that both hypotheses may be correct.

ARTERIOSCLEROSIS

Animal behavior experiments have linked psychological factors to both arteriosclerosis (e.g., Henry, Ely, Stephens, Ratcliffe, Santisteban, & Shapiro, 1971; Ratcliffe & Snyder, 1967) and atherosclerosis (e.g., Bassett & Cairncross, 1975, 1977; Lang, 1967; Paré, Rothfeld, Isom, & Varady, 1973; Uhley & Friedman, 1959). The term arteriosclerosis simply means hardening of the arteries, and includes a variety of conditions that cause the artery walls to become thick and hard. While atherosclerosis may be regarded as a form of arteriosclerosis, a distinguishing characteristic is that in atherosclerosis the inner layer of the arterial wall becomes thick and irregular due to an intimal lesion called an atheromatous plaque. Typically this plaque has a lipid core of free and ester cholesterol covered by a cap of fibrous tissue and may be associated with a necrotic process. Eventually the plaque may calcify.

The exact mechanisms by which plaques grow and progressively narrow the arterial lumen are not fully known. However, continued lipid and lipoprotein accumulation in the lesion, hemorrhage into a plaque, and fibrous organization of thrombi forming on the surface of the plaque have all been implicated. Once the arterial lumen is narrowed by at least 75%, regional blood flow may be compromised (Hollander, 1977).

The means by which catecholamines could mediate the relationship between behavioral stress and the development of atherosclerotic plaques are shown in Figure 2.1. According to Ross and Glomset (1976) the initiating event in the atherosclerotic process involves injury to the arterial endothelium. In the face of emotional stress, the resulting increases in blood pressure may produce damage to the endothelial lining of arterial vessels due to turbulence and shear stress. Catecholamines released during prolonged stress reactions might also insult the endothelium directly (Fuller & Langner, 1970; Raab, 1971; Schade & Eaton, 1977). Such effects appear to be modulated through changes of potassium and manganese thereby producing a low potassium to sodium ratio, which disturbs cell contractility and structure.

One of the basic characteristics of the intact endothelium is its nonreactivity to platelets. When small gaps develop in the endothelial lining, functional platelets seal these gaps (Wall & Harker, 1980). However, when more pronounced endothelial injury occurs, platelets adhere immediately to exposed subendothelial tissue structures. Adherent platelets recruit additional platelet constituents. The platelets also contain a growth factor that promotes smooth muscle proliferation (Kaplan, Brockman, Chernoff, Lesznik, & Drillings, 1979), which appears to be a key factor in the development of arteriosclerosis.

High levels of circulating catecholamines elicited during sympathetic nervous system activation also act to promote the mobilization of lipid stores from adipose tissues (Heindel, Oschi, & Jeanrenaud, 1975). These mobilized lipids

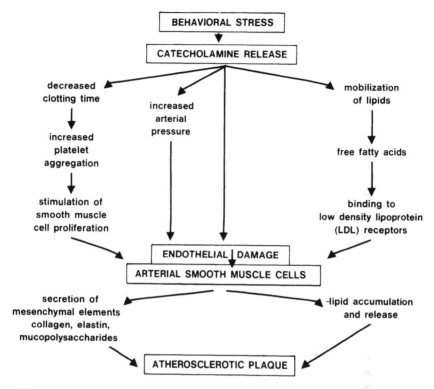

FIG. 2.1.   Mechanisms by which peripheral catecholamine release is hypothesized to mediate the relationship between behavioral stress and the development of atherosclerosis.

are hydrolyzed to free fatty acids for energy production in muscular activity (Zieler, Maseri, Klassen, Rabinowitz, & Burgess, 1968). Thus, sympathetic nervous system activation evoked by physical exertion or stress can lead to the effective utilization and rapid clearance of free fatty acids from the circulation. In contrast, the lesser metabolic requirements of emotional stress that is not accompanied by strong exertion can lead to some of the free fatty acids being converted to triglycerides by the liver. These are then circulated in the blood as a component of very low density lipoproteins (Schonfeld & Pfleger, 1971). Eventually some remnants of these lipoproteins are transported back to the liver where they are converted into low density lipoproteins and again released into the circulation. In humans the very low density lipoproteins are the major source of low density lipoproteins (Sigurdsson, Nicoll, & Lewis, 1975). And it is the low density lipoproteins that are the direct source of most lipid in atheroma (Miller, 1980). The lipid accumulating in greatest amount is cholesterol (Goldstein & Brown, 1975).

Thus far discussion has focused upon the role of catecholamines as putative mediators in atherosclerosis related to increased behavioral stress. The pituitary-adrenocortical system can also become activated during psychosocial stress leading to prolonged elevations of plasma corticosteroids (e.g., Bronson & Eleftheriou, 1965). This is of some interest as a putative atherogenic mechanism since cortisol has also been shown to potentiate diet-induced atherosclerosis in cynomologus monkeys (Sprague, Troxler, Peterson, Schmidt, & Young, 1980), and an association between elevated plasma cortisol and early atherosclerosis has been demonstrated by coronary angiography (Troxler, Sprague, Albanese, Fuchs, & Thompson, 1977). Other hormones that may become elevated during stress, and whose chronic elevation has been linked to arterial damage are growth hormone (Liddle, Island, & Meadar, 1962) and thyroxine (Hermann & Quarton, 1965; Levi, 1974). Thyroxine has also been shown to potentiate catecholamine sensitivity, and there is evidence that augmented levels of thyroid hormone can lead to an increase in the number of beta-adrenergic receptors present in the heart (Williams, Lefkowitz, Watanabe, Hathaway, & Besch, 1977).

Although the exact mechanisms by which emotional stresses induce arteriosclerosis and atherosclerosis remain speculative, there is some evidence that such associations do exist. The exact behavioral circumstances under which different kinds of degenerative arteriosclerotic changes occur still remain to be clarified. Ratcliffe (1968), for example, reported that an increase in the prevalence of arterial lesions found among mammals and birds dying at the Philadelphia Zoo was related to intraspecies social pressures. However, the instances of coronary heart disease that Ratcliffe and his collaborators related to psychosocial factors in zoo animals (Ratcliffe, 1968), chickens (Ratcliffe & Snyder, 1967) and swine (Ratcliffe, Luginbuhl, Schnarr, & Chacko, 1969) were associated only with arteriosclerotic stenosis of small intramural arteries and not with macroscopic lesions of the extramural coronary arteries or aorta. In contrast, Henry, Ely, Stephens, Ratcliffe, Santisteban, & Shapiro (1971) related arteriosclerosis of the aorta and intramural coronary vascular bed as well as glomerular mesangial changes to psychosocial factors in CBA mice. Finally, rats (Uhley & Friedman, 1959) and squirrel monkeys (Lang, 1967) subjected to atherogenic diets and psychological stress have shown elevated levels of serum cholesterol and intramural coronary atherosclerosis relative to control animals.

The experiment by Henry et al. (1971) is illustrative. Experimental mice were weaned at 12–14 days and reared in pint-size glass jars until they were 4 months of age. At that time groups of 30 to 50 experimental animals of both sexes were placed in a complex environment consisting of standard boxes joined by narrow interconnecting tubes to a single central feeding and watering area. The tubes were sufficiently narrow so that only one animal could pass through at a time. According to Henry et al. the formerly isolated animals were not able to adapt to the social demands that the system imposed, and in consequence experienced repeated confrontations leading to vigorous fighting. In contrast, control animals raised from birth in such an environment or reared together as siblings in stock boxes were less stimulated as evidenced by the absence of scarring and epilation. Other control animals were reared and maintained in jars all of their lives.

The major findings of the Henry et al. (1971) study were that relative to control animals, the experimental group showed more severe arteriosclerotic degeneration of the intramural coronary vessels and aorta as well as myocardial fibrosis and interstitial nephritis. In related experiments Henry and his collaborators found that mice raised similarly to those in the experimental condition of the Henry et al. (1971) study developed sustained hypertension (Henry, Meehan, & Stephens, 1967) in part mediated by increases in the adrenal medullary enzymes, tyrosine hydroxylase, and phenylethanolamine N-methyltransferase (Henry, Stephens, Axelrod, & Mueller, 1971). It thus appears likely that the arteriosclerosis observed by Henry et al. (1971) as a function of psychosocial stress was related to sympathetic nervous system activation and the release of catecholamines into the circulation.

Further insights into the relationships between morphological changes occurring in intramural coronary vessels as a function of behavioral stress have been provided by Bassett & Cairncross (1977). They observed that daily exposure of rats for up to 2 mos to a situation requiring escape from electric shock led to changes in the endothelial lining of the coronary vessels within the heart as well as to deposits of lipid in arteriole walls. The escape procedure involved a 4-sec duration light stimulus preceding the movement of a partition that dislodged the rat from a platform onto an electrified grid. Immediately after the rat was dislodged from the platform, the moveable partition promptly retracted and the animal was able to return to the platform. Electric shock was terminated by the return of the animal to the platform. Experimental rats received 7 light-shock exposures randomly placed throughout each 35-min test session. Escape sessions were repeated daily for periods of 1, 5, 10, 20, 40, or 60 days. For each of these time periods the experimental and control groups consisted of 12 animals each. Although not clearly specified, it appears that the control and experimental animals were treated similarly but in unspecified fashion, except that control animals were never placed in the experimental apparatus.

For each time period tested, 6 experimental and 6 control hearts were prepared for electron microscopy, and 6 experimental and 6 control hearts were prepared for light microscopy. Electron microscopic analysis consisted of examining 35 blood vessels from each left ventricular wall. The vessels were examined for the presence of junctional gaps between adjacent cells in the endothelial lining and for evidence of platelet aggregation. No distinction was made as to whether the vessels studied were arterioles, capillaries or venules. Since capillaries are most numerous, however, they probably had the greatest representation. Light microscopic analysis consisted of staining myocardial sections with Oil-red-O in isopropanol, which is a general lipid stain for neutral fats.

Bassett and Cairncross (1977) found normal junctions between endothelial cells in the coronary vasculature of control and in the 1, 5, and 10 day experimental group hearts. Junctions between endothelial cells in these animals usually involved either an extensive overlap between adjacent cells or the intrusion of a tongue from one cell into the groove of another. These junctions appeared to be sealed. Among the 20-day animals a single gap junction was observed. In contrast, half of the 40-day experimental and five of six 60-day experimental group animals showed junctional gaps. The 40 and 60 day experimental groups also showed a significantly higher number of platelets as compared to the control and other experimental groups. In control groups the platelets were always found away from the endothelial lining; whereas, both the 40 and 60 day experimental groups revealed platelets adhering to the endothelial lining with visible signs of aggregation.

At the time of sacrifice blood was collected in heparinized tubes and centrifuged in order to obtain cell free plasma for later corticosterone analysis. Control groups revealed mean plasma corticosterone levels of approximately 25 mg/100 ml of plasma. In contrast, the 1 and 5-day experimental groups revealed mean plasma corticosterone levels of about 90 mg/100 ml of plasma, which gradually decreased to about 44 mg/ml in the day 40 and day 60 experimental groups.

The findings of Bassett and Cairncross (1977) indicated that relatively prolonged exposure to behavioral stress may lead to pathological changes in the myocardium. At least some of these changes appear to be associated with junctional gaps in the endothelial lining of the coronary microcirculation and with increased platelet aggregation. Normally, the intact endothelium provides a barrier against the free exchange of large lipid molecules such as cholesterol between plasma and the arterial wall. When the endothelium becomes damaged, however, such molecules may equilibrate rapidly (Zilversmit, 1975). Bassett and Cairncross (1975, 1977) have suggested that in situations of prolonged stress, endogenous inflammatory substances can cause separation of adjacent endothelial cells (i.e. gap junctions). One source of these endogenous inflammatory substances may be mast cells, which are found around small as opposed to large blood vessels. Bassett and Cairncross (1975) found an increase in such mast cells in rats as a function of prolonged exposure to irregular, signalled foot shock. These mast cells hold and release histamine (Goth & Johnson, 1975), which can be triggered by catecholamines (Heitz & Brody, 1975) in response to sympathetic arousal.

An interesting aspect of the Bassett and Cairncross (1977) results, was the good correlation found between the adaptation of the steroid response as indicated by corticosterone levels and the onset of progressive changes in the coronary vasculature. Glucocorticoids, for example, have been found to protect against the effects of endogenous inflammatory substances, thereby preventing the leakage of macromolecules as well as thrombotic complications (Shimamoto,

1968). Interestingly, the intensity of the vascular permeability response to histamine is subject to the influence of adrenal cortical hormones. Corticosterone depresses vascular permeability elicited by intracutaneous histamine in rats; whereas, adrenalectomy enhances permeability (Garcia Leme & Wilhelm, 1975). It would therefore appear that in the Bassett and Cairncross (1977) experiment, prolonged exposure to behavioral stress resulted in junctional gaps and platelet adhesion in the coronary microcirculation that were associated with the deposition of lipids. These changes were likely to have been mediated by catecholamines. The relationships observed between corticosterone levels and the myocardial changes induced by stress, suggest that glucocorticoids could have a protective function against such alterations in myocardial morphology, since they only occurred after substantial adaptation of the steroid response took place.

Thus far, attention has been focused upon the singular role of behavioral stress in the development of arteriosclerosis. Several prospective studies that have indentified risk factors for CHD indicate that it has a multicausal origin (Kannel & Gordon, 1971; Rosenman, Brand, Jenkins, Friedman, Straus, & Wurm, 1975; Stamler & Epstein, 1970). Moreover, as the number of risk factors attributable to an individual increases arithmetically, the person's actual risk increases disproportionately (Lew, 1973; Stamler & Epstein, 1970). This suggests that in order to understand the etiology and pathogenesis of CHD in general, and the relationship between behavioral stress and the development of CHD in particular, one must study the interaction of risk factors.

An important interaction for promoting risk of atherosclerosis and CHD occurs between blood lipids and arterial pressure. This is of particular interest with regard to the study of stress-induced atherosclerosis since the catecholamines released by stress both mobilize lipids and increase arterial pressure. Prospective epidemiologic evidence indicates that at any blood lipid value, risk of CHD and atherothrombotic brain infarction is directly proportional to blood pressure level (Kannel & Dawber, 1973). Direct experimental confirmation of these findings has been provided by animal research in which lipid-induced atherosclerosis has been shown to be accelerated by systematically increasing blood pressure (Deming, Mosbach, Bevans, Daly, Akell, Martin, Brun, Halpern, & Kaplan, 1958; Moses, 1954; Bronte-Stewart & Heptinstal, 1954). Presumably, catecholamines and/or hemodynamic factors that insult the vascular epithelium can make it vulnerable to chemical factors such as elevated levels of lipids and low density lipoproteins (Ross & Glomset, 1976; Ross & Harker, 1976).

Thus far, it has not been possible to develop a nonhuman primate model in which behavior-induced increases in blood pressure have led to sustained hypertension associated with arteriosclerosis or atherosclerosis. In experiments conducted upon squirrel monkeys (Benson, Herd, Morse, & Kelleher, 1969; Herd, Morse, Kelleher, & Jones, 1969), rhesus monkeys (Forsyth, 1969), and baboons (Harris, Gilliam, & Brady, 1976), behavioral manipulations including button-press shock avoidance or the direct reinforcement of blood pressure elevations have led to pronounced increases of arterial pressure for 12 hrs per day or more during periods lasting many months. However, these experiments detected the development of neither atherosclerosis nor hypertension that was sustained for long periods outside of the experimental situation. The low fat, low cholesterol laboratory diets fed to the animals in these studies may have prevented such pathology by precluding interactions between increased arterial pressure on the one hand and elevated levels of serum cholesterol and low density lipoproteins on the other.

The effects of behavioral stress upon animals given an atherogenic diet has received at least some attention and is likely to receive a good deal more in the future. In one experiment rats fed a high lipid diet and exposed to unpredictable grid shocks for 2 or 8 days showed higher levels of accumulated cholesterol in aorta, kidney, liver, and serum as compared to control rats fed only the high lipid diet (Paré, Rothfeld, Isom, & Varaday, 1973). Similar results were obtained in animals subjected to 30 days of shock stress except that kidney tissue revealed much lower levels of accumulated levels of cholesterol, which did not differ significantly between stressed and unstressed animals. Since significant differences between stressed and unstressed rats tended to occur in the investigators' assessment of cholesterol clearance rather than in their assessment of cholesterol absorbtion, the investigators concluded that shock stress primarily influenced the ability of the animals to release and to clear cholesterol. The experimenters also interpreted the low level of cholesterol seen in the kidney after 30 days as reflecting better cholesterol clearance in this tissue than in aorta or liver.

These findings provide at least preliminary evidence that behavioral stress can interact with hypercholesteremia to influence cholesterol metabolism. Evidence also exists that behavioral stress superimposed upon an atherogenic diet can accelerate atherogenesis (Lang, 1967; Uhley & Friedman, 1959). In one study 15 adult experimental rats fed a diet high in fat and cholesterol were placed into a special cage for 6 hrs per day, 5 days per week for a period of 10 mos (Uhley & Friedman, 1959). The alternate charging of one half of the grid floor every 5 min throughout the 6 hr per day experimental period compelled the animals to move from one side of the cage to the other. In contrast, the 12 adult control rats, who were fed the same diet as the experimental rats, were never placed in the electrified special cage.

At the end of 10 mos, 7 experimental and 7 control rats survived. Although average body weight was the same in each group, total serum cholesterol and lipid levels were significantly higher in the experimental than in the control group. Moreover, the experimental animals showed significantly more sudanophilic staining in the intima of coronary artery vessels than did control animals. The authors contrast these findings with those of an earlier unpublished study in which rats were studied for a prolonged period of time using a similar protocol as the present study, but were not fed an atherogenic diet. Animals in the earlier study revealed neither hypercholesteremia nor discernible coronary atherosclerosis.

In another study examining the effects of behavioral stress in animals fed an atherogenic diet, 18 squirrel monkeys were divided into 3 groups, each consisting of 4 males and 2 females (Lang, 1967). Each of the monkeys in the first 2 groups were placed in an experimental chamber (Skinner box) for 1 hr per day, 5 days per week, for a period of 25 mos. During this period animals in one of these groups were merely restrained in the Skinner box; whereas, animals in the other group were each subjected to an unsignaled (Sidman) shock avoidance task in which pressing a lever and releasing it postponed shock for 30 to 50 sec. The monkeys in a third group, serving as cage controls, were left in their cages during the 25 mos of the experiment.

Examination of total serum cholesterol immediately prior to termination of the experiment indicated significantly higher cholesterol levels in the 2 groups just completing sessions in the Skinner box than in the cage control group. Postmortem microscopic examination revealed atherosclerosis of the coronary arteries in (a) 5 of 6 monkeys in the unsignaled avoidance group, (b) 4 of 6 monkeys that had been placed regularly in the Skinner box without the unsignaled avoidance training, and (c) 0 of 6 cage control monkeys. The coronary lesions were in the small intramyocardial arteries and consisted of both intracellular and extracellular intimal sudanophilic accumulations.

The experiments examining the effects of environmental stress upon animals subjected to a high fat–high cholesterol diet indicate that such stress can exacerbate atherosclerosis (Lang, 1967; Paré et al., 1973; Uhley & Friedman, 1959). These studies also revealed a positive relationship between stress-induced elevations in total serum cholesteral and the development of atherosclerosis. Although direct linkages among behavioral stress, the release of catecholamines during sympathetic arousal, hemodynamic changes, diet, lipid mobilization, lipid utilization, and the development of atherosclerosis have not yet been examined in the same experiment, the studies by Uhley and Friedman (1959), Lang (1967) and Paré et al. (1973) suggest that such experiments would be feasible and potentially valuable. In particular, these studies point to the need for direct comparisons to be made between behaviorally stressed animals on atherogenic versus nonatherogenic diets.

An examination of the experiments just described also points to the need for experiments to be conducted in order to ascertain how specific behavioral stresses are related to the development of atherosclerosis. Although the Uhley and Friedman (1959) experiment convincingly related behavioral stress to the development of coronary atherosclerosis, lack of information concerning the living conditions of the control and experimental rats, the psychosocial responses of the experimental animals in and out of the stressful situation, the age and sex of the subjects, etc., leave unclear what it was about the behavioral manipulation that exacerbated the atherosclerosis. In the Lang (1967) experiment it appears that behavioral factors associated with the almost daily capturing and handling of the squirrel monkeys and/or keeping the monkeys in a restricted environment for an hour per day completely overshadowed the unsignaled avoidance contingency. Thus, it was not clear in either the Uhley and Friedman or the Lang experiment exactly what the behavioral stress was that actually exacerbated the atherosclerosis. Interestingly, whereas behavioral factors such as handling may have exacerbated atherosclerosis in squirrel monkeys, cholesterol fed rabbits that were regularly handled and petted in the laboratory were shown to have fewer intimal sudanophilic lesions than rabbits that were not handled (Nerem, Levesque, & Cornhill, 1980). Such discrepancies emphasize the need for considering the effects of species, age, sex, psychosocial groupings, and variables associated with behavioral development when assessing how specific behavioral variables may contribute to the development of atherosclerosis.

Individual differences in autonomic reactivity to behavioral challenge have also been implicated in the development of CHD. Human research, for example, has shown that individuals displaying the Type A coronary prone behavior pattern elevate heart rate and/or systolic pressor responses relative to their non-coronary prone, Type B counterparts in the face of behavioral challenge (e.g., Dembroski et al., 1979; Glass et al., 1980; Manuck and Garland, 1979). In a recent study Manuck and Kaplan (1981) have documented a positive relationship between behaviorally-induced heart rate reactivity and coronary artery atherosclerosis in cynomolgus monkeys. Prior to sacrifice Manuck and Kaplan fitted 26 male, cynomolgus monkeys with EKG telemetry devices. The monkeys had previously been fed a moderately atherogenic diet for 20 mos. Heart rate reactivity was assessed during a behavioral challenge consisting of the prominent display by the experimenter of a large "monkey glove" such as was usually used prior to the capture and physical handling of the animals.

At necropsy, the coronary arteries were fixed, and sections were taken from the left main, left anterior descending, left circumflex, and right coronary arteries. Atherosclerosis, recorded as the intimal area for each section with a digitizer, was compared between animals identified as the 8 highest and 8 lowest heart rate responders to the behavioral challenge. The results revealed that relative to the low heart rate reactors, the high heart rate responders exhibited significantly greater atherosclerosis in their coronary arteries. Although preliminary and retrospective in nature, these results suggest that heart rate reactivity to stimulus situations perceived as being aversive may be related to the severity of atherosclerosis.

SUDDEN CARDIAC DEATH

Sudden cardiac death refers to natural death, due to cardiac causes that occurs between a few seconds and several hours after the onset of symptoms (Moss, 1980; Titus, 1978). Various major studies have used, 1, 2, 6, or 24 hrs as the criterion. Friedman, Manwaring, Rosenman, Donlon, Ortega, & Grube (1973) have further subdivided sudden cardiac death into instantaneous (less than 30 sec after the onset of symptoms) and noninstantaneous (minutes to hours) categories. In general, many fewer discrepancies in pathophysiological findings appear among studies when a criterion of 6 hrs or less is used than when a 24 hr period is included (Titus, 1978). According to Moss most investigators in the field now use a 1-hr period. In any event, the key features of sudden cardiac death are that (a) natural death due to cardiac causes occurs shortly after the onset of terminal symptoms, (b) time and mode of death are unexpected, and (c) the patient may or may not have had known preexisting CHD.

Although victims of sudden cardiac death may or may not have had known preexisting CHD, in the vast majority of cases, severe occlusive atherosclerosis of the major epicardial coronary arteries antedated the terminal event. In this respect, atherosclerosis of the epicardial coronary vessels is the major predisposing factor. In most cases, therefore, sudden cardiac death, which is natural, unexpected death due to cardiac causes, can be equated with sudden coronary death, which is death associated with coronary artery disease.

Coronary atherosclerosis appears to be the major predisposing cause of sudden coronary death; the terminal pathophysiological event is ventricular fibrillation. The precipitating causes of the ventricular fibrillation are not completely known. Evidence of myocardial ischemia is common, but in most cases this is not attributable to acute coronary arterial events such as recent changes in the atherosclerotic lesion or the development of thrombi (Lie & Titus, 1975; Reichenbach, Moss, & Meyer, 1977). Many, but not all victims of sudden coronary death, have identifiable myocardial infarcts. Scars of old infarcts are common and are found in nearly half of the victims. Acute infarcts less than 48 hrs old that are already healing are also common (Titus, 1978). The findings of Myers and Dewar (1975) that victims of sudden coronary death were more likely to have been subjected to an acute psychological stressor than were victims of a nonfatal infarct are compatible with animal studies also suggesting that activation of the sympathetic nervous system and the neurogenic release of catecholamines are important factors in precipitating ventricular fibrillation.

Current evidence suggests that sympathetic nervous system arousal and the release of catecholamines can interact with a variety of predisposing factors (e.g., atherosclerosis; left ventricular hypertrophy; the effects of prior infarcts) to result in ventricular fibrillation and sudden coronary death. The state of the coronary vessels, condition of the heart and its conduction system, ability of the heart to extract oxygen, duration of the psychological stress and its severity, all appear to be important variables.

Although sudden coronary death usually occurs against a backdrop of atherosclerosis, stress-induced damage to the myocardium can occur in the absence of pronounced coronary atherosclerosis. This cardiomyopathy may be of minor functional importance or it can be associated with a lethal event. In stressed young rats, for example, the lesions may be histologically manifested as scattered necrosis of small fiber groups, which are invisible to the naked eye, and which may heal without leaving a trace (Selye, 1961). In contrast, acute behavioral experiments in pigs have revealed severe macroscopically-evident instances of cardiopathy, ventricular arrhythmias and in some instances sudden cardiac death (Johansson, Jonsson, Lannek, Blomgren, Lindberg, & Poupa, 1974). To the extent that (a) healed or healing myocardial infarcts antedating the onset of terminal symptoms are found in most instances of sudden coronary death (Titus, 1978), and (b) evidence of catecholamine-induced necrosis apparently occurs in many instances of sudden coronary death (Eliot & Todd, 1976), animal studies of stress-induced myocardial necrosis may generate useful information whether or not they occur against a backdrop of atherosclerosis or ultimately result in acute myocardial infarction or sudden coronary death.

STRESS-INDUCED MYOCARDIAL DAMAGE

Evidence of myocardial degeneration has been observed as a function of frightening sensory stimuli in restrained wild rats (Raab, Chaplin, Bajusz, 1964), unsignaled, unpredictable foot-shock in domestic rats (Miller & Mallov, 1977), shocks delivered by an animal prod in swine muscularly weakened by a muscle relaxant (Johansson et al., 1974), behavioral stress associated with the trapping, handling and transport in baboons (Groover, Seljeskog, Haglin, & Hitchcock, 1963), and shock avoidance conditioning in squirrel monkeys (Corley, Shiel, Mauck, Clark & Barker, 1977). Myocardial degeneration has also been observed as a function of relatively long-term psychosocial stress in mice (Henry, Ely, Stephens, Ratcliffe, Santisteban, & Shapiro; 1971), rabbits (Weber & Van der Walt, 1973), and baboons (Lapin & Cherkovich, 1971).

Evidence of myocardial necrosis was produced in both captured wild rats and domestically reared laboratory rats after exposure to tape recordings of cats hissing and rats squealing during fighting (Raab et al., 1964). The tapes were played for 15-min durations every half hour for 3 or 7 days. Control rats were never exposed to the recordings and never showed evidence of myocardial necrosis. Although descriptions of experimental procedures pertaining to housing, maintenance, histology, and even how many days animals were actually run were only sketchily presented, it appears that 69% of the wild rats showed scattered myocardial necrosis. In contrast, only a few domestic rats showed such necrosis and this required pretreatment with a sensitizing dose of fluorocortisol for 7 successive days prior to exposure to the noise stimuli. Based upon the photomicrographs presented, it appears that at least some of the small necrotic foci were located subendocardially. Also, the necrosis included instances of coagulation necrosis and coagulative myocytolysis. The investigators ascribed the stress-induced scattered myocardial lesions that occurred in the absence of vascular abnormalities to "localized states of anoxia in the ventricular tissue under the metabolic (increased oxygen consumption) and microcirculatory (subendothelial vascular compression, shortened diastone) influence of liberated adreno- and sympathogenic catecholamines (p. 668).''

A word about the inner third of the left ventricle (subendocardium) is in order, since it is nearly always involved in acute myocardial infarction, and since it contains unique features predisposing it to myocardial necrosis (Eliot, 1979). First, it has the lowest partial pressure of oxygen of any part of the heart. Second, it's oxygen demands are the highest, because it's myofibril lengths are the longest and are subjected to mechanical stress. Third, it's blood flow is dependent upon diastole, which becomes shortened during tachycardia. Fourth, increased afterload (which is the resistance against which the ventricle contracts) brought about by sympathetically-induced increases in arterial pressure, increase myocardial oxygen demands. Fifth, endogeneous catecholamines liberated during stress, which increase ventricular contractility and rate also increase myocardial oxygen demand. Therefore, to the extent that myocardial necrosis is observed in the inner third of the left ventricular myocardium following behavioral stress, sympathetic arousal and the release of catecholamines would appear to be implicated.

In the experiment by Raab et al. (1964) both coagulation necrosis and coagulative myocytolysis were observed. Briefly, coagulation necrosis refers to myocardial cellular death in a state of lost contractility; whereas, coagulative myocytolysis refers to myocardial cellular death while the cell is hypercontracted. In the former case hypoxia of cardiac muscle related to increased myocardial oxygen demand leads to ischemic necrosis characterized by a loss of glycogen, interstitial edema, exudation, and polymorphonuclear leukocyte infiltration. Coagulation necrosis appears not to damage the myofibrils with the exception of a stretching of the filaments by surrounding viable cells. This gives rise to the elongated, thin wavy fibers seen microscopically in certain victims of sudden coronary death (Eliot, 1979). Coagulation necrosis, with its attendant features has also been produced directly in the animal laboratory by infusion of sympathomimetic agents (Ferrans, Hibbs, & Black, 1964; Ferrans, Hibbs, Walsh, & Burch, 1969).

As previously mentioned, coagulative myocytolysis refers to myocardial cellular death while the cell is hypercontracted. Aside from the hypercontraction, the hallmark of this form of myocardial necrosis is a breakdown of anomalous contraction bands, which begin to be absorbed within about 8 hrs, resulting in a vacuolated appearance. Coagulative myocytolysis is rapid in onset and in disappearance, leaving little detectable histologic evidence within 24 hrs of its onset. The lesions are distributed as widely scattered foci located predominantly in the inner third of the left ventricle. Coagulative myocytolysis occurs in approximately three-quarters of sudden coronary deaths in which coronary obstruction is not demonstrated (Baroldi, Radice, Schmid & Leone, 1974; Baroldi, 1975; Lie & Titus, 1975). It has been produced in the animal laboratory by infusion of sympathomimetic agents and is attributed to a direct effect on the myocardial cell (hyperfunctional overdrive) rather than as a secondary effect of ischemia (Eliot,

Todd, Clayton, & Pieper, 1978). Although coagulative necrosis and coagulative myocytolysis may occur differentially as a function of the condition of the heart and vasculature as well as duration and intensity of sympathetic arousal, experiments such as those conducted by Raab et al. (1964) indicate that both types of myocardial degeneration can exist in the same heart.

Severe myocardial damage attributable to acute behavioral stress has also been documented in 6-mos-old swine (Johansson et al., 1974; Jonsson & Johansson, 1974). Experimental animals were injected intravenously with succinylcholine, a curare-like compound that blockades motor end-plates, at a dosage that produced muscular weakness without respiratory distress. The animals were then shocked on a hind limb with an animal prod 5 or 6 times during the next 15 to 20 min. Pigs that survived the session were shot through the brain and killed instantly 16 to 48 hrs later. Control animals, sacrificed in the same manner, were neither injected with succinylcholine nor shocked.

Johansson et al. (1974) found that of 23 experimental swine, 2 died during the experimental session and another 3 hrs later. These 3 animals revealed multiple intramural, subepicardial, and subendocardial hemorrhages. In 14 other hearts from experimental animals, small subendocardial hemorrhages were seen in the left ventricle mainly marked on the papillary muscles and the trabeculae carneae. Six experimental animals showed circumscribed pale areas in the posterior wall of the left ventricle. Myocardial degeneration and necrosis were found in all 23 experimental animals, but in none of the 9 control animals. Damaged muscle cells were found throughout the left ventricle, but were most prominent in the subendocardium, particularly in the papillary muscles. Many foci were minute consisting of only 1 or 2 muscle cells; other foci measured about 1 mm in diameter and were composed of several damaged cells.

In the Jonsson and Johansson (1974) study, which looked at ultrastructural changes in the hearts of many of the same animals described by Johansson et al. (1974), the experimental animals revealed evidence of both coagulative necrosis and coagulative myocytolysis. At the periphery of necrotic foci, myofibrils were contracted. Within the necrotic areas changes included complete lysis of the myofilaments. Ultrastructural alterations included severe swelling of the tubules of the sarcoplasmic reticulum, loss of glycogen, damage to myofilaments, mitochondrial damage, increase in the number of lipid droplets and infiltration of mononuclear cells. In the Jonsson and Johansson study electron densities of various size and appearance were found in areas of total myocardial necrosis. Such densities presumably consist of calcium salts. These as well as the other ultrastructural findings resembled those seen after infusion of catecholamines (Ferrans et al., 1969).

Findings that accumulations of tissue-bound calcium occur in regions of myocardial necrosis, provided a basis for the development of radiopharmaceutical procedures to assess myocardial damage. Clinical studies with human patients (Parkey, Bonte, Meyer, & Graham, 1974), as well as experimental studies with dogs (Zweiman, Joman, O'Keefe, & Idoine, 1975), rabbits (Dewanjee & Kahn,

1976) and rats (Lessem, Pollimeni, & Page, 1977) determined that the uptake of the radionuclide technetium - 99 m was dramatically increased in infarcted myocardium relative to normal myocardium when the radionuclide was coupled to phosphate complexes that have a high affinity for tissue-bound calcium. The use of technetium-99-m-stannous pyrophosphate (Tc-99m-PP) or technetium-99m-methylene diphosponate (Tc-99m-MDP) has been used in behavioral experiments in rats to assess diffuse as well as more focal myocardial damage (Miller, 1978; Miller, Gilmour, Grossman, Mallov, Wistow, & Rohner, 1977; Miller & Mallov, 1977).

Miller et al. (1977) placed rats into 1 of 4 treatment conditions: (a) control; (b) epinephrine injection through a cutaneous incision; (c) a 2-hr session in which a 1 mA grid shock was given at variable intervals around a mean of 24 sec; or (d) a 12-hr grid shock session. Then, 18 hrs after epinephrine injection or 8 hrs after termination of the shock conditions, each animal received an intravenous injection of Tc-99m-PP or Tc-99m-MDP. After 100 or 300 min the animals were sacrificed. Hearts were removed, washed, blotted, weighed and counted in a scintillation counter. Subsequently, sections were prepared for light microscopy and stained with hematoxylin and eosin.

Neither the catecholamine injection nor grid shock conditions produced mortality prior to the time of sacrifice. The epinephrine injections produced large and relatively uniform, grossly visible foci of damage along the posterior interventricular septum and base of the left ventricle. Intermittent foot shock resulted in myocardial injury that was not macroscopically evident following 2 hrs of stress. Following 12 hrs of foot shock, however, widely scattered small foci of grossly visible injury were evident. In terms of whole-heart radionuclide concentrations, higher scintillation counts were obtained 300 than 100 min after injection. Tc-99m-MDP produced higher counts than Tc-99m-PP. Whole heart concentrations of MDP were an order of magnitude greater in the epinephrine injection condition than in the 12 hr foot shock condition. Concentration of MDP was in turn much greater in the 12 than in the 2 hr foot shock condition, and the MDP concentration in the 2 hr foot shock condition was significantly greater than in the control condition. The use of Tc-99m-MDP would therefore appear to provide a reasonably sensitive radiobioassay for quantitatively assessing diffuse myocardial damage in behavioral experiments.

In another study Miller and Mallov (1977) showed that radionuclide accumulation occurred only in nonanesthetized rats suggesting that the myocardial damage was CNS-mediated. They also showed that the heightened uptake was not due to increased muscle activity accompanying the stress, since levels of Tc-99m-MDP in the myocardium of restrained rats also given a dose of d-tubocurarine that minimized movement without impairing respiration, did not differ significantly from those in nonrestrained, noncurarized rats. In contrast, animals receiving foot shock showed significantly greater uptake than animals not receiving foot shock whether or not they were restrained and curarized. More recently, Miller (1978) found that the uptake of Tc-99m-MDP is greatly reduced if foot shocks are preceded by a warning signal than if foot shocks are presented unsignaled. The studies by Miller and his colleagues would therefore appear to provide a firm link between psychological aspects of stress (e.g., stimulus predictability) and the extent of myocardial injury.

Another series of studies, which was conducted by Corley and his associates, has also demonstrated a relationship between behavioral aspects of stress (e.g., use of an available instrumental response in an aversive situation) and myocardial damage in squirrel monkeys (Corley, Mauck, & Shiel, 1975; Corley, Shiel, Mauck, Clark, & Barber, 1977; Corley, Shiel, Mauck & Greenhoot, 1973). In the first of these studies, chair-restrained monkeys were trained to press a response lever to postpone tail shock in an unsignaled (Sidman) avoidance situation (Corley et al., 1973). By pressing the lever every few seconds the monkey could thereby avoid being shocked for prolonged periods. Once the animals were trained on the avoidance task, 8-hr avoidance sessions were continually alternated with 8 hrs of rest. The experiment was terminated and the animals were sacrificed when avoidance animals ceased responding in the experimental session. All 8 monkeys subjected to the avoidance situation showed microscopic evidence of at least scattered myofibrillar degeneration; whereas, control animals never shocked in the experimental situation showed no evidence of myocardial pathology. Because no controls for shock were used, however, it is not possible to relate specifically the myocardial damage to the avoidance contingency as opposed to the shocks, the shocks associated with chair-restraint, etc.

In a subsequent experiment Corley et al. (1975) subjected squirrel monkeys to an "avoid-yoke" procedure in which one member of a pair was trained to manipulate a lever to avoid tail shock. Each time that the "avoid" animal failed to meet the schedule requirement, both this animal and its "yoked" partner received shock. Thus, both animals always received the same number and temporal pattern of shocks, but only the avoid animal had control over whether shock would occur.

Corley et al. (1975) observed physical deterioration and severe bradycardia with ventricular arrest in 5 of 6 yoked monkeys, causing termination of the experiment. None of the yoked monkeys and only 1 of 6 avoid monkeys showed evidence of myocardial damage. Although these results seem paradoxical with regard to the earlier Corley et al. (1973) study, it should be recalled that the inability of the avoid monkeys to lever-press was the criterion for termination in the earlier study; whereas, physical debilitation in 5 of 6 yoked monkeys led to termination in the later study. Presumably, if the avoid animals in the second study were continued in the experiment until they ceased pressing, myocardial damage would have been seen at necropsy.

In order to test the hypothesis that myocardial lesions could be produced preferentially in the avoid animals of avoidance-yoke pairings, Corley et al. (1977) increased the severity of the stress associated with the avoidance situation. Instead of chairing and training the avoidance monkey before exposure to prolonged shock avoidance sessions, the monkeys were subjected to a 24-hr shock avoidance session without prior training. Briefly, 11 pairs of male monkeys were examined. Both monkeys were restrained at the neck and waist, but only the avoid animal had access to the response lever. In order to escape or to avoid a 1 sec. 4 mA shock the avoid monkey had to make a lever press response that postponed shock for 40 sec. If no response was made, shock reoccurred at 5-sec intervals. However, shock was also terminated automatically after 20 successive shocks without a response, which indicated that the monkey was unable to respond. The yoked monkey in each pair received each shock delivered to the avoid monkey, but had no control over shock occurrence.

Several animals died in the course of the experiment and the remaining animals were sacrificed from 24-146 hrs after initiation of the experimental session in order to assess the permanence of the myocardial damage observed. Cardiac tissue sections were made through the midportion of the left ventricle in all animals, and fuchsin stains (e.g., Masson's trichrome) were used to identify areas of myocardial damage. An important result of the experiment was that although both avoidance and yoked monkeys showed selective staining of myocardial cells, called fuchsinophilia, the staining was significantly more pronounced in the avoidance monkeys. It also seemed to represent a persistent morphologic effect, since it was readily observable in monkeys killed 5 days after the termination of the stress session.

Selye (1958) first described fuchsinophilia as an early indicator of myocardial damage, and subsequent research specifically related it to myofibrillar degeneration (Reichenbach & Benditt, 1968). According to Fleckenstein, Janke, Doring, and Leder (1975), extreme stress causes a release of toxic levels of catecholamines. This, in turn, causes myocardial cells to hypercontract and to become overloaded with calcium which, if not reversed, leads to myofibrillar degeneration. In any event, the effects of intense behavioral stress associated with pronounced sympathetic arousal tends to lead to calcium related changes observable in damaged myocardial fibers that are evidenced as (a) changes in elecron density that can be photographed under the electron microscope (Jonsson & Johansson, 1974), (b) increases in radioactive counts when radionuclides are coupled to phosphate complexes having a high affinity for tissue-bound calcium (Miller et al., 1977), or (c) fuchsinophilia (Corley et al., 1977). In the last study, myocytolysis and necrosis were also presented as additional evidence of permanent stress-induced myocardial damage.

ARRHYTHMIAS

Although atherosclerosis is an important substrate for increased mortality due to CHD, and both atherosclerosis and cardiomyopathy are associated with the vast majority of coronary fatalities, the terminal event precipitating a massive myocardial infarction and/or coronary-related death is a fatal arrhythmia. In most instances the arrhythmia is ventricular fibrillation. This rhythm disorder is characterized by irregular, continuous, uncoordinated twitching of the ventricular muscle fibers. The result is abrupt cessation of cardiac pumping such that there is no longer any output of blood from the heart. Irreversible brain damage ensues within several minutes unless the fibrillation is reversed.

Although acute or chronic myocardial ischemia most often seems responsible for initiating the sequences of events that lead to ventricular fibrillation, other factors must also be taken into account. There are several reasons for believing that these factors are associated with transient, potentially reversible disruptions of the heart's electrical activity. First, patients who have been resuscitated from sudden cardiac death do not immediately reexperience ventricular fibrillation, although this may recur at a later time. Second, in most victims of sudden coronary death, an acute coronary arterial event that can be recognized by morphological study is not present (Titus, 1978). Thus, changes in an atherosclerotic lesion or obstructing thrombi are usually not evident. It therefore appears that while myocardial ischemia creates the biochemical, hormonal and metabolic conditions that set the stage for ventricular fibrillation, other factors associated with central and autonomic nervous system functioning may momentarily destabilize the heart, precipitating ventricular fibrillation.

The sequences of events leading up to ventricular fibrillation have been modelled in animal behavior experiments. Such experiments have implicated behavioral stress in the precipitation of ventricular fibrillation. In one study, for example, the left anterior descending coronary artery was occluded in conscious pigs (Skinner, Lie, & Entman, 1975). For some animals occlusion occurred without prior adaptation to the laboratory situation; whereas, for other animals as many as 8 daily adaptation sessions were conducted before a 20-min occlusion session took place. Each adaptation session consisted of tying the animal's feet together, transporting it from the vivarium to the laboratory, attaching the recording wires and occluder tubes, and then leaving the animal undisturbed for 1 hr before returning it to its home cage. The experimental session included the above steps through the attachment of the occluder tubes, which were then used to ligate the coronary artery.

Skinner et al. (1975) found that animals receiving the 8 adaptation sessions did not reveal ventricular fibrillation during the 20 min coronary occlusion period; some of these animals also did not show fibrillation during the next 24 hrs of monitoring. In contrast, the animals that were not adapted to the experimental procedures revealed ventricular fibrillation 9-14 min following occlusion. Usually this fibrillation was preceded by ventricular arrhythmias (e.g., extrasystoles, premature ventricular contractions) occurring during the first few minutes of acute coronary occlusion. A period of normal sinus rhythm was reinstated between the initial arrhythmias and the onset of fibrillation. It is not clear from the authors' description of the experiment, however, if the ventricular arrhythmias occurring at the onset of occlusion were observed in adapted as well as in unadapted pigs. Nevertheless, the experiment did demonstrate that the behavioral stress of an experimentally naive pig being tied up, transported from the vivarium to the laboratory, and then being prepared for experimentation was sufficient to trigger ventricular fibrillation following the occlusion of a major coronary artery. Adaptation to these stressful procedures prior to occlusion delayed or prevented the fibrillation.

In order to study cardiac vulnerability to ventricular fibrillation, Lown and his coworkers have attempted to develop indices of electrical instability of the heart and its predisposition to malignant arrhythmias (Lown, Regis, DeSilva, Reich & Murawski, 1980). An assumption made in such experiments is that the nonobtrusive measures of electrical instability of the heart and ventricular fibrillation thresholds share a common electrophysiologic basis. To the extent that this assumption is correct, and to the extent to which the nonobtrusive measures in turn are derived from measures reflecting normal physiological processes, the nonobtrusive measures can be used as a marker of cardiac vulnerability for ventricular fibrillation without the animal's heart having to undergo the fibrillation.

Prior to the development of nonobtrusive measures, it was found that a single pulse of electrical stimulation to the ventricle during the occurrence of the T wave of the electrocardiogram could trigger ventricular fibrillation (Wiggers & Wegria, 1939/1940). The current intensity required to induce fibrillation was used as a quantitative estimate of the propensity of the ventricle to fibrillate. Subsequently, Han (1969) found that the current intensity required to produce fibrillation could be substantially reduced if trains of pulses rather than single pulses were presented during diastole.

In related work, Han and Moe (1954) found that if 3 stimuli are presented in close succession during diastole at low current intensities they will elicit 3 extrasystoles. If, however, current intensity is progressively increased towards the ventricular fibrillation threshold, there comes a point where the 3 stimuli will elicit 4 or more responses (repetitive extrasystoles). This repetitive extrasystole threshold has since been used as an estimate of the propensity of the ventricle to fibrillate. Advantages of this measure are that it (a) appears not to substantially alter cardiac function, (b) does not seem to influence the animal's behavior, and (c) has been reported to be a constant 66% of the current required to reach the ventricular fibrillation threshold (Matta, Verrier, & Lown, 1976).

In one experiment using the repetitive extrasystole threshold as an endpoint, platinum stimulating electrodes were placed at the apex of the right ventricle in dogs (Lown, Verrier, & Corbalan, 1973). A week after surgery, initial stimulation parameters were obtained for each animal. The amplitude of the first stimulus (S_1) was set at twice the current intensity required to propagate an extrasystole during diastole. The pulse was discharged progressively earlier in the cycle, in 10 msec steps, until a response no longer occurred. This defined the effective refractory period for a stimulus of twice threshold intensity. The delay of S_1 was set at 10 msec beyond the effective refractory period. A similar procedure was used to determine the current intensity and delay for S_2 and for S_3. The 3 pulses thus resulted in a sequence of 3 early extrasystoles. Current of S_3 was then increased in increments of 5-mA until a repetitive ventricular response occurred. At times when sequential pulsing was taking place the heart was artificially placed at 200 beats per min.

In the main experiment 5 dogs were each tested in 2 different environments (Lown et al., 1973). One environment, which was designed to minimize discomfort and behavioral stress consisted of a cage to which the dog was acclimatized for 1 hr per day for 3 days before testing. The other environment was one in which the animal was restrained in a sling during each of 3 daily sessions. During each of these sessions the animal received an electric shock while in the sling. On days 4 and 5 the animals were examined in each environment; no cutaneous shocks were presented. The current intensity required to elicit a repetitive response to S_3 was 3 times greater in the cage (43 mA) than in the sling (15 mA) environment. Lown et al. (1973) suggested that the lower repetitive extrasystole threshold obtained in the behaviorally stressing situation was due to increased sympathetic activity as exemplified by a rapid unpaced heart rate and somatic tremor. According to Lown et al. (1980), placing dogs in the behaviorally stressful environment described above also resulted in elevated plasma catecholamines. In other experiments conducted by Lown's group, dogs showed decreases in ventricular effective refractory period (Lawler, Botticelli, & Lown, 1976) or in repetitive extrasystole thresholds (Lawler, 1975) during a signaled avoidance task. Although based on indirect evidence, possibly unrelated to pathology, the findings of Lown and his coworkers are consistent with the view that sympathetic activation associated with behavioral stress reduces the threshold for ventricular fibrillation. Presumably such changes under conditions such as myocardial ischemia could lead to ventricular fibrillation itself.

The situation appears to be more complex, however, since under certain conditions increases in cardiac contractility and heart rate may be associated with reductions rather than increases in ventricular arrhythmias, even under conditions of myocardial ischemia. In one study, for instance, chair-restrained rhesus monkeys received Pavlovian conditioning in which 1 tone preceded tail shock and another preceded food (Randall & Hasson, 1978). After the completion of training a major coronary (e.g. left anterior descending; left circumflex) artery was occluded with a snare. This produced cardiac arrhythmias, primarily premature ventricular ectopic complexes.

Responses during conditioning included increases in heart rate, cardiac contractility (dP/dt), and arterial pressure. In general, ventricular arrhythmias only increased during conditioning trials when heart rate and contractility fell within a restricted and rather well-defined range (e.g., 152-188 beats/min). In some cases, for example, large increases in heart rate as a conditioned response were not associated with increases in the frequency of ventricular arrhythmias, but smaller mangitude increases of heart rate in the same animal were.

The basic findings of the study were consistent with the view that moderate elevations in sympathetic drive potentiated the occurrence of ventricular arrhythmias; whereas, more marked increases resulted in a rapid sinus pacemaker frequency that then dominated the cardiac rhythm. This interpretation is also consistent with previous reports that (a) ventricular extrasystoles are suppressed during exercise in most people (e.g., Lamb & Hiss, 1962; Pickering, Johnston, & Honour, 1978), and (b) patients with premature ventricular contractions during rest can learn to supress their arrhythmias via operantly conditioned increases in heart rate (Pickering & Miller, 1977).

The results of the experiments reviewed in this section thus far suggest that the relationship between behaviorally induced sympathetic arousal and the elaboration of ventricular arrhythmias is not a simple one, even under circumstances of myocardial ischemia. In the study by Skinner et al. (1975), for example, acute behavioral stress in pigs with an occluded coronary artery invariably produced ventricular fibrillation; whereas, in the study by Randall and Hasson (1978) aversive Pavlovian conditioning trials associated with coronary occlusion in rhesus monkeys that already had developed conditioned responses sometimes reduced the frequency of ventricular arrhythmias below basal levels, even though the conditioned responses included increases in cardiac contractility, heart rate, and arterial pressure. While the 2 studies obviously differed in terms of species and stimulus conditions, an attempt to resolve the paradox might also be presented in terms of neural versus hormonal catecholaminergic innervation of the heart. According to this hypothesis acute, severe, unpredictable stress leads to the release of epinephrine from the adrenal medulla, which in an ischemic heart can induce ventricular fibrillation; whereas, during exercise or in well-learned behavioral situations in which synergistic parasympathetic and sympathetic interactions occur, rapid sinus pacemaker frequency may come to dominate the cardiac rhythm and in some instances even override ischemia-related arrhythmias. This would be especially likely if the sympathetic innervation of the heart during exercise and during well-learned behavioral situations were both mediated by the cardiac accelerator nerves.

The above hypothesis is suggested by several lines of research. These include experiments describing the distribution of β adrenoceptors at the heart (e.g., Baker & Potter, 1980) and experiments examining the differential release of catecholamines during exercise versus behavioral stress (Dimsdale & Moss, 1980) and life-threatening circumstances. In an important series of experiments Baker and Potter determined that the β-adrenoceptors are not distributed in the same manner as the noradrenergic innervation of the heart by the cardiac accelerator nerves. Thus, the ratio of receptors to endogenous norepinephrine in the dog and rat heart was found to be almost 6 times higher in the left ventricle, which is only minimally innervated neuronally than in the maximally innervated right atrium. Baker and Potter therefore concluded that most cardiac adrenoceptors are not at nerve endings, but are localized where they can respond optimally to circulating epinephrine, the distribution being similar to that of the coronary blood flow. According to Baker and Potter, receptors at nerve endings in the heart are activated by neurally released norepinephrine. Circulating levels of this catecholamine, however, rarely approach concentrations that can normally be expected to affect most cardiac adrenoceptors. In contrast, during life-threatening situations (e.g., hemorrhage, severe acidosis, hypoglycemia, hypoxia, and the discharge of pheochromocytomas) circulating plasma levels of epinephrine reach concentrations that are adequate for this catecholamine to activate beta-adrenoceptors throughout the heart. To these situations also may be added acute psychological stress (Glass et al., 1980) and smoking (Volle & Koelle, 1975).

In terms of the hypothesis presented to reconcile the findings of the Skinner et al. (1975) and Randall and Harris (1978) studies, it is to be assumed that the acute, severe, unpredictable stress involved in transporting bound, experimentally naive pigs to the laboratory in the former study led to the release of epinephrine from the adrenal medulla inducing ventricular fibrillation in the ischemic heart. In contrast, it is to be assumed that the well-learned, predictable Pavlovian conditioning stimulus in the latter experiment elicited the release of norepinephrine from terminals in the vicinity of the S-A and A-V nodes producing rapid sinus pacemaker activity that then dominated the cardiac rhythm and in some instances overrode the ischemia-related arrhythmias. While the basic hypothesis presented is speculative, it is in principle testable. Moreover, the results of pharmacologic manipulations in the Randall and Hasson study can readily be accomodated by the hypothesis.

Randall and Hasson (1978) found that administration of the beta-adrenergic blocking agent propranolol, but not the parasympathetic antagonist atropine, eliminated conditioned increases in ventricular arrhythmias. This suggests that it was the release of catecholamines at the heart that produced the arrhythmias. Administration of the alpha-adrenergic blocking agent phenylephrine in sufficient dose to mimic the magnitude of the pressor response did not influence the frequency or arrhythmias, since this manipulation did not influence the beta-adrenoceptors of the heart. However, infusion of norepinephrine did increase the frequency of arrhythmias. This should be expected, because exogenous norepinephrine should influence the beta-adrenoceptors throughout the heart even though endogenous norepinephrine would only have an effect at neuronal end-terminals.

Although an explanation of discrepant incidences in ventricular fibrillation in terms of differential release of catecholamines from the cardiac accelerator nerves and the adrenal medulla may be useful, it still can not account for some other circumstances in which ventricular fibrillation either does or does not occur. Thus, for example, there appear to be some instances in which coronary death related to behavioral stress is preceded by ventricular fibrillation and other instances in which death is preceded by sinus bradycardia terminating in ventricular standstill. At least in some circumstances the explanation of the discrepancy may be due to sympathetic-parasympathetic interactions although in other cases involving massive myocardial infarction the discrepancy is explicable in terms of location of the lesion.

In the experiment by Johansson et al. (1974), previously described, pigs were subjected to "restraint-stress" (prevention of escape behavior by myorelaxant) in conjunction with electric shock. Severe cardiopathy was observed in all experimental animals. Of 3 animals that died suddenly, death was immediately preceded by ventricular fibrillation in 1 case and by sinus bradycardia terminating in ventricular standstill in 2 others. Major electrocardiographic changes included T wave inversion in all experimental animals and ventricular tachycardia in 14 of 23 animals.

In the experiment by Corley et al. (1977), also previously described, squirrel monkeys were subjected to 24 hrs of unsignaled escape/avoidance or to a yoked condition. Four deaths were associated with the experimental stress. Of these, 2 avoidance monkeys and 1 yoked monkey succumbed during the experimental session; another avoidance monkey seemed to show some recovery from the obvious effects of the stress, but died suddenly 48 hrs later. For the 3 monkeys that succumbed during the session, heart rate declined from over 200 beats/min to ventricular asystole within 5–10 min. The cardiovascular changes and stress-induced deaths did not appear to be related to the extent of myofibrillar degeneration that was observed in the myocardia of these animals as opposed to those who survived. Other instances in which severe behavioral stress has led to pronounced bradycardia followed by cardiac arrest have been reported for the rat by Richter (1957) and for the tree shrew by Von Holst (1972).

BEHAVIORAL PROCESSES, PHYSIOLOGIC RESPONSES, AND THE SPECIFICITY OF CARDIOVASCULAR PATHOLOGY

The results of animal behavior experiments have incontrovertably linked severe, behavioral stress with the development of cardiovascular pathology. More specifically, these studies have implicated behaviorally aversive situations in the development of atherosclerosis, cardiomyopathy and ventricular arrhythmias, and have suggested that sympathetic nervous system activity resulting in the peripheral release of catecholamines may be an important mediator. To a limited extent behavioral contingencies such as the predictability or unpredictability of aversive stimulation have also been related to the severity of cardiopathology (e.g., Miller, 1978). More provocative are distinctions that can be made among specific types of pathology, their association with separate identifiable psychological processes, and their putative mediation by different physiological events.

The possibility has been suggested, for example, that differences in perceived control over aversive situations may lead to separate patterns of autonomic response, which in turn may result in alternate manifestations of cardiovascular pathology (Schneiderman, 1978).

There is some evidence indicating that individuals confronted with an aversive situation tend to reveal one pattern of autonomic reactivity if fight, flight or other appropriate active coping responses are being attempted, but another pattern if coping responses seem unavailable. The former pattern, sometimes referred to as the defense reaction has been described extensively (Abrahams, Hilton, & Zbrozyna, 1960; Cannon, 1929; Djojosugito, Folkow, Kylstra, Lisander, & Tuttle, 1970; Hess, 1957). It is characterized by increased striate muscle activity, heart rate, cardiac output and vasodilation in skeletal muscle. The second pattern, which occurs in aversive situations in which an active coping response does not seem available is characterized by extreme vigilance, an inhibition of movement, an increase in sympathetic nervous system activity, but also a vagally mediated decrease in heart rate. This pattern can occur in anticipation of an aversive situation where coping is possible (Adams, et al., 1968; Anderson & Tosheff, 1973) or it can occur in more extreme form as part of a conservation withdrawal reaction (Engel & Schmale, 1972; Henry & Stephens, 1977; Selye, 1950). Examples of the 2 patterns of response, one associated with active coping and the other with anticipation of an aversive situation, have both been described within individual experiments (Adams, et al., 1968; Anderson & Tosheff, 1973).

Anderson and Tosheff (1973), for example, examined the cardiovascular responses of dogs during daily 1-hr sessions of unsignaled shock-avoidance as well as during the 1 hr preceeding this session when the animals were kept in a restraint harness in the experimental chamber. In terms of the coping versus noncoping distinction, the animal in the shock-avoidance situation can be said to have a coping response in its repetoire that allows it to successfully avoid noxious stimulation. Typically this involves a motor response requiring an expenditure of energy. In contrast, the animal restrained in the harness prior to an avoidance session learns to stay passively in the apparatus until the aversive conditioning session is begun.

Anderson and Tosheff (1973) found that placing the animals in a restraint harness for a 1-hr period immediately preceding the avoidance contingency was associated with a preparatory cardiovascular response pattern consisting of progressive decreases in heart rate and cardiac output accompanied by a progressive increase in total peripheral resistance. This yielded a net elevation in blood pressure. Once the avoidance period began, heart rate and cardiac output increased substantially. This further elevated blood pressure even though total peripheral resistance decreased below the level observed at the beginning of the preavoidance period.

A similar difference in cardiovascular response patterns has been described between cats immediately before and during fighting (Adams, et al., 1968). Preparation for fighting, both in the shorter periods preceding fighting and in longer trials during which animals were prevented from fighting by a barrier, was associated with bradycardia, decreased cardiac output, hind-limb vasoconstriction and increased total peripheral resistance. In contrast, during actual fighting, heart rate, cardiac output and hind-limb blood flow increased, while total peripheral resistance decreased.

The finding that 2 basic patterns of cardiovascular response can be found to hold across species and across experimental situations is consistent with Hilton's (1975) observations that (a) the central nervous system is organized to produce integrated patterns of response rather than changes in single, isolated variables, and (b) the repertoire of patterned cardiovascular responses is very small, thus facilitating the job of examining the neuraxis for pathways mediating these patterns. In recent work in my laboratory we have identified regions of the hypothalamus that appear to be involved in the mediation of the 2 patterns of cardiovascular response under consideration (Gellman, Schneiderman, Wallach, & LeBlanc, 1981).

Electrical microstimulation of the medial hypothalamus of the rabbit, particularly the ventromedial hypothalamic nucleus, elicited circling movements, hind-limb thumping and increases in heart rate and blood pressure (Gellman et al., 1981). In contrast, stimulation of electrode sites only slightly more lateral in the anterior and posterior hypothalamus resulted in tonic immobility except for a raising of the ears and orienting-like slow movements of the head; an increase in blood pressure and a decrease in heart rate mediated by the vagus nerves were also noted. In preliminary work we have also observed that stimulation of the ventromedial hypothalamus in the rabbit leads to increases in serum catecholamines, and damage to the endothelium of the aorta, which is observable under the electron microscope. These findings are consistent with results reported by Soviet investigators.

In one study Sudakov and Yumatov (1978) found that stimulation of the ventromedial hypothalamus of rabbits produced a pressor response and an increase in plasma epinephrine that was abolished by adrenalectomy. In another study Ulyaninsky, Stepanyan, and Krymsky (1978) found that intermittent electrical stimulation of the ventromedial hypothalamus in rabbits for up to 2 weeks elicited cardiac arrhythmias (atrial fibrillation, ventricular extrasystoles, and ventricular fibrillation) associated with increased catecholamine content in the blood and myocardium. On the first day of stimulation 5 of 43 experimental animals went into ventricular fibrillation and died. Fibrillation was preceded by ventricular extrasystoles in 4 of 5 animals. The fifth animal did not have a prodromal arrhythmia prior to ventricular fibrillation. In rabbits in which stimulation of the hypothalamus resulted in pronounced rhythm disorders, the ultrastructure of the myocardial cells exhibited foci of hypercontraction. There was also obvious swelling and destruction of the mitochondria as well as the presence of lipid droplets.

Just as electrical stimulations of the different regions of the hypothalamus have been shown to elicit alternate behavioral and cardiovascular responses as well as instances of cardiovascular pathology, animal behavior studies have also produced results suggesting that alternate behavioral contingencies associated with specific cardiovascular responses may lead to different forms of cardiovascular pathology.

In a study by Corley et al. (1975), for example, squirrel monkeys were subjected to an avoid-yoke procedure. Recall that in this procedure the shock-avoidance animal has control over shock delivery, whereas the yoked animal does not. The animals were initially given daily 1-hr sessions until fewer than 10 shocks per hr were administered. Then, 8-hr experimental sessions were continually alternated with 8-hr rest periods. The experiment was terminated when either the shock-avoidance animal or its yoked partner was too weak to continue.

Corley et al. (1975) found that in 5 of 6 pairs of monkeys, the experiment had to be terminated because of physical deterioration in the yoked animal. Typically, severe bradycardia, characterized by a decline in heart rate below 100 beats per min, occurred during the final session in the yoked monkeys. This progressed to asystole and death in 2 animals, results which might conceivably have also been observed in the other deteriorated yoked animals had they not been sacrificed soon after the session.

The results of the study by Corley et al. (1975) seem paradoxical, when compared with a previous study by Corley et al. (1973). In the former study, monkeys on a shock-avoidance schedule developed pronounced myofibrillary degeneration, which was not seen in the latter study. However, a critical difference existed between the 2 studies, since the former experiment, which did not have a yoked condition, depended upon the inability of the avoidance animal to lever-press as the criterion for termination. When one considers the outcomes of the 2 studies together, it becomes apparent that cardiopathy, when it developed, differed between animals as a function of experimental contingency. Thus, squirrel monkeys, subjected to unsignaled avoidance, developed myofibrillar degeneration if run long enough; whereas yoked animals ultimately revealed bradycardia and ventricular arrest without evidence of myofibrillar degeneration. Differences have also been observed between shock avoidance and yoked monkeys in terms of blood pressure, with only the former developing hypertension (Forsyth, 1969; Herd, Morse, Kelleher, & Jones, 1969).

The observations of Corley et al. (1975) concerning the yoked animals is particularly interesting in light of other findings. In rats, for example, stomach ulcers have been found to be more extensive in yoked than in avoidance animals (Weiss, 1968). Profound bradycardia, similar to that observed by Corley's group has also been observed in other situations where animals received severe, unavoidable stress. Richter (1957), for instance, found that rats that died after being subjected to severe unavoidable water stress did not drown due to asphyxiation, but instead revealed a pronounced vagally mediated bradycardia that immediately preceded death.

Another behavioral situation in which severe unavoidable stress has been reported to lead to profound bradycardia and ultimately death has been reported by Von Holst (1972). Ordinarily, when tree shrews fight, the subjugated animal must leave the territory. Von Holst prevented this by placing the subjugated animal in a cage that was separated only by a wire mesh from the victor. The subjugated animals in this experiment hardly moved, and spent almost all day lying motionless in the corner of the cage. They were obviously sympathetically aroused as evidenced by the sustained erection of their tail hairs. Nevertheless, they also showed bradycardia responses. Many of these subjugated animals eventually sank into a coma and died in uremia due to renal insufficiency. The time period varied from a couple of days to 2 weeks. At necropsy, there was evidence of an acute decrease in renal blood flow with tubular necrosis and glomerular ischemia.

The evidence just reviewed tentatively suggests that when animals having a coping response in their repertoire develop behaviorally-induced cardiovascular pathology, this may occur in the form of hypertension and cardiomyopathy; whereas, in animals lacking a coping response, severe behavioral stress may lead to profound bradycardia and ventricular arrest without evidence of pronounced myofibrillar degeneration.

If one assumes that dominant animals are able to cope, whereas submissive animals are subjected to more unavoidable stresses, experiments by Henry and his collaborators may also be interpreted in terms of a coping versus noncoping framework. In one study, for example, Henry, Ely, and Stephens (1972) examined changes that occur in adrenal weight and blood pressure as a function of dominant and submissive roles assumed by mice in normally socialized colonies. During early stages of colony differentiation, dominant mice show increased release of catecholamines as compared with subordinates. In contrast, the subordinates reveal a relative increase in adrenocortical activity. These biochemical changes eventually vanish after about 5 mos, but are replaced by a chronic increase in blood pressure for the dominant and an increase in adrenal weight for the submissive animals. The results of the experiments by Henry and his collaborators therefore appear to be consistent with the view that dichotomous physiological and morphological changes occur as a function of coping versus noncoping behaviors during potentially threatening situations.

Although the notion is attractive that different psychological processes such as coping versus noncoping may lead to alternate physiological responses, and that these in turn can result in differentiated forms of pathology, this formulation can at present only be offered as a tentative working hypothesis. Problems concerning experimental methodology and the accommodation of discrepant findings reduce both the precision and robustness of the formulation. For example, while it is tempting to attribute the differences in cardiovascular performance observed during the avoidance-yoke procedure to control over shock delivery, and hence coping capability, it should also be noted that (a) the occurrence of shock is more predictable in the avoidance than in the yoked condition, and (b) more physical exertion is required in the lever-press, shock-avoidance than in the yoked condition.

Because of a lack of well-controlled, programmatic research, the boundaries of the coping versus noncoping formulation have not been adequately documented. Whereas the Corley et al. (1973, 1975) experiments suggest that shock-avoidance animals are likely to develop myofibrillar degeneration and yoked animals to develop profound bradycardia followed by ventricular standstill, a more recent study by Corley, Shiel, Mauck, Lark, and Barber (1977) has documented an experimental situation in which both avoidance and yoked animals show evidence of myocardial degeneration and cardiac arrest. In this study pairs of avoidance and yoked squirrel monkeys were exposed to a 24-hr experimental session. Unlike the previous experiments in the series, the avoidance animals in this last study were not gradually shaped to avoid shock over a number of relatively short sessions. The length of experimental session, too, which was 24 hrs in the most recent study, was likely to have had an effect.

The major findings of the experiment by Corley et al. (1977) were that (a) myocardial degeneration and cardiac arrest were more readily induced in avoidance than in yoked monkeys; (b) heart rates declined from over 200 beats per min to ventricular asystole within 5-10 min for the 1 yoked and 2 avoidance animals that succumbed during the 24 hr session; and (c) the 2 avoidance monkeys that died during the experiment apparently ceased responding (lost coping ability?) before heart rate began to drop. It would therefore appear that under conditions of very intense, acute but extended (e.g., 24 hr) stress (a) sympathetic arousal and the profuse release of catecholamines can lead to cardiomyopathy even if active coping is not attempted, and (b) ability to cope may become impaired even if a coping mechanism is initially used by the animal. Examples of cardiomyopathy as well as profound bradycardia leading to ventricular asystole in the same animal have been reported by Johansson et al. (1974) as well as by Corley et al. (1977).

CONCLUSIONS

The animal behavior literature has definitively established that relatively prolonged and/or intense exposure to behaviorally stressful stimuli can lead to pathological changes in the myocardium including coronary atherosclerosis and myocardial damage. Peripheral release of catecholamines has been identified as an important putative mechanism mediating such pathologies. The release of epinephrine by the adrenal medulla in animals with impaired coronary circulation has been related to ventricular arrhythmias including ventricular fibrillation in behavioral experiments.

For the most part, available evidence suggests that psychological stress is more of a precipitating than a predisposing factor in the development of atherosclerosis as well as in the initiation of ventricular fibrillation. The effects of behavioral stressors upon animals given an atherogenic diet have already received some attention, and are certain to receive a good deal more in the near future.

Although experiments have causally related behavioral stress to atherogenesis, cardiomyopathy, and lethal ventricular arrhythmias, the exact relationships between specific behavioral variables and CHD have not yet been clearly specified. One pervasive deficiency in experimental design has been a lack of stimulus control. Consequently, the exact roles of stimulus predictability, availability of coping responses, and the effortfulness of these responses have not yet been related to the development of CHD with adequate precision. Other deficiencies have often included insufficient information about the animals being studied, particularly concerning home cage living conditions, life history, relative maturity, psychosocial behavior, and sex.

Attempts to explicate putative mechanisms that might be mediating pathological processes have also been hampered until fairly recently by a lack of comprehensive physiological, biochemical and morphological analyses. However, recent advances in technique and the application of these techniques to the study of relationships between behavior and the development of CHD augur well for the future. Thus, for example, use of a tethering procedure (e.g. Byrd, 1979) in conjunction with computer analyses permits 24 hr per day recordings of blood pressure. In addition, the concurrent use of a remotely controlled permanently implanted venous catheter permits blood samples to be obtained covertly without the animal being aware of the procedure (Daniel S. Mitchell, personal communication). This is an important advantage when studying behaviorally induced changes in epinephrine, norepinephrine, and other neuroendocrine and humoral agents whose plasma concentrations are known to be altered rapidly in the behaving animal. The development of methods for precisely monitoring plasma catecholamines, lipoprotein fractions, renin, cortisol and electrolytes should also permit detailed examination of the biochemical mechanisms that might be mediating behaviorally-induced pathology. Similarly, recent advances in technology now permit detailed examination of the state of the systemic circulation, coronary vessels, condition of the heart and its conduction system, and the ability of the heart to extract oxygen during behavioral experiments. Use of computer analyses in the development of ethograms has made it possible to study individual differences in behavior that may influence the development of CHD. Thus, for example, Coelho and Bramblett (1980) and Bramblett, Coelho and Mott (1981) have begun to analyze nonhuman primate behavior categories such as tension, threat, attack, subordination, and affinity, and to relate prevailing behavioral patterns to levels of serum cholesterol. Similar work relating the effects of social interaction to coronary atheroclerosis in nonhuman primates has been in progress at the Bowman Gray school of medicine for several years (e.g., Hamm, 1980; Kaplan, Manuck, & Clarkson, 1981). Finally, as the present chapter has indicated, electron microscopy (e.g., Bassett & Cairncross, 1977; Jonsson and Johansson, 1974) and other advanced morphological techniques (e.g., Miller & Mallov, 1977) are now being used to specify important relationships between behavior and CHD. Whereas, previous research was largely content to relate severe behavioral stress with the development of cardiovascular pathology, it now appears that the time is ripe for relating separate identifiable psychological processes to specific types of pathology and examining their putative mediation by different biochemical and physiological events.

REFERENCES

Adams, D. B., Baccelli, G., Mancia, G., & Zanchetti, A. Cardiovascular changes during naturally elicited fighting behavior in the cat. *American Journal of Physiology,* 1968, *216,* 1226–1235.

Abrahams, V. C., Hilton, S. M. & Zbrozyna, A. Active vasodilation produced by stimulation of the brain stem: Its significance in the defense reaction. *Journal of Physiology* (London), 1960, *154,* 491–513.

Anderson, D. C., & Tosheff, J. Cardiac output and total peripheral resistance changes during preavoidance periods in the dog. *Journal of Applied Physiology,* 1973, *34,* 650–654.

Baker, S. P., & Potter, L. T. Biochemical studies of cardiac β-adrenoceptors, and their clinical significance. *Circulation Research,* 1980, *46,* (Supp. I), 34–42.

Baroldi, G. Different types of myocardial necrosis in coronary heart disease. A pathophysiologic review of their functional significance. *American Heart Journal,* 1975, *89,* 742–752.

Baroldi, G., Radice, F., Schmid, G., & Leone, A. Morphology of acute myocardial infarction in relation to coronary thrombosis. *American Heart Journal,* 1974, *87,* 65–75.

Bassett, J. R. & Cairncross, K. D. Morphological changes induced in rats following prolonged exposure to stress. *Pharmacology, Biochemistry and Behavior,* 1975, *3,* 411–429.

Bassett, J. R. & Cairncross, K. D. Changes in the coronary vascular system following prolonged exposure to stress. *Pharmacology, Biochemistry and Behavior,* 1977, *6,* 311–318.

Benson, H., Herd, J. A., Morse, W. H., & Kelleher, R. T. Behavioral induction of arterial hypertension and its reversal. *American Journal of Physiology,* 1969, *217,* 30–34.

Blumenthal, J. A., Williams, R. B., Jr., Kong, Y., Schanberg, S. M., & Thompson L. W. Type A Behavior Pattern and Coronary Atherosclerosis, *Circulation,* 1978, *58,* 634–639.

Bramblett, C. A., Coehlho, A. M., Jr., & Mott, G. E. Behavior and Serum Cholesterol in a Social Group of Cercopithecus aethiops. *Primates,* 1981, *22,* 96–102.

Bronson, F. H., & Eleftheriou, B. E. Adrenal response to fighting in mice: separation of physical and psychological causes. *Science,* 1965, *147,* 627–628.

Bronte-Stewart, V., & Heptinstal, R. H. The relationship between experimental hypertension and cholesterol-induced atheroma in rabbits. *Journal of Pathology,* 1954, *68,* 407–414.

Byrd, L. D. A tethering system for the direct measurement of cardiovascular function in the caged baboon. *American Journal of Physiology: Heart and Circulatory Physiology,* 1979, *5,* H775–H779.

Cannon, W. B., & de la Paz, D. Emotional stimulation of adrenal secretion. *American Journal of Physiology*, 1911, *28*, 64–70.

Cannon, W. R. *Bodily changes in pain, hunger, fear and rage* (2nd Ed.). New York: Appleton, 1929.

Caraffa-Braga, E., Granata, L., & Pinotti, O. Changes in blood-flow distribution during acute emotional stress in dogs. *Pfluegers Archiv der gesamte Physiologie*, 1973, *339*, 203–216.

Carruthers, M. E. Aggression and atheroma. *Lancet*, 1969, *2*, 1170–1171.

Coelho, A. M., & Bramblett, C. A. *Species specificity in stress modeling in nonhuman primates.* Presented at a pre-meeting workshop on stress, American Society of Primatologists, Winston-Salem, North Carolina, 1980.

Corley, K. C., Mauck, H. P., & Shiel, F. O'M. Cardiac-responses associated with ''yoked-chair'' shock avoidance in squirrel monkeys. *Psychophysiology*, 1975, *12*, 439–444.

Corley, K. C., Shiel, F. O'm., Mauck, H. P., Clark, L. S., & Barker, J. V. Myocardial degeneration and cardiac arrest in squirrel monkey: physiological and psychological correlation. *Psychophysiology*, 1977, *14*, 322–328.

Corley, K. C., Shield, F. O'M., Mauck, H. P., & Greenhoot, J. Electrocardiographic and cardiac morphological changes associated with environmental stress in squirrel monkeys. *Psychosomatic Medicine*, 1973, *35*, 361–364.

Dawber, T. R., Meadors, C. F., & Moore, F. E. Epidemiological approaches to heart disease: The Framingham study. *American Journal of Public Health*, 1951, *41*, 279–290.

Dembroski, T. M., MacDougall, J. M., Herd, J. A. & Shields, J. L. Effect of level of challenge on pressor and heart rate responses in Type A and Type B subjects. *Journal of Applied Social Psychology*, 1979, *9*, 209–228.

Deming, Q. B., Mosbach, E. H., Bevans, M. D., Daly, M. M., Akell, L. L., Martin, E., Brun, L. M., Halpern, E., & Kaplan, R. Blood pressure, cholesterol content of serum and tissues and atherosclerosis in the rat. *Journal of Experimental Medicine*, 1958, *107*, 581–590.

Dewanjee, M. K., & Kahn, P. C. Mechanism of localization of 99m Tc-labeled pyrophosphate and tetracycline in infarcted myocardium. *Journal of Nuclear Medicine*, 1976, *17*, 639–646.

Dimsdale, J. E., & Moss, J. M. Plasma catecholamines in stress and exercise. *Journal of the American Medical Association*, 1980, *243*, 340–342.

Djojosugito, A. M., Folkow, B., Klystra, P., Lisander, B., & Tuttle, R. S. Differentiated interaction between the hypothalamic defense reaction and baroreceptor reflexes. 1. Effects on heart rate and regional flow resistance. *Acta Physiologica Scandinavica*, 1970, *78*, 376–383.

Eliot, R. S. *Stress and the Major Cardiovascular Disorders.* New York, Futura Publishing Co., 1979.

Eliot, R. S., & Todd, G. L. Stress-Induced Myocardial Necrosis. *The Journal of the South Carolina Medical Association*, 1976, 33–37. (Supplement).

Eliot, R. S., Todd, G. L., Clayton, F. C., & Pieper, G. M. Experimental catecholamine-induced acute myocardial necrosis. In V. Manninen and P. I. Halonen (Eds.). *Advances in Cardiology, Volume 25*, Basel: S. Karger AG, 1978.

Engel, G. L., & Schmale, A. H. Conservation-withdrawal: A primary regulatory process for organismic homeostasis. *Physiology, Emotion & Psychosomatic Illness*, Ciba Foundation Symposium, 1972, *8*, 57–76.

Ferrans, V. J., Hibbs, R. G., Black, W. C., & Weilbaecher, D. G. Isoproterenol-induced myocardial necrosis: A histochemical and electron microscopic study. *American Heart Journal*, 1964, *68*, 71–90.

Ferrans, V. J., Hibbs, R. G., Walsh, J. J., & Burch, G. E. Histochemical and electron microscopical studies on the cardiac necroses produced by sympathomimetic agents. *Annals of the New York Academy of Science*, 1969, *156*, 309–332.

Fleckenstein, A., Janke, J., Doring, H. J., & Leder, O. Key role of Ca in the production of noncoronarogenic myocardial necroses. In A. Fleckenstein & G. Rona (Eds.), Recent advances in studies on cardiac structure and metabolism, Volume 6. *Pathophysiology and morphology of myocardial cell alteration.* Baltimore, University Park Press, 1975.

Forsyth, R. P. Blood pressure responses to long term avoidance schedules in the restrained rhesus monkey. *Psychosomatic Medicine,* 1969, *31,* 300–309.

Friedman, M., Manwaring, J. H., Rosenman, R. H., Donlon, G., Ortega, P., & Grube, S. M. Instantaneous and sudden deaths: clinical and pathological differentiation in coronary artery disease. *Journal of the American Medical Association,* 1973, *225,* 1319–28.

Friedman, B., Oester, Y. T. & Davis, O. F. The effect of arterenol and epinephrine on experimental arteriopathy. *Archives Internationales de Pharmacodynamie et de Therapie,* 1955, *102,* 226–234.

Fuller, G., & Langner, R. Elevation of aortic proline hydroxylase: A biochemical defect in experimental atherosclerosis. *Science,* 1970, *168,* 987–989.

Garcia Leme, J. & Wilhelm, D. L. The effects of adrenolectomy and corticosterone on vascular permeability responses in the skin of the rat. *British Journal of Experimental Pathology,* 1975, *56,* 402–407.

Gellman, M., Schneiderman, N., Wallach, J. & LeBlanc, W. Cardiovascular responses elicited by hypothalamic stimulation in rabbits reveal a mediolateral organization. *Journal of the Autonomic Nervous System,* 1981, *4,* 301–317.

Glass, D. C., Krakoff, L. R., Contrada, R., Hilton, W. F., Kehoe, K., Mannucci, E. G., Collins, C., Snow, B., & Elting, E. Effect of harassment and competition upon cardiovascular and plasma catecholamine responses in Type A and Type B individuals. *Psychophysiology,* 1980, *17,* 453–463.

Goldstein, J. L., & Brown, M. S. Lipoprotein receptors, cholesterol metabolism and atherosclerosis. *Archives of Pathology,* 1975, *99,* 181–192.

Goth, A., & Johnson, A. R. Current concepts on the secretory function of mast cells. *Life Sciences,* 1975, *16,* 1201–1214.

Graham, J. D. P. High blood pressure after battle. *Lancet,* 1945, *248,* 239–240.

Groover, M. E., Seljeskog, L. L., Haglin, J. J., & Hitchock, C. R. Myocardial infarction in the Kenya baboon without demonstrable atherosclerosis. *Angiology,* 1963, *14,* 409–416.

Guideri, G., Barletta, M., Chau, R., Green, M. & Lehr, D. Method for the production of severe ventricular dysrhythmias in small laboratory animals. In P. Roy & G. Rona (Eds.), *The Metabolism of Contraction,* Baltimore, University Park Press, 1975.

Haft, H. I., & Fani, K. Intravascular platelet aggregation in the heart induced by stress. *Circulation,* 1973, *48,* 164–169.

Hamm, T. E. A nonhuman primate model of the effect of sex and social interaction on coronary artery atherosclerosis. Unpublished doctoral dissertation. Bowman Gray School of Medicine of Wake Forest University, 1980.

Han, J. Ventricular vulnerability during acute coronary occlusion. *American Journal of Cardiology,* 1969, *24,* 857–862.

Han, J., & Moe, G. K. Nonuniform recovery of excitability in ventricular muscle. *Circulation Research,* 1964, *14,* 44–60.

Harris, A. H., Gilliam, W. J., & Brady, J. V. Operant conditioning of large magnitude, 12-hour duration, heart rate elevations in the baboon. *Pavlovian Journal of Biological Science,* 1976, *11,* 86–92.

Heindel, J. J., Orci, L., Jeanrenaud, B. Fat mobilization and its regulation by hormones and drugs in white adipose tissue. In E. J. Masoro, (Ed.), *International Encyclopedia of Pharmacology and Therapeurics. Pharmacology of Lipid Transport and Atherosclerotic Processes,* 24, 175–373, Oxford: Pergamon, 1975.

Heitz, D. C., & Brody, M. J. Possible mechanism of histamine release during active vasodilation. *American Journal of Physiology,* 1975, *228,* 1351–1357.

Henry, J. P., & Stephens, P. M. *Stress, Health and the Social Environment: A Sociobiologic Approach to Medicine.* New York: Springer-Verlag, 1977.

Henry, J. P., Ely, D. L., & Stephens, P. M. Changes in catecholamine-controlling enzymes in response to psychosocial activation of the defence and alarm reactions. In *Physiology, Emotion and Psychosomatic Illness, Ciba Foundation Symposium 8.* Amsterdam. Associated Scientific Publishers, 1972, pp. 225–251.

Henry, J. P., Ely, D. L., Stephens, P. M., Ratcliffe, H. L., Santisteban, G. A. & Shapiro, A. P. The role of psychosocial factors in the development of arteriosclerosis in CBA mice. *Atherosclerosis,* 1971, *14,* 203–218.

Henry, J. P., Meehan, J. P., & Stephens, P. M. The use of psychosocial stimuli to induce prolonged systolic hypertension in mice. *Psychosomatic Medicine,* 1967, *29,* 408–432.

Henry, J. P., Stephens, P. M., Axelrod, J., & Mueller, R. A. Effect of psychosocial stimulation on the enzymes involved in the biosynthesis and metabolism of noradrenaline and adrenaline. *Psychosomatic Medicine,* 1971, *33,* 227–237.

Herd, J. A., Morse, W. H., Kelleher, R. T., & Jones, L. G. Arterial hypertension in the squirrel monkey during behavioral experiments. *American Journal of Physiology,* 1969, *217,* 24–29.

Hermann, H. T., & Quarton, G. C. Psychological changes and psychogenesis in thyroid hormone disorders. *Journal of Clinical Endocrinology and Metabolism,* 1965, *25,* 327–338.

Hess, W. R. *Functional Organization of the Diencephalon.* New York: Grune & Stratton, 1957.

Hilton, S. M. Ways of viewing the central nervous control of the circulation—old and new. *Brain Research,* 1975, *87,* 213–219.

Hollander, W. Biochemical pathology of atherosclerosis and relationship to hypertension. In J. Genest, E. Koiw, & O. Kuchel (Ed.), *Hypertension: Physiopathology and Treatment.* New York: McGraw-Hill, 1977.

Jenkins, C. D. Recent evidence supporting psychologic and social risk factors for coronary disease. *New England Journal of Medicine,* 1976, *294,* 1033–1038.

Jonsson, L., & Johansson, G. Cardiac muscle cell damage induced by restraint stress. *Virchows Archiv B Cell Pathology,* 1974, *17,* 1–12.

Johansson, G., Jonsson, L., Lannek, N., Blomgren, L., Lindberg, P., & Poupa, O. Severe stress-cardiopathy in pigs. *American Heart Journal,* 1974, *87,* 451–457.

Kannel, W. B., & Dawber, T. R. Hypertensive cardiovascular disease. The Framingham study. In. G. Onesti, K. E. Kim, & J. H. Moyer (Eds.), *Hypertension: Mechanisms and Management.* New York: Grune & Stratton, 1973.

Kannel, W. B., & Gordon, T. *The Framingham Study: An Epidemiological Investigation of Cardiovascular Disease,* Sec. 27, US Government Printing Office. No. 1740–0329, 1971.

Kaplan, J. R., Manuck, S. B., & Clarkson, T. B. Social factors and coronary artery atherosclerosis in cynomolgus monkeys. Paper presented at the annual meetings of the American Heart Association, Dallas, TX, 1981.

Kaplan, K. L., Brockman, J., Chernoff, A., Lesznik, G. R., & Drillings, M. Platelet alpha granule proteins. Studies on release and subcellular localization. *Blood,* 1979, *53,* 604–618.

Krantz, D. S., Sanmarco, Selvester, R. H., & Matthews, K. A. Psychological correlates of progression of atherosclerosis in men. *Psychosomatic Medicine,* 1979, *41,* 467–475.

Lamb, L. E., & Hiss, R. G. Influences of exercise on premature contractions. *American Journal of Cardiology,* 1962, *10,* 209–216.

Lang, C. M. Effects of psychic stress on atherosclerosis in the squirrel monkey (*Saimiri sciureus*). *Proceedings of the Society of Experimental Biology and Medicine,* 1967, *126,* 30–34.

Lapin, B., & Cherkovich, G. M. Environmental change causing the development of neuroses and corticovisceral pathology in monkeys. In L. Levi (Ed.), *Society, Stress and Disease: The Psychosocial Environment and Psychosomatic Diseases.* London. 1971.

Lawler, J. E., Botticelli, L. G., & Lown, B. Changes in cardiac refractory period during signalled avoidance in dogs. *Psychophysiology*, 1976, *13*, 373–377.

Levi, L. Psychosocial stress and disease: A conceptual model. In E. K. E. Gunderson & R. H. Rahe (Eds.), *Life Stress and Illness*, Springfield, Illinois: Charles C. Thomas, 1974.

Lessem, J., Pollimeni, P., & Page, F. Tc-99m pyrophosphate image of rat ventricular infarcts: Correlation of time course with microscopic pathology. *American Journal of Cardiology*, 1977, *39*, 279–285.

Levy, M. N. Neural mechanisms in cardiac arrhythmias. *The Journal of Laboratory and Clinical Medicine*, St. Louis, *90*, 589–591, 1977.

Lew, E. A. High blood pressure, other risk factors and longevity: The Insurance viewpoint. In Laragh, J. H. (Ed.), *Hypertension manual: Mechanisms, Methods, and Management*. New York: Dun-Donnelly (Yorke Medical Books), 1973, pp. 43–145.

Liddle, G. W., Island, D., & Meadar, C. K. Normal and abnormal regulation of corticotropin secretion in man. *Recent Progress in Hormone Research*, 1962, *18*, 125–132.

Lie, J. T., & Titus, J. L. Pathology of the myocardium and the conduction system in sudden coronary death. *Circulation*, *52*, 41, 1975.

Lown, B. Sudden cardiac death: the major challenge confronting contemporary cardiology. *American Journal of Cardiology*, 1979, *43*, 313–328.

Lown, B., DeSilva, R. A., Reich, P., & Maurawski, B. J. Psychophysiologic Factors in Sudden Cardiac Death. *American Journal of Psychiatry*, 1980, 137:11, 1325–1335.

Manuck, S. B. & Kaplan, J. R. *Behaviorally-induced heart rate reactivity and coronary artery atherosclerosis in monkeys*. Paper presented at the annual meeting of the Society for Psychophysiological Research, Washington, D.C., 1981.

Mason, J. W., Mangan, G. F., Brady, J. V., Conrad, D., & Rioch, D. M. Concurrent plasma epinephrine, norepinephrine, and 17-hydroxycorticosteroid levels during conditioned emotional disturbances in monkeys. *Psychosomatic Medicine*, *23*, 344–353, 1961.

Matta, R. J., Verrier, R. L., & Lown, B. The repetitive extrasystole threshold as an index of vulnerability to ventricular fibrillation. *American Journal of Physiology*, 1976, *230*, 1469–1473.

Miller, D. G. Effect of signaled versus unsignaled stress on rat myocardium. *Psychosomatic Medicine*, 1978, *40*, 432–434.

Miller, G. J. High density lipoproteins and atherosclerosis. *Annual Review of Medicine*, 1980, *31*, 97–108.

Miller, D. G., Gilmour, R. F., Grossman, E. D., Mallov, S., Wistow, B. W., & Rohner, R. F. Myocardial uptake of Tc99m skeletal agents in the rat after experimental induction of microscopic foci of injury. *Journal of Nuclear Medicine*, 1977, *18*, 1005–1009.

Miller, D. G., & Mallov, S. The quantitative determination of stress-induced myocardial damage in rats. *Pharmacology, Biochemistry and Behavior*, 1977, *7*, 139–145.

Moses, C. Development of atherosclerosis in dogs with hypercholesterolemia and chronic hypertension. *Circulation Research*, 1954, *2*, 243–248.

Moss, A. J. Prediction and prevention of sudden cardiac death. *Annual Review of Medicine*, 1980, *31*, 1–14.

Myers, A., & Dewar, H. A. Circumstances attending 100 sudden deaths from coronary disease with coroner's necropsies. *British Heart Journal*, 1975, *37*, 1133–43.

Nerem, R. M., Levesque, M. J., & Cornhill, J. F. Social environment as a factor in diet induced atherosclerosis. *Science*, 1980, *208*, 1475–1476.

Paré, W. P., Rothfeld, B., Isom, K. E., & Varady, A. Cholesterol synthesis and metabolism as a function of unpredictable shock stimulation. *Physiology and Behavior*, *1973*, *11*, 107–110.

Parkey, R. W., Bonte, F. J., Meyer, S. L., & Graham, K. D. A new method for radionuclide imaging of acute myocardial infarction in humans. *Circulation*, 1974, *50*, 540–546.

Pickering, T. G., Johnston, J., & Honour, A. J. Suppression of ventricular extrasystoles during sleep and exercise, and effects of autonomic drugs. In P. J. Schwartz, A. M. Brown, A. Malliani,

& A. Zanchetti (Eds.), *Neural Mechanisms in Cardiac Arrhythmias*. New York: Raven, 1978.

Pickering, T. G., & Miller, N. E. Learned voluntary control of heart rate and rhythm in two subjects with premature ventricular contractions. *British Heart Journal*, 1977, *49*, 152–159.

Raab, W. Emotional and sensory stress factors in myocardial pathology. *American Heart Journal*, 1966, *72*, 538–564.

Raab, W. Cardiotoxic biochemical effects of emotional-environmental stressors: Fundamentals of psychocardiology. In L. Levi (Ed.). *Society, Stress and Disease*. London: Oxford, 1971.

Raab, W., Chaplin, J. P., & Bajusz, E. Myocardial necroses produced in domesticated rats and in wild rats by sensory and emotional stresses. *Proceedings of the Society of Experimental Biology and Medicine*, 1964, *116*, 665–669.

Randall, D. C., & Hasson, D. M. Incidence of cardiac arrhythmias in monkey during classic aversive and appetitive conditioning. In P. J. Schwartz, A. M. Brown, A. Malliani & A. Zanchetti (Eds.), *Neural Mechanisms in Cardiac Arrhythmias*. New York: Raven, 1978.

Ratcliffe, H. L. Environment, behavior, and disease. In E. Stellar & J. M. Sprague (Eds.), *Physiological Psychology, vol. 2*. New York: Academic Press, 1968.

Ratcliffe, H. L., Luginbuhl, H., Schnarr, W. R. & Chacko, K. Coronary arteriosclerosis in swine. *Journal of Comparative and Physiological Psychology*, 1969, *68*, 385–392.

Ratcliffe, H. L. & Snyder, R. L. *Arteriosclerotic Stenosis of the Intramural Coronary Arteries of Chickens: Further Evidence of a Relation to Social Factors*. From the Penrose Research Laboratory, Zoological Society of Philadelphia and the Department of Pathology, University of Pennsylvania, 1967. Pgs. 357–365.

Reichenbach, D. D., & Benditt, E. P. Myofibrillar degeneration: A response of the myocardial cell to injury. *Archives of Pathology*, 1968, *85*, 189–199.

Reichenbach, D. D., Moss, N. S., & Meyer, E. Pathology of the heart in sudden cardiac death. *American Journal of Cardiology*, 1977, *39*, 865–872.

Richter, C. P. On phenomenon of sudden death in animals and man. *Psychosomatic Medicine*, 1957, *19*, 191–198.

Rona, G., Chappel, C. I., Balasy, T., & Caudry, R. An infarct-like myocardial lesion and other toxic manifestations produced by isoproterenol in the rat. *Archives of Pathology*, 1959, *67*, 443–455.

Rosenman, R. H., Brand, R. J., Jenkins, C. D., Friedman, M., Straus, R., & Wurm, M. Coronary heart disease in the Western Collaborative Group Study: Final follow-up experience of 8 ½ years. *Journal of the American Medical Association*, 1975, *233*, 872–877.

Ross, R., & Glomset, J. A. The pathogenesis of atherosclerosis. New England *Journal of Medicine*, 1976, *295*, 369–377.

Ross, R., & Harker, L. Hyperlipidemia and atherosclerosis. *Science*, 1976, *193*, 1094–1100.

Russek, H. I. Emotional stress as a cause of coronary heart disease. *Journal of the American College Health Association*, 1973, *22*, 120–123.

Selye, H. *The Physiology and Pathology of Exposure to Stress*, Montreal: Acta, Inc., 1950.

Selye, H. *The Chemical Prevention of Cardiac Necroses*. New York: The Ronald Press, Co., 1958.

Selye, H. *The Pluricausal Cardiopathies*. Springfield, Illinois: Charles C. Thomas, 1961.

Schade, D., & Eaton, R. The regulation of plasma ketone body concentration by counter regulatory hormones in man. I. Effect of norepinephrine in diabetic man. *Diabetes*, 1977, *26*, 989.

Schneiderman, N. Animal models relating behavioral stress and cardiovascular pathology. In T. M. Dembroski, S. M. Weiss, J. L. Shields, S. G. Haynes, & M. Feinleib, (Eds.), *Coronary-Prone Behavior*. New York: Springer-Verlag, 1978.

Schonfeld, G., & Pfleger, B. Utilization of exogenous free fatty acids for the production of very low density lipoprotein triglyceride by livers of carbohydrate-fed rats. *Journal of Lipid Research*, 1971.

Shimamoto, T. Experimental study on atherosclerosis: an attempt at its prevention and treatment. *Acta Pathologica,* Japan, 1969, *19,* 15–43.

Sigurdsson, G., Nicoll, A., & Lewsi, B. Conversion of very low density lipoprotein to low density lipoprotein. *Journal of Clinical Investigation,* 1975, *56,* 1481–90.

Skinner, J. E., Lie, J. T., & Entman, M. L. Modification of ventricular fibrillation latency following coronary artery occlusion in the conscious pig: The effects of psychological stress and beta-adrenergic blockade. *Circulation,* 1975, *51,* 656–667.

Sprague, E. A., Toxler, R. G., Peterson, D. F., Schmidt, R. E., & Young, J. T. Effect of cortisol on the development of atherosclerosis in cynomolgus monkeys. In S. S. Kalter (Ed.), *The Use of Nonhuman Primates in Cardiovascular Diseases.* Austin: University of Texas Press, 1980.

Stamler, J., & Epstein, F. Coronary heart disease. Risk factors as guides to preventive action. *Preventive Medicine,* 1970, *1,* 27–36.

Sudakov, K. V., & Yumatov, E. A. Acute Psychosocial Stress as the Cause of Sudden Death. *USA-USSR First Symposium on Sudden Death,* Yalta, USSR, 405–416, 1978.

Titus, J. L. Pathology of Sudden Cardiac Death. In *USA-USSR First Symposium on Sudden Death,* Yalta, USSR, 309–318, 1978.

Troxler, R. G., Sprague, E. A., Albanese, R. A., Fuchs, R., & Thompson, A. J. The association of elevated plasma cortisol and early atherosclerosis as demonstrated by coronary angiography. *Atherosclerosis,* 1977, *26,* 151–162.

Uhley, H. N., & Friedman, M. Blood lipids, clotting and coronary atherosclerosis in rats exposed to a particular form of stress. *American Journal of Physiology,* 1959, *197,* 396–398.

Ulyaninsky, L. S., Stepanyan, E. P., & Krymsky, L. D. Cardiac Arrhythmia of Hypothalamic Origin in Sudden Death. *USA-USSR First Symposium on Sudden Death,* Yalta, USSR, 417–429, 1978.

Volle, R. L., & Koelle, G. B. Ganglionic stimulating and blocking agents. In L. S. Goodman & A. Gilman (Eds.), *The Pharmacological Basis of Therapeutics* (5th Ed.). New York: MacMillan, 1975.

Von Holst, D. Renal failure as the cause of death in Tupaia belangeri (tree shrews) exposed to persistent social stress. *Journal of Comparative Physiology,* 1972, *78,* 236–273.

Wall, R. T., & Harker, L. A. The endothelium and thrombosis. *Annual Review of Medicine,* 1980, *31,* 361–71.

Weber, H. W., & Van der Walt, J. J. Cardiomyopathy in crowded rabbits: A preliminary report. *South African Medical Journal,* 1973, *47,* 1591–1595.

Weiss, J. M. Effects of coping behavior on development of gastroduodenal lesions in rats. *Proceedings of the 75th Annual Convention of the American Psychological Association,* 263–264, 1968.

Wiggers, C. J., & Wegria, R. Ventricular fibrillation due to single, localized induction and condenser shocks applied during the vulnerable phase of ventricular systole. *American Journal of Physiology,* 1939/1940, *128,* 500–508.

Williams, L. T., Lefkowitz, R. J., Watanabe, A. M., Hathaway, D. R., & Besch, H. R. Thyroid hormone regulation of beta-adrenergic receptor number: possible biochemical basis for the hyperadrenergic state in hyperthyroidism. *Clinical Research,* 1977, *25,* 458.

Zierler, K. L., Maseri, A., Klassen, D., Rabinowitz, D., & Burgess, J. Muscle metabolism during exercise in man. *Transcripts of the Association of American Physicians,* 1968, *81,* 266–269.

Zilversmit, D. B. Mechanisms of cholesterol accumulation in the arterial wall. *American Journal of Cardiology,* 1975, *35,* 559–566.

Zweiman, F. E., Joman, B. L., O'Keefe, A., & Idoine, J. Selective uptake of ^{99m}Tc and ^{67}Ga in acutely infarcted myocardium. *Journal of Nuclear Medicine,* 1975, *16,* 975–979.

3 Perspectives on Coronary-Prone Behavior

Theodore M. Dembroski and James M. MacDougall
Eckerd College

J. Alan Herd
Baylor College of Medicine

Jim L. Shields
National Heart, Lung, and Blood Institute

ORIGIN AND DEVELOPMENT OF THE TYPE A CONCEPT

Cardiovascular related diseases are the leading causes of death in western industrialized societies; and even in their nonlethal manifestations, these diseases produce immense economic, social, and psychological suffering. Despite decades of intense biomedical research, knowledge of the etiology of coronary heart disease (CHD) remains so limited that most new cases cannot be predicted from the best combination of the traditional risk factors of elevated levels of blood pressure, serum cholesterol, and smoking (Jenkins, 1976; Keys, Taylor, Blackburn, Brozek, Anderson, & Simonson, 1971).

The pandemic of CHD largely emerged during the twentieth century. This emergence and recently reported slight declines in coronary related *deaths* cannot readily be attributed to changes in diet, diagnostic procedures, genetic factors, age structure of the population, or physical exercise (Gordon & Thom, 1975; Mann, 1977; Michaels, 1966; Rosenman, 1978a; White, 1974). Nor can changes in disease rates be completely related to alterations in the incidence of the traditional known risk factors of age, serum cholesterol, systolic blood pressure, and cigarette smoking (Corday & Corday, 1975; Mann, 1977; Rosenman, 1978a). Moreover, the same combination of risk factors that is predictive of

CHD in the United States is associated with different rates of incidence and prevalence of CHD in other cultures (Keys, 1970; Gordon, Garcia-Palmieri, Kagan, Kannel, & Schiffman, 1974). Thus, the search has continued for additional risk factors in the multiple risk factor approach to understanding, predicting, and controlling CHD.

To date, one important outcome of this search has been the realization that a complex interplay of constitutional, environmental, and behavioral factors participate in the etiology of CHD. In fact, there is growing suspicion that behavioral factors may play a prominent and perhaps focal role in hastening the development of CHD and in precipitating clinical events.

Conceptually, it is possible to divide coronary-prone behaviors into two general categories. The first category includes consummatory behaviors that increase risks through ingestion of substances which insult either acutely or chronically, directly or indirectly, the cardiovascular system. Examples of such consummatory behaviors include cigarette smoking, immoderate alcohol consumption, use of certain drugs, and excessive dietary intake of saturated fat, cholesterol, calorie-dense carbohydrates and the like. The importance of these behavioral factors, together with a sedentary lifestyle, is underscored by the efforts of Federal agencies, health organizations, and private medical groups to persuade people to eliminate or modify these behaviors to a degree that will reduce traditional risk factors in a clinically significant fashion (Farquhar, 1978; Keys, et al., 1971; MRFIT, 1976). Secondary prevention through persuading people to have their blood pressure checked and to seek and maintain pharmacologic regimens of hypertension control are attempts at risk factor reduction that are also logically linked to the first class of coronary-prone behaviors.

A second category of coronary-prone behaviors may contribute to the etiology of CHD through a different set of pathways. These behaviors and pathways, which are the central focus of this chapter, can be generally subsumed under the broad concept of "stress" as a psychological and physiological response to social and environmental events. The importance of the relationship between emotional behavior and sudden death has long been recognized by physicians. Nearly two thousand years ago Celsus (30 A.D.) linked behavioral states and cardiovascular reactivity by recognizing that ". . . fear and anger and any other state of the mind may often be apt to excite the pulse." (Cited in Buell & Eliot, 1979.) This fact did not escape William Harvey (1628), the father of cardiovascular physiology, when he commented over three hundred years ago, "Every affection of the mind that is attended with either pain or pleasure, hope or fear, is the cause of an agitation whose influence extends to the heart." Both Heberden (1772) in England, who was one of the first to clearly describe the symptoms of angina pectoris, and a contemporary, Fothergill (1781), implicated emotional states, particularly anger, as predisposing factors in CHD. Wardrop (1851) also concurred with his predecessors, and the physician Trousseau (1882) extended these observations to suggest that outbursts of anger may aggravate heart disease to such an extent as to precipitate sudden death. Anecdotal evidence supporting his assertion was already available from the violent and firey tempered John Hunter (1729–1793), a great pioneer in cardiovascular surgery and pathology. Hunter suffered from emotion-related bouts of angina and had stated, "My life is at the mercy of any rascal who chooses to put me in a passion." Dr. Hunter died shortly after participating in a vociferous and heated faculty meeting at the Royal College of Physicians in Glasgow, Scotland. As Sir William Osler described it, "In silent rage and in the next room gave a deep groan and fell down dead" (cited in DeBakey & Gotto, 1977).

The focus of these anecdotal accounts has been on the emotions, with particular emphasis on hostility and anger in exciting clinical symptoms or precipitating sudden death; however, in describing individuals prone to CHD, the German physician Von Dusch (1868) included not only emotions but also other behavioral attributes such as vigorous voice stylistics and hard-driving job involvement. Similarly, William Osler (1892) was eloquently succinct in attributing CHD to ". . . the high pressure at which men live and the habit of working the machine to its maximum capacity." He described his typical coronary patient as ". . . not the delicate, neurotic person . . . but the robust, the vigorous in mind and body, the keen and ambitious man, the indicator of whose engine is always at full speed ahead."

During the twentieth century, psychiatrists began to turn their attention to the psychological characteristics of coronary patients. In this connection, the Menningers (1936) led the way by describing their coronary patients as possessing strongly aggressive attributes. Other psychiatrists in the 1940's offered descriptions of those who were coronary-prone as evidencing hard-driving achievement oriented behavior (Dunbar, 1943); as chronically performing in a tough-minded manner in the interest of achieving power and prestige while being insensitive to nuances in the environment (Kemple, 1945); and compulsively engaging in a never-ending struggle for mastery (Arlow, 1945; Gildea, 1949).

Despite the wealth of clinical impressions regarding the relationship between behavioral characteristics and CHD, systematic and programmatic research in the area was not launched until the 1950's. Two pioneering cardiologists, Drs. Meyer Friedman and Ray Rosenman (1959), began an orderly analysis of coronary-prone behavior by (a) providing a conceptual definition of a coronary-prone behavior pattern; (b) developing a reliable means of assessing the pattern; and (c) launching research studies to investigate the validity of the concept of coronary-prone behavior. The conceptual definition they evolved and to which they applied the label of the Type A pattern, considered coronary-prone behaviors as an action-emotion complex consisting of high levels of achievement concerns, hard-driving job involvement, competitiveness, aggressiveness, hostility, time-urgency, and impatience. The action-emotion complex was seen as emerging most often in response to environmental challenges or provocations common in Western industrialized existence. Because they observed that Type A individuals often spoke in a loud, explosive, rapid, and accelerated fashion, they developed a structured interview (SI) to assess the Type A pattern. In this interview, exaggerated voice and psychomotor mannerisms as well as subjective self reports were used to classify persons as extreme Type A_1, incompletely developed Type A_2, or the converse Type B_3 and B_4 patterns, which were characterized by the relative absence of Type A attributes. The label Type X was reserved for a small percentage of subjects who possessed equal amounts of Type A and B behaviors. Initial prevalence studies revealed that the Type A pattern was substantially more characteristic of coronary patients than others (Friedman & Rosenman, 1959; Rosenman & Friedman, 1961); but the bulk of the evidence linking the Type A pattern with clinical CHD was derived from the prospective Western Collaborative Group Study (WCGS) (Rosenman, Friedman, Straus, Wurm, Kositchek, Hahn, & Werthessen, 1964).

Over 3,000 middle-aged males free of CHD symptoms were followed for eight and one-half years. The results revealed that Type A subjects were about twice as likely as Type B subjects to manifest the major clinical symptoms of CHD (for a review of the WCGS, see Brand, 1978). Other researchers have corroborated and extended the findings of Friedman and Rosenman. For example, although the Rosenman-Friedman interview was the primary means of assessing Type A in the WCGS, a questionnaire called the Jenkins Activity Survey (JAS), which was developed to duplicate the interview designation of Type A and B was also used in the WCGS (Jenkins, Rosenman, & Friedman, 1967). Research using the JAS, SI and other questionnaires designed to assess Type A attributes has firmly established over the past two decades an association between Type A behaviors and clinical CHD (for reviews, see Jenkins, 1976; 1978; Rosenman & Friedman, 1974; Zyzanski, 1978). Independently of traditional risk factors, Type A behaviors have been related to (a) the incidence and prevalence of clinical CHD in both men and women (Brand, Rosenman, Jenkins, Sholtz, & Zyzanski, 1978; Haynes, Feinleib, & Kannel, 1980); (b) recurrent clinical events (Brand, Rosenman, Scholtz, & Friedman, 1976; Jenkins, Zyzanski, & Rosenman, 1976); (c) angiographically confirmed severity of atherosclerosis (Blumenthal, Williams, Kong, Schanberg, & Thompson, 1978; Frank, Heller, Kornfeld, Sporn, & Weiss, 1978; Friedman, Rosenman, Straus, Wurm, & Kositchek, 1968; Williams, Haney, Lee, Kong, Blumenthal, & Whalen, 1980); and (d) most recently in a preliminary report, the progression of atherosclerosis in men (Krantz, Sanmarco, Selvester, & Matthews, 1979).

As Jenkins (1978) has cogently argued, establishment of the Type A pattern as an independent risk factor for CHD has proceeded in an orderly manner, employing rigorous criteria similar to those used by epidemiologists to identify elevations of age, serum cholesterol, blood pressure, and cigarette smoking as risk factors for CHD. Recently, the National Heart, Lung and Blood Institute assembled a review panel representing a variety of biomedical and behavioral specialties to critically examine the evidence for the association between Type A behavior and CHD. The following is the opening paragraph of the panel's final report.

> The Review Panel accepts the available body of scientific evidence as demonstrating that Type A behavior (as defined by the SI, JAS, and Framingham scale) is associated with an increased risk of clinically apparent CHD in employed, middle-aged U.S. citizens. This increased risk is over and above that imposed by age, systolic blood pressure, serum cholesterol, an smoking and appears to be of the same order of magnitude as the relative risk associated with any of these other factors.[1]

Although a general association between the Type A pattern and CHD has been demonstrated, many problems remain in need of solution. For example, the fact remains that the Type A pattern is a relatively poor predictor of CHD, a characteristic which is equally shared with the traditional risk factors for the disease. Despite this, the Type A pattern as classically measured by the SI and JAS is likely to remain with us for some time to come because of the data base established in the WCGS. In other words, it is unlikely any time soon that another prospective study will be launched to examine potential behavioral predictors among symptom-free individuals. In the meantime, a promising first step in further refinement of the definition of coronary-prone behaviors was illustrated by Matthews, Glass, Rosenman, & Bortner (1977) who showed that some components of the Friedman-Rosenman Type A pattern appear to have greater strength of association with CHD than others. The attributes primarily reflected potential for hostility, competitiveness, impatience, irritability, and vigorous voice stylistics. Interestingly, there was no linear relationship reported between SI-derived categories of Type A (i.e., different levels of Type A behaviors) and CHD in the WCGS. It is possible that the lack of a dose-response relationship between levels of Type A and CHD was due to inappropriate weighting of certain components of the Type A pattern in designating subjects as more or less extreme Type A. Present efforts at component scoring of the SI to provide continuous variables for the total pattern and its components can be used to reexamine this issue with extant WCGS data. Along the same line, other as yet unidentified attributes remain to be specified and their relationship to *different* manifestations of CHD established (e.g., angina vs. myocardial infarction). To the extent that additional variables can be derived from the SI, the WCGS data should prove invaluable to future research.

---

[1]*Coronary-prone behavior and coronary heart disease: A critical review.* Report of the Coronary-Prone Behavior Review Panel submitted to the National Heart, Lung, and Blood Institute, National Institutes of Health, December 1978. The authors express gratitude to the members of the Review Panel, whose thoughtful discussions helped clarify some of the ideas expressed in this review. In this connection, Dr. Stephen Weiss, who coordinated this meeting, deserves special thanks and credit.

In approaching this research, it would be desirable to investigate the interactions between the Type A pattern and its components, other psychological and behavioral attributes, and environmental circumstances to determine which combinations are more strongly related to manifestations of CHD. Williams et al., (1980), for example, showed that hostility (MMPI defined) and the Type A pattern (SI defined) each made independent contributions in predicting angiographically documented severity of atherosclerosis. Research of this kind can be extended in a number of ways. For example, use of the MMPI offers the opportunity of exploring interactions of Type A behaviors with other psychological attributes. Similarly, component analyses of the interviews in the Williams et al. sample could determine whether the same factors that predicted CHD in the Matthews et al. component analyses of the WCGS interviews also predict severity of atherosclerosis.

Despite the conceptual emphasis on the importance of the environment in evoking Type A behavior, most research in the area has not included adequate measures of environmental demand. Correction of this deficiency should receive high priority, since measurement of both Type A attributes and environmental demand offers promise for improved prediction. As noted above, it is possible that several different types of behavior may eventually qualify as coronary-prone and that combinations of such behaviors including environmental circumstances that participate in evoking them, may jointly increase risk for CHD. Such considerations lead to the clear recognition that the conceptual and operational definitions of coronary-prone behavior are presently in an evolving state and eventually will only partially overlap with the original Friedman and Rosenman conceptualization of the Type A pattern. For this reason, future research should include component scoring of the SI and JAS as well as assessment of other potentially promising attributes.

In this connection, research both in the United States and abroad has consistently replicated the finding of an association between Type A attributes and CHD, but since most of this research has been conducted with white male adults, it is unknown whether Type A behaviors are distributed in the United States and other cultures. Cross-cultural research offers yet another opportunity for identifying behaviors that are coronary-prone (for a discussion of these issues, see Cohen, 1978).

Type A behavior appears to be related primarily to CHD, although some evidence suggests that it may be related to violent death, mild forms of illness, and alcoholism as well (Glass, 1977; Rose, Jenkins, & Hurst, 1978). Much more work is clearly needed to determine the nature of such relationships and the possible mechanisms involved. In addition, this work should be extended to determine whether Type A behaviors are related to a variety of other diseases, e.g., migraine, noncoronary arteriosclerosis, ulcer, etc. Here component analyses of Type A and examination of other psychological attributes, e.g., neuroticism, depression, etc., may reveal interesting interactions between behaviors and diseases.

Although the Type A pattern has been shown to precede the onset of CHD, it is not certain whether other as yet unidentified factors jointly influence the development of both Type A behavior and CHD. In this regard, there are no longitudinal data evaluating Type A behavior over the life span and, as yet, only meager data are available regarding the precise mechanisms involved in the development of the pattern (for a discussion of these issues, see Matthews, 1978). Generally, the behavior of Type A and Type B individuals appears to differ in predictable ways (Glass, 1977); however, since most of this research used JAS-defined Type A and B subjects, and since the JAS and SI methods of assessment only partially overlap (MacDougall, Dembroski, & Musante, 1979— see below), construct validity studies are needed to determine the behavioral characteristics of SI defined A's and B's. Similar work will be necessary to establish the validity of important behavioral elements identified through component scoring analyses in association research. The critical role of the environmental setting in evoking Type A behaviors appears well established, but work is just beginning bearing on perceptual and cognitive information processing differences between the Types (Matthews & Brunson, 1979; Streufert, Streufert, Dembroski, & MacDougall, 1979), and how such differences may influence psychological, behavioral, and physiological processes and vice versa.

At present, Type A is usually conceptualized as a behavior pattern rather than a personality construct. Some prefer it this way: "The behavior pattern is a *consistent syndrome* of behaviors (traits) that can be specified and quantified. It is theoretically more sound to refer to it as a 'behavior type' than as a 'personality type.''' (Caffrey, 1978). Others bemoan the lack of theoretical guidance in the area. Referring to the Type A concept, Scherwitz, Leventhal, Cleary, and Laman (1978) remark: "It does not provide a theory or picture of the behavioral mechanisms underlying the behavior, and does not provide a theory to explain how behavioral mechanisms underlying the Type A concept relate to the physiological mechanisms causing CHD." Based on their work with self-referencing in Type A's (i.e., the use of I, me, mine, my), they suggest that the construct of self-involvement may be central in explaining the relation between Type A behavior and CHD. On the other hand, based on his extensive laboratory studies, Glass (1977) conceptualizes the Type A pattern as a style of response evoked by environmental stressors in individuals who possess a heightened need to master or control their environment. The fact is that a variety of theoretical approaches to the problem of the relations between behavior and disease can be applied to the Type A area (cf. Buell & Eliot, 1979; Dembroski, MacDougall, & Shields, 1977; Eliot, 1979; Greenspan, 1979; Herd, 1978; House, 1974; Schwartz, 1977). In any event, the development of a more theoretical approach to Type A must necessarily proceed in an orderly programmatic manner including the establishment of (a) conceptual and operational definitions of constructs derived from the new theory; (b) the reliability and validity of such constructs and their relation to the Type A pattern and its components; and (c) association of constructs with traditional risk factors, potentially damaging physiologic conditions, severity of atherosclerosis, and prevalence, incidence and recurrence of clinical CHD. At least in the short run, what is more likely to develop than any "grand theory or picture" of Type A is a series of minitheories that will address the various components of the Type A pattern and other behavioral attributes that have been demonstrably related to clinical CHD or potentially damaging physiologic reactions.

PATHOPHYSIOLOGY AND THE TYPE A PATTERN

A plausible hypothesis is that the Type A behavior pattern contributes to the development of coronary artery disease and/or the precipitation of clinical events via the repeated and excessive activation of sympathetic autonomic and neuroendocrine mechanisms (Friedman, 1978). As yet, however, there is only indirect evidence to support such an hypothesis. Studies with animal subjects have demonstrated that chronic exposure to aversive physical or social stress produces a broad range of cardiovascular pathologies, including arterial hypertension, elevated serum cholesterol levels, arteriosclerosis, and myofibrillary degeneration of the heart (Benson, Herd, Morse, & Kelleher, 1969; Corley, Shiel, Mauck, & Greenhoot, 1973; Forsyth, 1971; Henry, Ely, Stephens, Radcliffe, H. L., Santisteban, G. A., & Shapiro, A. P., 1971; Herd, Morse, Kelleher, & Jones, 1969; Lang, 1967; Schneiderman, 1978). Interestingly, such effects generally emerge only when animals are permitted the opportunity to actively cope with the stressor (Schneiderman, 1978). When no effective coping strategy is possible or the animal lacks adequate dominance to affect control, physiopathology becomes manifest in gastrointestinal ulceration, renal defects, bradycardia and hypotension, and ventricular arrest (Corley, Mauck, & Shiel, 1975; Von Holst, 1972; Weiss, 1968).

Even if one assumes that a differential tendency toward sympathetic nervous system arousal contributes to greater levels of CHD in Type A individuals, it remains crucial to elucidate the pathways through which such arousal might act to promote disease processes. Several mechanisms are plausible. For example, high circulatory levels of catecholamines act to promote mobilization of lipid stores from adipose tissue. Normally, such mobilization is prompted by demands of physical exertion or cold stress, and the mobilized lipids are hydrolyzed to free fatty acids for energy production in muscular activity (Heindel, Orci, & Jeanrenaud, 1975; Zierler, Maseri, Klassen, Rabinowitz, & Burgess, 1968). Those free fatty acids not used for production of energy are taken up by adipose tissues and the liver. Those taken up by the liver subsequently are secreted in the form of triglyceride-rich particles called very low density lipoproteins (VLDL). These lipoproteins circulate in the blood and transport triglycerides to skeletal muscle, heart muscle, and adipose tissue. Upon removal and hydrolysis of a portion of the triglycerides contained in VLDL, the lipoprotein remnants are transported back to the liver where they are further degraded. Part of the remnant is utilized further by the liver and part is released into the circulation as low density lipoprotein (LDL) (Eisenberg, Bilheimer, Levy, & Lindgren, 1973). This LDL is the source for lipoproteins and cholesterol that may be deposited in walls of arteries. The rate of VLDL production by the liver is limited in part by circulating levels of free fatty acids. Therefore, increased rates of lipid mobilization without comparable increases in extraction and utilization by skeletal and heart muscle could increase levels of VLDL circulating in peripheral blood, thereby elevating levels of LDL and causing large amounts of lipoprotein and cholesterol to enter walls of large arteries forming plaques and atheroma. Elevations of triglycerides and cholesterol in serum have been observed in untyped individuals subjected to a variety of stressors (Friedman, Rosenman, & Carroll, 1958; Peterson, Keith, & Wilcox, 1962; Taggart, Carruthers, & Somerville, 1973), and preferentially in Type A individuals in the course of normal day-to-day activities (Friedman, 1978; Rosenman & Friedman, 1961).

Other related physiological processes also may play a role in atherogenesis. These include (a) catecholamine-enhanced rates of platelet aggregation and thrombosis (Davies & Reinert, 1965; Davis, 1974; O'Brien, 1963); (b) sympathetic nervous system induced increases in blood pressure and flow turbulence which may damage vessel walls (Ross & Glomset, 1976); (c) direct pathogenic effects of VLDL on the vascular endothelium (Ross & Harker, 1976); and (d) direct lesions of blood vessels of the heart produced by chronically elevated levels of circulating catecholamines (Haft, 1974). All of these processes may increase the severity of atherosclerosis and all may occur with greater severity in Type A than Type B subjects (Dembroski, MacDougall, & Shields, 1977; Friedman, 1977; Friedman, St. George, Byer, & Rosenman, 1960; Friedman, Byers, Diamant, & Rosenman, 1975; Glass, Krakoff, Hilton, Kehoe, Mannucci, Collins, Snow, & Elting, 1980).

In the presence of severe coronary atherosclerosis, stress-induced activation of the sympathetic nervous system could cause myocardial damage even without acute coronary thrombosis (Eliot, 1979; Hellstrom, 1973; Kuller, Lilienfield, & Fischer, 1966; Raab, 1971), and protraction of this cycle may lead to enhanced susceptability to gross infarction or ventricular arrhythmias. Even mild emotional stress in persons with coronary heart disease can produce serious arrhythmias and intense emotions can trigger fatal ventricular fibrillation (Eliot, 1979; Malik, 1973; Myers & Dewar, 1975). Interestingly, Type A individuals have a higher risk of sudden cardiac death than Type B individuals (Friedman, Manwaring, Rosenman, Donlon, Ortega, & Grube, 1973).

In summary, a considerable body of research supports the proposition that Type A and B subjects differ in levels of activity on a number of physiological dimensions potentially related to the genesis of CHD and the precipitation of acute clinical events. However, it must be emphasized that no programmatic research exists which unequivocally links these physiological differences to cardiovascular pathology. Although involvement of the ANS and adrenal-hypothalamic-pituitary axis is consistent with the bulk of the data thus far collected, until prospective studies can demonstrate that autonomic sympathetic and related neuroendocrine reactivity *per se* is a risk factor for the development of CHD, one must be cautious in ascribing causal status to this pathway. (For an excellent account of the relationship between stress and pathophysiological mechanisms in CHD, see Eliot, 1979.)

SOCIAL PSYCHOPHYSIOLOGY OF TYPE A

Given the *tentative assumption* that chronic activation of ANS and neuroendocrine mechanisms contributes to the behavior-disease linkage, a logical next step is to identify the specific behavioral characteristics of the Type A individual which, in concert with appropriate environmental triggers, are responsible for percipitating and maintaining such arousal. Such an analysis is essential for several reasons. First, it is likely that many aspects of the Type A pattern are not by themselves pathological and, indeed, may even be protective in effect (e.g., job involvement). Second, even the potentially damaging components of the pattern are likely to operate only under certain environmental circumstances, whose characteristics have yet to be determined. Third, it is very plausible that as yet unrecognized behavioral and/or constitutional factors which are correlated with the Type A pattern may generate some or indeed all of the risk now attributed to Type A. And fourth, an important question concerns the degree to which physiopathology may arise from a tendency of susceptible Type As to show quantitatively larger autonomic responses to a given stressor versus the possibility that Type As simply generate a cummulatively larger total amount of autonomic activity through behavioral protraction or initiation of stressful interactions with the environment. The issue is thus one of specificity. Most Type As will not develop CHD and some Type Bs will. The task is to identify the particular features of the behavior pattern and environmental setting which together predispose constitutionally susceptible individuals to recurring and excessive physiological arousal and mobilization of metabolic substrates beyond the actual physical demands of the situation.

One approach to this problem is to subject Type A and B persons to a variety of controlled social situations while monitoring their physiological responses. Such social psychophysiological research offers the dual advantages of identifying those aspects of the environment which are most likely to trigger excessive autonomic arousal in Type A compared with Type B persons, while simultaneously identifying the behavioral characteristics and constitutional factors which mediate excessive arousal. Research of this type rests on the assumptions that those behavioral-environmental interactions salient to the disease process can be effectively modeled in the laboratory and that primarily non-invasive measures of cardiovascular reactivity can be used to index more fundamentally important neuroendocrine and sympathetic nervous system reactions.

An additional assumption in this work, and one whose validity has recently been called into question, concerns the equivalence of techniques used to assess the Type A pattern. With a few exceptions, investigators have employed either the SI developed by Rosenman and Friedman (Rosenman, 1978b) and modified for students (Dembroski, 1978), or the JAS modified for students (Krantz, Glass, & Snyder, 1974). The former measurement procedure is clearly the more desirable of the two since it constituted the primary assessment technique in the WCGS and thus has the strongest epidemological linkage to CHD (Brand et al., 1978). The latter device, however, is enormously easier to use and does not require extensive training of the investigators. Unfortunately, data clearly show that the JAS provided little or no independent predictivity for CHD in the WCGS beyond a capacity to duplicate the SI designations (Brand et al., 1978). Moreover, as mentioned earlier, the JAS does not agree well with SI categorical determination of Type A, particularly with college students (Chesney, Black, Chadwick, & Rosenman, 1981; MacDougall et al., 1979; Matthews & Saal, 1978; Scherwitz, Berton & Leventhal, 1978). In spite of these limitations, the JAS has been the assessment technique of choice in over 50% of the studies described below. Our own psychophysiological work (Dembroski, MacDougall, Shields, Petitto, & Lushene, 1978) and that of Glass and his coworkers (personal communication) have consistently revealed that where the two instruments are used in a single study, the JAS is found to be a poorer predictor of physiological reactivity. Insofar as these social psychophysiological studies derive much of their interest from their potential ability to clarify the relationship between Type A and CHD, the use of the JAS as the sole measure of Type A attributes is not an optimal strategy. This is particularly true when studies attempt to delineate environmental factors critical in evoking excessive arousal in Type As compared with Bs, and the *lack* of an A-B difference may have theoretical import, at least to the degree that the findings reflect factors other than measurement error. In this regard, the exclusive use of other Type A assessment techniques, such as the Vickers scale (1973) or the Bortner performance test (Bortner, 1969) is even more hazardous, since these instruments have not been systematically validated against CHD endpoints at all.

Overall, our perception of the matter is that globally defined Type A, as assessed by the SI, is weakly to moderately correlated with physiological hyperreactivity in some of the laboratory paradigms used thus far, and then only under certain circumstances (e.g., ego involving instructions). In any given sample of subjects classified as Type A and B according to this technique, there is a reasonable probability that the Type A sample will contain a sufficiently larger number of higher responders to yield an overall group difference. Where other assessment techniques are employed, it is possible that the ratio of high responders in the A relative to the B group will be diminished to the point that many studies will report either numerically smaller differences between the Types, or will fail to find differences at all in some samples. An alternative and even more disturbing possibility is that findings obtained with other procedures may not be relevent to Type A as operationally defined in the WCGS, yet will be equated with this construct. The simplest immediate solution to this problem is to employ *both* the SI and JAS (and any promising new measures) in all social psychophysiological research and to compare the results within the same sample. With adequate sample sizes, it would be possible under these conditions to ascertain whether the two assessment techniques contribute independently to predicting physiological reactivity.

With these cautionary notes in mind, let us examine the psychophysiological studies available to date. For expository convenience these studies can be grouped into several general and somewhat overlapping categories, reflecting the experimenter's attempts to analyze the role of various situational and/or person variables in evoking A-B differences in physiological reactivity.

Performance Challenges.   The largest category is comprised of those studies which have subjected Type A and B subjects to performance challenges of various sorts. The rationale for such a manipulation is straightforward in that Type A behavior has been conceptually defined as a coping strategy aroused by the need to master the demands of everyday life (Glass, 1977), and competitiveness is a major trait characterization of Type As in virtually all of the writings of Friedman and Rosenman. This type of research has utilized both task and social-competitive challenges to performance competency. In the former, the experimenters have challenged the subjects to perform well relative to explicit or implied performance standards, while in the latter type of study, subjects are placed in active competition with another subject or confederate.

Concerning first task manipulations of performance challenge, an initial demonstration study by Dembroski et al. (1977) revealed that behaviorally extreme SI-defined Type As showed greater SBP and HR increases than Bs while working on a choice reaction time task under high challenging instructions. This effect was partially replicated by Manuck, Craft, and Gold (1978), who found greater SBP (but not HR) increases in JAS-defined Type As relative to Bs when working on a difficult cognitive task under high incentive conditions. More systematic experiments concerning the effect of performance challenge have manipulated the level of challenge within a study. Dembroski, MacDougall, Herd, and Shields (1979a) found that SI-defined Type As and Bs showed relatively small differences in SBP and HR reactivity on both cold pressor and reaction time tasks when the instructions emphasized the simplicity of the tasks, but when the same tasks were given with instructions which emphasized the demanding nature of the tasks and the need for will power to do well, the reactivity differences between the Types were markedly increased. Somewhat similar effects have been reported by Pittner and Houston (1980) and Goldband (1980) when the nature of the task and the instructions have been designed to manipulate the degrees of ego involvement of the subjects. Briefly, in the Pittner and Houston study, Vickers scale and JAS-defined Type As showed greater SBP, DBP, and HR responses than Bs on a task involving threats to self esteem, but not on a task involving threat of shock. Similarly, Goldband found evidence that JAS-defined Type As decrease their forearm pulse transit times (PTT - a measure which may be correlated with average blood pressure) under competitive-time urgent instructions versus neutral instructions, while the PTT response of Type Bs was unaffected by the manipulation. Interestingly, some data from both of the latter studies suggest that under conditions of low challenge, Type As may psychologically disengage from the task to the extent of showing slightly lower reactivity than the Type Bs.

In the context of research of this sort, three studies have directly compared the SI and JAS with respect to the ability of these instruments to differentiate high versus low responders, and in each case, the SI was found to be a better predictor of SBP and HR increases (Dembroski et al., 1978; Dembroski et al., 1979a; Glass, personal communication). There is some suggestion, however, that paper and pencil measures of Type A (JAS and Vickers scale) occasionally are somewhat more sensitive to differences in magnitude of DBP increase (Dembroski et al., 1978; Pittner & Houston, 1980), suggesting again the possibility that the different measuring instruments are assessing distinguishable patterns of physiological reactivity. Finally, it should be noted that at least two studies have not found overall A-B differences in physiological arousal to performance challenge. In one study only the JAS was used and blood pressure was not assessed (Price & Clark, 1978); but Scherwitz et al. (1978) using *both* the SI and JAS found no reactivity differences between As and Bs across a broad variety of tasks. When subjects were subdivided on a dimension called ''self-involvement,'' it was reported that high self-involved Type As showed higher blood pressure levels than low self-involved Type As. Unfortuantely, inspection of these authors' data indicate that the difference in levels existed in baseline and was not differentially influenced by the various tasks. Our own work and that carried out in Krantz's laboratory (personal communication) have not confirmed the hypothesis that self involvement *per se* is a crucial mediating factor linking Type A and physiological reactivity.

Studies which have manipulated performance challenge through *social competition* are logical outgrowths of an earlier study by Friedman et al. (1975), which demonstrated greater behavioral arousal and serum norepinephrine release in Type A compared to Type B males when the subjects were directly competing in a stressful problem solving task for a valuable prize. More recently, Van Egeren (1979a, b; unpublished manuscript) has conducted a series of studies demonstrating that JAS-defined Type As tend to show greater social competition and larger vasomotor (digital pulse measure), heart rate, and ECG changes when working on a variety of one-to-one mixed-motive competitive games. In this connection, Dembroski, MacDougall, and Lushene (1979b) have shown that male Type As evidence greater SBP and DBP increases in response to the social challenge of both the SI and a difficult quiz over American history. The differential SBP response was also observed in Type A females in a similar test paradigm (MacDougall, Dembroski, & Krantz, 1981—see below for a more extended discussion). Krantz, Schaeffer, Davia, Dembroski, MacDougall, and Shaffer (1981) have also found significantly greater HR and marginally significant BP responses in As relative to Bs in the same paradigm using patients about to undergo angiographic testing. Finally, in a recent study by Glass et al. (1980), SI-defined Type As and Bs were tested on a challenging solitary performance task, in face-to-face competition with a confederate of the experimenter, and in face-to-face competition coupled with verbal harrassment by the confederate. Similar to the Dembroski et al. (1978) findings, Type As showed greater increases in SBP, HR, and plasma epinephrine in response to the solitary performance challenge, and also in the verbal harrassment condition, but not under conditions of simple face-to-face competition (see work by Glass cited in this chapter). This latter result suggests that Type Bs are quite capable of evidencing large changes in physiological reactivity under appropriate conditions and that overall differences between the Types may be evident only under conditions of moderate and intense challenge. In this regard, the simple face-to-face competition condition described by Glass et al. (1980) appears appreciably more challenging than the manipulations employed by Van Egeren and those used in our own published work. Recent unpublished research in our laboratory has confirmed the Glass et al. finding that face-to-face competition for substantial monetary rewards produces very large levels of cardiovascular reactivity in both Type A and B subjects, but relatively small A-B differences in the size of the changes. The A-B difference observed under the harrassment condition used by Glass et al. is intriguing and may reflect the additional tapping of a hostility dimension which is more prevalent in the Type A subjects. This would suggest again that both competitive involvement and potential for hostility may contribute independently to enhancing CHD risks for Type A individuals.

In addition to social or performance challenge manipulations, two studies have examined the effect of manipulations of external incentives (money) on the performance and physiological reactivity of Type A and B subjects. Manuck and Garland (1979) used independent groups of JAS-defined Type A and B male subjects who completed timed concept formation problems under either a "no reward" condition (although apparently involving challenging instructions) or a condition in which money was given for correct answers. While the authors noted an overall A-B difference in SBP and DBP elevations, the interaction of Type A-B and the incentive manipulation was not significant for any physiological measure. To the extent that *trends* were apparent in the data, it seemed that Type As responded with equal amounts of reactivity under both levels of incentive, while Type Bs showed a tendency toward higher reactivity only under the explicit incentive condition. These physiological data were paralleled by behavioral and self-report data indicating that the Type As were maximally involved regardless of the incentive condition.

As one of the conditions in the study previously described, Glass et al. (1980) first tested their subjects under instructional conditions which emphasized the need to do well and then half-way through the test altered the task to a high-incentive condition where criterion performance allegedly could lead to a $25.00 gift certificate. As noted before, significant A-B differences in SBP, DBP, and serum epinephrine increases were noted for the overall task, but the incentive shift had no differential effect on the magnitude of the change in these measures shown by the two Types. A marginally significant interaction of Type A-B by incentive was noted, however, such that the incentive shift produced a slight increase in HR for the Type As and a slight drop for the Bs.

In all, the data concerning the effect of performance challenge on the physiological responsivity of Type A subjects are relatively consistent. Seemingly, to the degree that Type As (defined by both the SI and paper-pencil instruments) become involved in the task, either through instructional manipulations or social challenge, they tend to show greater levels of cardiovascular and catecholaminic responsivity than do Type Bs. With respect to the existing data, monetary incentives, at least when added to already established levels of competitive involvement, seem to have minor effects. The fact that Type B subjects can be induced to show equally large responses under relatively intense competitive challenge (Glass et al., 1980) argues that the differences between the types may be primarily in the threshold of challenge needed to secure competitive engagement.

In view of these differences in physiological reactivity between the Types, one might expect to find equally consistent differences in self reports of emotional-motivational states and actual performance. In fact, this has not been the case. Examination of the studies cited above reveals that Type As and Bs do not show consistent differences in self reports of anxiety, irritation and the like. This finding can be interpreted in three ways. Either Type As do not in fact experience subjectively greater emotional arousal in response to challenge manipulation, or they deny it publicly, or they have habituated to such elevated arousal states to an extent that the subjective impact has become equal to the lower arousal states of the Type B subjects. With regard to actual quality of task performance of the Types, most studies have found few differences, although occasionally, Type As have been found to be somewhat superior, probably as a result of their greater task involvement (Frankenhaeuser, Lundberg, & Forsman, 1980a; MacDougall et al., 1981; Manuck & Garland, 1979).

Uncontrollable Stressors. Several psychophysiological studies concerned with the Type A-B dimension have attempted to evaluate the degree to which Type A subjects are differentially reactive in the face of uncontrollable stressors of either a physical or psychological nature. From Glass's theoretical perspective, such stressors should be highly effective in evoking both behavioral and physiological reactivity in Type A subjects, since Type As are viewed as possessing a strong need to be in control of events and threats to such control are seen as the elicitors of the behavior pattern itself. An early and frequently cited study by Caplan and Jones (1975) actually found no significant differences in HR between subjects classified as A or B according to the Vickers scale in response to the stress of an untimely closing of a university computer center, although a trend was present for Type As to report more subjective stress. Weidner and Matthews (1978) using female subjects reported limited data suggesting that Type A subjects were somewhat more prone than their Type B counterparts to evidence greater SBP elevations in the face of predictable but non-controllable noise. Surprisingly, however, the effect was not observed in the unpredictable-noncontrollable noise condition, possibily because the Type Bs were equally highly reactive under this condition. Most recently, Lovallo and Pishkin (1980) using the SI to categorize subjects as Type A or B, found no differences in BP (measured before and after, but not during the task) or HR in response to uncontrollable noise, task failure, or combinations of the two. However, Type As did show higher task-induced changes in skin conduction levels, spontaneous skin potential production, and in serum triglicerides. An interesting and quite different study found that SI-defined Type As compared with Bs showed greater SBP elevations in response to the physiological and psychological stress of coronary bypass surgery (Kahn, Kornfeld, Frank, Heller, & Hoar, 1980). This effect is particularly noteworthy because the subjects were under general anesthesia and the differences between the Types thus presumably reflected the operation of mechanisms which were at least in part independent of conscious mediation.

Frankenhaeuser's group in Sweden has recently begun studying physiological responses of individuals categorized as Type A or B using a modified form of the JAS. Frankenhaeuser, Lundberg, and Forsman (1980b) have reported that although not differing in the magnitude of response to the demands of performing mental arithmetic under noise stress, the Types did differ in physiological response to a subsequent 1-hour period of forced inactivity. Specifically, Type As compared with Bs reported the experience to be more stressful and secreted greater amounts of epinephrine and cortisol (urine determinations). Frankenhaeuser and her colleague have suggested a distinction between "effort without distress," which is associated primarily with sympathetic adrenal-medullary responses and *suppression* of adrenal cortical secretions (cortisol), and "effort with distress" arising primarily from uncontrollable demands and accompanied by *both* sympathetic and adrenal cortical activity. In combination with the Frankenhaeuser et al. data noted above, two other experiments by Lundberg and Forsman (1979) and Frankenhaeuser et al. (1980a) suggest that JAS-defined Type As are prone to show larger adrenal cortical responses than Bs where the test situation is ambiguous and/or uncontrollable in nature. By contrast, when the task is highly controllable, even if quite demanding, adrenal cortical response differences between the types are diminished. This research points up clearly the need for investigators to expand the range of physiological parameters employed in assessing A-B differences in response to situational stress. A cautionary note is in order, however, in evaluating the work of the Swedish group. The version of the JAS used by this group is even further removed from the primary interview definition of Type A, and there is a strong need to replicate their findings using SI typed subjects.

In all, the data relating uncontrollable stress to physiological reactivity in Type A and B subjects are somewhat ambiguous. Although Type As overall appear to be more physiologically reactive than Type Bs, the differences are not consistent across studies either with respect to the nature of the imposed stressor or the type of physiological response involved. Our suspicion is that the potential effect of uncontrollable stressors such as noise, heat, or forced restriction of activity on the physiological responses of Type A subjects is mediated by the subject's perception of the threat to competent performance imposed by the stressor and/or the degree to which the manipulation is seen as capricious or unnecessary. Moreover, the laboratory studies thus far conducted have been of a relatively brief duration, and it is possible that larger differences would emerge after longer periods of exposure to stress. In this regard, at least some of the early work of Glass (1977) and his colleagues suggests that JAS-defined Type A subjects may, if given the choice, continue to subject themselves to the stressful situation after the Type Bs have dropped out. In this case, even though absolute differences in physiological response between the Types may not be significant in the short run, the behavioral characteristics of the Type As might insure larger net amounts of a stress-induced physiological reactivity. This possibility is, of course, equally applicable to the behavior of Type As in other circumstances in which net differences in reactivity have been observed.

Naturalistic Physiological Studies.   In addition to the Caplan and Jones (1975) study noted above, five other studies have attempted to relate the Type A-B dimension to levels of autonomic reactivity assessed in the course of normal day-to-day activities. Such studies are significant, first because they may be directly related to the earlier biochemical research of Friedman and his co-workers which demonstrated differences between *extreme* As and Bs in serum catecholamines during the working day, but not at night (Friedman, St. George, Byers, & Rosenman, 1960), and second, because they bear upon the validity of laboratory simulation research for evaluating physiological reactivity differences in Type A and B subjects. In one large-scale study which addressed this issue,

DeBaker, Kornitzer, Kittel, Bogaert, Van Durme, Vincke, Rustin, Degre, & DeSchaepdrijver (1979) found no evidence that Belgian white-collar factory workers classified as Type A by the SI showed higher work-day levels of urinary catecholamines, heart rate, or ECG abnormalities than their Type B counterparts. But, unlike Friedman et al. (1960), these researchers did not use preselected extreme As and Bs. By contrast, Manuck, Corse, and Winkelman (1979) have reported that Type A lawyers (JAS-defined) showed higher peak levels and greater day-to-day variability in both SBP and DBP across a 6-week work day study than did Type Bs. This effect was not replicated, however, by Rose et al. (1978) for JAS-defined Type A and B air traffic controllers; and in a study by Stokols, Novaco, Stokols, and Campbell (1978), the highest levels of casual SBP were obtained for JAS-defined *Type Bs* under high commuting stress. (In this study, Type As did show larger SBP levels than Bs under intermediate levels of commuting stress.) Finally, Waldron, Hickey, McPherson, Butonsky, Gruss, Overall, Schmader, & Wohlmuth, (1980) found that JAS scores of male college students (but not females) were weakly related to diastolic blood pressure levels during periods of academic stress and disruption.

Overall, these data are both inconclusive and confusing. The Manuck et al. (1979) findings are consistent with the hypothesis that Type As are more physiologically reactive in the course of their day-to-day activities; however, JAS scores for this sample were not related to levels of physiological reactivity observed on a difficult and presumably challenging cognitive task which previously had yielded blood pressure differences in Type A and B college students. The negative findings of the DeBaker et al. group are particularly striking in view of the fact that the study was large in scope, apparently well controlled, and utilized the SI as the primary method of assessment. Apart from the fact that extreme As and Bs were not preselected and exclusively used in this study, we have no convincing explanation for this inconsistency with Friedman's earlier work. It is, of course, possible that either the SI is not an entirely appropriate assessment device for detecting Type A behavior in Belgian males, or the absolute levels of situational stress in the Belgian factories were sufficiently low that A-B differences were greatly attenuated. In all, however, it remains to be demonstrated that the ANS hyperreactivity of Type A subjects seen in the laboratory can be consistently related to similar responses in day-to-day life.

Other Person Variables.   As noted above, the Matthews et al. (1977) reanalysis of the WCGS interview data revealed that only certain components of the Type A pattern correlated significantly with CHD. These included potential for hostility, competitive drive, impatience, and vigorous voice stylistics. Subsequent research by Dembroski et al. (1978; 1979a) confirmed that these components in general and hostility in particular were also most strongly related to blood pressure elevations in response to performance challenge. Indeed, in the latter study, high hostile Type As showed large blood pressure elevations even under conditions of very mild challenge, while low hostile Type As showed elevations only when the challenge was made quite intense. More recent data on female subjects exposed to either social or performance challenge showed that ratings of potential for hostility were significantly correlated with SBP elevations even when global assessments of Type A were not (MacDougall et al., 1981). These data are consistent with earlier findings implicating hostility as a contributor to higher blood pressure responses of individuals to stress (Harburg, 1962; Hokanson, 1961), and, as noted above, with the finding that Type A and hostility may evidence independent associations with severity of coronary atherosclerosis (Williams et al., 1980).

A second important person variable which has only recently begun to receive attention is the sex of the individual. The majority of studies concerned with the psychophysiological responses of Type A and B persons have used male subjects. This strategy reflects the fact that (a) CHD is enormously more prevalent in males; (b) the major assessment devices (SI & JAS) were all developed and standardized on male populations; and (c) the WCGS utilized males exclusively in establishing the prospective link between Type A and CHD. Nonetheless, Type A has been related to CHD in females (Rosenman & Friedman, 1961; Haynes et al., 1980; Williams et al., 1980) and it is important to explore whether Type A females are similar to their male counterparts in showing greater cardiovascular responses to stress. Nine social psychophysiological studies have utilized female subjects. Weidner and Matthews (1978) used females exclusively and, as noted above, found greater SBP increases in Type As (JAS-defined) in one of their uncontrollable noise stress conditions. Van Egeren (1979a, b; unpublished manuscript) has reported that JAS-defined Type A male and female subjects were similar in showing larger vasomotor, heart rate, and ECG changes than Type B subjects in the course of various mixed-motive games. In one study by Lundberg and Forsman (1979) both male and female Type A students showed larger cortisol responses than Bs while working on a prolonged vigilance task. By contrast, Manuck et al. (1978) failed to find JAS-defined A-B differences in blood pressure reactivity in women in the same paradigm in which large differences were observed in male Type A and B subjects. A similar result was reported recently by Waldron et al. (1980). A partial resolution of these inconsistencies is offered by a recent study by MacDougall et al. (1981) who found that SI-defined A and B females showed no physiological reactivity differences on a psychomotor performance task which previously had been demonstrated to yield large A-B differences in males, but did differ in SBP elevations in the face of interpersonal confrontations with another female. A plausible explanation is that female Type A subjects are potentially more physiologically reactive than their Type B counterparts, but the type and range of situational events which trigger such responses may be narrower or, perhaps, just different from those which are relevant to male Type As. In particular, we hypothesize that even extreme Type A women are much less susceptible to being caught up in the competitive, job or school performance demands of contemporary society, but instead respond primarily to verbal social competition and interpersonal stress (MacDougall et al., 1981).

Other person variables potentially relevant to the physiological response of the Type A individuals which have received experimental attention include involvement with self (Scherwitz et al., 1978); task involvement (Manuck & Garland, 1979); sensory intake and rejection (Williams, 1978); cognitive complexity (Streufert et al., 1979); need for control (Glass, 1977); and locus of control (Manuck et al., 1978). At the present time, however, it is clear that none of these constructs has received sufficient experimental attention to warrent inclusion as a mediator variable linking Type A with autonomic hyperractivity.

SUMMARY AND CONCLUSIONS

Dynamic rather than static physiologic differences apparently mediated primarily through sympathetic adrenal-medullary and, possibly, adrenal-cortical function appear to distinguish As from Bs, but much work is necessary before the specific environmental circumstances in interaction with particular Type A attributes and other person variables can be identified as responsible for the physiologic arousal differences reported between As and Bs. In short, the Type A pattern is by no means equivalent to physiologic reactivity. In this regard, it is critical that researchers carefully consider the characteristics of (a) environmental factors, e.g., level of challenge or sensory intake versus rejection tasks (Williams, 1978); (b) person variables, e.g., JAS- versus SI-defined As or high versus low hostile As (Dembroski et al., 1978; 1979a, b); and (c) measurement of different physiologic parameters, e.g., catecholamines versus cortisol (cf. Glass et al., 1980 vs. Frankenhaeuser et al., 1980a) blood pressure versus skin resistance (cf. Manuck et al., 1978 vs. Price & Clarke, 1978), including timing of the measurements, e.g. blood pressure before, after, *and* during activity (cf. Lovallo & Pishkin, 1979 vs. Glass et al., 1980). Extant research already suggests that there will be wide variation in research results depending on the presence or absence of any of the above variables. In any case, the most fruitful psychophysiological approach clearly is the use of multiple conditions and measures, including studies in the natural environment.

What is clear is that there are substantial individual differences in physiologic reactivity. Research suggests that some individuals respond to even mild environmental challenge with excessive physiological response, while others show such arousal only when specifically challenged, and some may show enhanced arousal only in response to chronic and high levels of environmental challenge (Dembroski et al., 1979a). The ultimate aim of research here should be to refine the definition of environmental-behavioral-physiologic processes that in combination can be used to increase the understanding, prediction, and possibly control of CHD. For example, research of this sort might be expected to evolve psychophysiological maneuvers that may transcend the error involved in current behavioral assessment procedures by serving as a more reliable and stronger predictor of CHD. In fact, we have proposed a testable model in this regard (Dembroski et al., 1979a), in which levels of propensity for physiologic reactivity and differential exposure to various levels of environmental challenge can be used in combination to predict levels of risk for CHD. It is our belief that more research emphasis on the above combinations should be included in paradigms investigating the A-B phenomenon. Two reasons dominate our thinking in this regard. First, there is a clear trend for researchers to find disproportionate numbers of Type As in their samples, which seriously questions the specificity value of Type A (see Chesney et al., 1981; MacDougall et al., 1979), and second, as noted above, there are wide individual differences in physiologic reactivity within both Type As *and* Type Bs. The major assumption underlying all of this work is that exaggerated physiologic response to everyday life events may hasten the onset of CHD. Therefore, direct study of physiologic reactivity as an individual difference variable in and of itself *and* the characteristics associated with such a propensity offers a more promising approach to understanding the behavior-physiologic response-disease relationship than primary focus on the A-B variable. We clearly are not recommending abandonment of the A-B phenomenon. After all, Type A is at least as potent a risk factor for CHD as the traditional risk factors and, indeed, interesting differences may yet be uncovered between Type A and B subjects who are both identified as high physiologic reactors by some standard maneuver. Rather, we are suggesting a better balance between future study of the two individual difference variables of Type A on the one hand and dispositional high physiologic response on the other.

ACKNOWLEDGMENTS

Preparation of this manuscript was supported by research grant HL-22809 awarded to the first two authors by the National Heart, Lung, and Blood Institute of the National Institutes of Health.

REFERENCES

Arlow, J. A. Identification of mechanisms in coronary occlusion. *Psychosomatic Medicine*, 1945, *7*, 195–209.

Benson, H., Herd, J. A., Morse, W. H., & Kelleher, R. T. Behavioral induction of arterial hypertension and its reversal. *American Journal of Physiology*, 1969, *217*, 30–34.

Blumenthal, J. A., Williams, R., Kong, Y., Schanberg, S. M., & Thompson, L. W. Type A behavior and angiographically documented coronary disease. *Circulation*, 1978, *58*, 634–639.

Bortner, R. W. A short rating scale as a potential measure of Pattern A behavior. *Journal of Chronic Diseases*, 1969, *22*, 87–91.

Brand, R. J. Coronary-prone behavior as an independent risk factor for coronary heart disease. In T.

M. Dembroski, S. M. Weiss, J. L. Shields, et al. (Eds.), *Coronary-prone behavior*. New York: Springer-Verlag, 1978.

Brand, R. J., Rosenman, R. H., Jenkins, C. D., Sholtz & Zyzanski Comparison of coronary heart disease prediction in the Western Collaborative Group Study using the structured interview and the Jenkins Activity Survey assessments of the coronary-prone Type A behavior pattern. Paper presented at the conference on Cardiovascular Disease Epidemiology of The American Heart Association, Orlando, March, 1978.

Brand, R. J., Rosenman, R. H., Sholtz, R. I., & Friedman, M. Multivariate prediction of coronary heart disease in the Western Collaborative Group Study compared to the findings of the Framingham Study. *Circulation*, 1976, *53*, 348–355.

Buell, J. C., & Eliot, R. S. Stress and Cardiovascular disease. *Modern Concepts of Cardiovascular Disease*, 1979, *4*, 19–24.

Caffrey, B. Psychometric procedures applied to the assessment of the coronary-prone behavior pattern. In T. M. Dembroski, S. M. Weiss, J. L. Shields, S. G. Haynes, & M. Feinleib (Eds.), *Coronary-prone behavior*. New York: Springer-Verlag, 1978.

Caplan, R. D., & Jones, K. W. Effects of work load, role ambiguity, and Type A personality on anxiety, depression, and heart rate. *Journal of Applied Psychology*, 1975, *60*, 713–719.

Chesney, M. A., Black, G. W., Chadwick, J. H., & Rosenman, R. H. Psychological correlates of the coronary-prone behavior pattern. *Journal of Behavioral Medicine*, 1981, *4*, 217–230.

Cohen, J. B. The influence of culture on coronary prone behavior. In T. M. Dembroski, S. M. Weiss, J. L. Shields, Haynes, S. & Feinleib, M. (Eds.), *Coronary-prone behavior*. New York: Springer-Verlag, 1978.

Corday, E., & Corday, S. R. Prevention of heart disease by control of risk factors: The time has come to face the facts. *American Journal of Cardiology*, 1975, *35*, 330–333.

Corley, K. C., Mauck, H. P., & Shiel, F. O'M. Cardiac responses associated with "yoked-chair" shock avoidance in squirrel monkeys. *Psychophysiology*, 1975, *12*, 439–444.

Corely, K. C., Shiel, F. O'M., Mauck, H. P., & Greenhoot, J. Electrocardiographic and cardiac morphological changes associated with environmental stress in squirrel monkeys. *Psychosomatic Medicine*, 1973, *35*, 361–364.

Davies, R. F., & Reinert, H. Arteriosclerosis in the young dog. *Journal of Atherosclerosis Research*, 1965, *5*, 181–188.

Davis, R. Stress and hemostatic mechanisms. In R. S. Eliot (Ed.), *Stress and the heart*, Mount Kisco, N. Y.: Futura, 1974, 97–122.

DeBacker, G., Kornitzer, M., Kittel, F., Bogaert, M., Van Durme, J. P., Vincke, J., Rustin, R. M., Degre, C., & DeSchaepdrijver, A. Relation between coronary-prone behavior pattern, excretion of urinary catecholamines, heart rate, and heart rhythm. *Preventive Medicine*, 1979, *8*, 14–22.

DeBakey, M. & Gotto, A. *The living heart*. New York: Charter Books, 1977.

Dembroski, T. M. Reliability and validity of methods used to assess coronary-prone behavior. In T. M. Dembroski, S. M. Weiss, J. L. Shields, Haynes, S. & Feinleib, M. (Eds.) *Coronary-prone behavior*. New York: Springer-Verlag, 1978.

Dembroski, T. M., MacDougall, J. M., Herd, J. A., & Shields, J. L. Effects of level of challenge on pressor and heart rate responses in Type A and B subjects. *Journal of Applied Social Psychology*, 1979a, *9*, 209–228.

Dembroski, T. M., MacDougall, J. M., & Lushene, R. Interpersonal interaction and cardiovascular response in Type A subjects and coronary patients. *Journal of Human Stress*, 1979b, *5*, 28–36.

Dembroski, T. M., MacDougall, J. M., & Shields, J. L. Physiologic reactions to social challenge in persons evidencing the Type A coronary-prone behavior pattern. *Journal of Human Stress*, 1977, *3*, 2–10.

Dembroski, T. M., MacDougall, J. M., Shields, J. L., Petitto, J., & Lushene, R. Components of the Type A coronary-prone behavior pattern and cardiovascular responses to psychomotor performance challenge. *Journal of Behavioral Medicine*, 1978, *1*, 159–176.

Dunbar, F. *Psychosomatic diagnosis*. New York: Paul B. Hoeber, 1943.

Eisenberg, S., Bilheimer, D. W., Levy, R., & Lindgren, F. T. On the metabolic conversion of human plasma very low density lipoprotein to low density lipoprotein. *Biochemical et Biophysica Acta*, 1973, *326*, 361–377.

Eliot, R. S. *Stress and the major cardiovascular diseases*. Mt. Kisco, N. Y.: Futura, 1979.

Farquhar, J. W. The community-based model of life style intervention trials. *American Journal of Epidemiology*, 1978, *108*, 103–111.

Forsyth, R. P. Regional blood-flow changes during 72-hour avoidance schedules in the monkey. *Science*, 1971, *173*, 546–548.

Fothergill, J. *Complete collection of the medical and philosophical works*. London: 1781.

Frank, K. A., Heller, S. S., Kornfeld, D. S., Sporn, A. A., & Weiss, M. B. Type A behavior pattern and coronary angiographic findings. *Journal of the American Medical Association*, 1978, *240*, 761–763.

Frankenhaeuser, M., Lundberg, U. & Forsman, L. Dissociation between sympathetic-adrenal and pituitary-adrenal responses to an achievement situation characterized by high controllability: Comparison between Type A and Type B males and females. *Biological Psychology*, 1980, *10*, 79–91. (a)

Frankenhaeuser, M., Lundberg, U., & Forsman, L. Note on arousing Type A persons by depriving them of work. *Journal of Psychosomatic Research*, 1980, *24*, 45–47.(b)

Friedman, M. Type A behavior pattern: Some of its pathophysiological components. *Bulletin of the New York Academy of Medicine*, 1977, *53*, 593–604.

Friedman, M. Type A behavior: Its possible relationship to pathogenetic processes responsible for coronary heart disease. In T. M. Dembroski, S. M. Weiss, J. L. Shields, S. G. Haynes, & M. Feinleib (Eds.), *Coronary-prone behavior*, New York: Springer-Verlag, 1978.

Friedman, M., Byers, S. O., Diamant, J., & Rosenman, R. H. Plasma catecholamine response of coronary-prone subjects (Type A) to a specific challenge. *Metabolism*, 1975, *4*, 205–210.

Friedman, M., Manwaring, J. H., Rosenman, R. H., Donlon, G., Ortega, P., & Grube, S. M. Instantaneous and sudden death: Clinical and pathological differentiation in coronary artery disease. *Journal of the American Medical Association*, 1973, *225*, 1319–1328.

Friedman, M., & Rosenman, R. H. Association of a specific overt behavior pattern with increases in blood cholesterol, blood clotting time, incidence of arcus senilis and clinical coronary artery disease. *Journal of the American Medical Association*, 1959, *169*, 1286–1296.

Friedman, M., Rosenman, R. H., & Carroll, V. Changes in the serum cholesterol and blood clotting time in men subjected to cyclic variation of occupational stress. *Circulation*, 1958, *17*, 852–861.

Friedman, M., Rosenman, R. H., Straus, R., Wurm, M., & Kositchek, R. The relationship of behavior pattern A to the state of the coronary vasculature: A study of fifty-one autopsy subjects. *American Journal of Medicine*, 1968, *44*, 525–537.

Friedman, M., St. George, S., Byers, S. O., & Rosenman, R. H. Excretion of catecholamines, 17-ketosteroids, 17-hydroxycorticoids, and 5-hydroxyindole in men exhibiting a particular behavior pattern (A) associated with high incidence of clinical coronary artery disease. *Journal of Clinical Investigation*, 1960, *39*, 758–764.

Gildea, E. Special features of personality which are common to certain psychosomatic disorders. *Psychosomatic Medicine*, 1949, *11*, 273.

Glass, D. C. Personal communication.

Glass, D. C. *Behavior patterns, stress and coronary disease*. Hillsdale, N.J.: Lawrence Erlbaum Associates, 1977.

Glass, D. C., Krakoff, L. R., Contrada, R., Hilton, W. F., Kehoe, K., Mannucci, E. G., Collins, C., Snow, S., & Elting, E. Effect of harassment and competition upon cardiovascular and catecholominic responses in Type A and B individuals. *Psychophysiology*, 1980, *17*, 453–463.

Goldband, S. Stimulus specificity of physiological response to stress and the Type A coronary-prone personality. *Journal of Personality and Social Psychology*, 1980, *39*, 670–679.

Gordon, T., Garcia-Palmieri, M. R., Kagan, A., Kannel, W. B., & Schiffman, J. Differences in coronary heart disease in Framingham, Honolulu, and Puerto Rico. *Journal of Chronic Diseases*, 1974, *27*, 329–344.

Gordon, T., & Thom, T. The recent decrease in CHD mortality. *Preventive Medicine*, 1975, *4*, 115–125.

Greenspan, K. Biologic feedback and cardiovascular disease. *Psychosomatics*, 1979, *19*, 1–8.

Haft, J. I. Cardiovascular injury induced by sympathetic catecholamines. *Progress in Cardiovascular Diseases*, 1974, *17*, 73–86.

Harburg, E. *Covert Hostility: Its social origins and relationship to compliance.* Unpublished doctoral dissertation, University of Michigan, 1962.

Harvey, W. *De motu cordis*, 1628. Quoted in R. Hunter & D. MacAlpine (Eds.), *Three hundred years of psychiatry 1535–1860*, London: Oxford University Press, 1963.

Haynes, S. G., Feinleib, M., & Kannel, W. B. The relationship of psychosocial factors to coronary disease in the Framingham study: Eight year incidence of coronary heart disease. *American Journal of Epidemiology*, 1980, *111*, 37–58.

Heberden, W. Some account of a disorder of the breast. *Medical Transactions Royal College of Physicians*, 1772, *2*, 59.

Heindel, J. J., Orci, L., & Jeanrenaud, B. Fat mobilization and its regulation by hormones and drugs in white adipose tissue. In E. J. Macow (Ed.), *International encyclopedia of pharmacology and therapeutics: Pharmacology of lipid transport and atherosclerotic process*, Oxford: Pergamon Press, 1975.

Hellstrom, H. R. Vasospasm in ischemic heart disease—A hypothesis. *Perspectives in Biology and Medicine*, 1973, Spring, 427–440.

Henry, J. P., Ely, D. L., Stephens, P. M., Radcliffe, H. L., Santisteban, G. A., & Shapiro, A. P. The role of psychosocial factors in the development of arteriosclerosis in CBA mice. *Atherosclerosis*, 1971, *14*, 203–218.

Herd, J. A. Physiological correlates of coronary prone behavior. In T. M. Dembroski, S. M. Weiss, J. L. Shields, S. G. Haynes, & M. Feinleib (Eds.), *Coronary-prone behavior.* New York: Springer-Verlag, 1978.

Herd, J. A., Morse, W. H., Kelleher, R. T., & Jones, L. G. Arterial hypertension in the squirrel monkey during behavioral experiments. *American Journal of Physiology*, 1969, *217*, 24–29.

Hokanson, J. E. Vascular and psychogalvanic effects of experimentally aroused anger. *Journal of Personality*, 1961, *29*, 30–39.

House, J. S. The effects of occupational stress on physical health. In O'Tolle, J. (Ed.), *Work and the quality of life: Resource papers for work in America.* Cambridge: MIT press, 1974, 146–170.

Jenkins, C. D. Recent evidence supporting psychologic and social risk factors for coronary disease. *New England Journal of Medicine*, 1976, *294*, 987–994; 1033–1038.

Jenkins, C. D. Behavioral risk factors in coronary artery disease. *Annual Review of Medicine*, 1978, *29*, 543–562.

Jenkins, C. D., Rosenman, R. H., & Friedman, M. Development of an objective psychological test for the determination of the coronary-prone behavior pattern in employed men. *Journal of Chronic Diseases*, 1967, *20*, 371–379.

Jenkins, C. D., Zyzanski, S. J., & Rosenman, R. H. Risk of new myocardial infarction in middle-aged men with manifest coronary heart disease. *Circulation*, 1976, *53*, 342–347.

Kahn, J. P., Kornfeld, D. S., Frank, K. A., Heller, S. S., & Hoar, P. F. Type A behavior and blood pressure during coronary artery/bypass surgery. *Psychosomatic Medicine*, 1980, *42*, 407–414.

Kemple, C. The Rorschach method and psychosomatic diagnosis. *Psychosomatic Medicine*, 1945, *7*, 85.

Keys, A. Coronary heart disease in seven countries: XIII Multiple variables. *Circulation*, 1970, *41*, *42*, 138–144.

Keys, A., Taylor, H. L., Blackburn, H., Brozek, J., Anderson, J. T., & Simonson, E. Mortality and coronary heart disease among men studied for 23 years. *Archives of Internal Medicine*, 1971, *128*, 201–214.

Krantz, D. S., Schaeffer, M., Davia, J., Dembroski, T., MacDougall, J., & Shaffer, R. Extent of coronary atherosclerosis, Type A Behavior, and Cardiovascular response to social interaction. *Psychophysiology*, 1981, *18*, 654–664.

Krantz, D. S., Glass, D. C., & Snyder, M. L. Helplessness, stress level, and the coronary-prone behavior pattern. *Journal of Experimental Social Psychology*, 1974, *10*, 284–300.

Krantz, D. S., Sanmarco, M. E., Selvester, R. H., & Matthews, K. A. Psychological correlates of progression of atherosclerosis in men. *Psychosomatic Medicine*, 1979, *41*, 467–475.

Kuller, L., Lilienfield, A., & Fischer, R. Epidemiological study of sudden and unexpected deaths due to arteriosclerotic heart disease. *Circulation*, 1966, *34*, 1056–1068.

Lang, C. M. Effects of psychic stress on atherosclerosis in the squirrel monkey (*Saimiri sciureus*). *Proceedings of the Society for Experimental Biology and Medicine*, 1967, *126*, 30–34.

Lovallo, W. R., & Pishkin, V. A psychophysiological comparison of Type A and B men exposed to failure and uncontrollable noise. *Psychophysiology*, 1980, *17*, 29–36.

Lundberg, U., & Forsman, L. Adrenal-medullary and adrenal-cortical responses to understimulation and overstimulation: Comparison between Type A and Type B persons. *Biological Psychology*, 1979, *9*, 79–89.

MacDougall, J. M., Dembroski, T. M., & Krantz, D. S. Effects of types of challenge on pressor and heart rate responses in Type A and B women. *Psychophysiology*, 1981, *18*, 1–9.

MacDougall, J. M., Dembroski, T. M., & Musante, L. The structured interview and questionnaire methods of assessing coronary-prone behavior in male and female college students *Journal of Behavioral Medicine*, 1979, *2*, 71–83.

Malik, M. A. O. Emotional stress as a precipitating factor in sudden deaths due to coronary insufficiency. *Journal of Forensic Sciences*, 1973, *18*, 47–52.

Mann, G. V. Diet-heart: End of an era. *New England Journal of Medicine*, 1977, *297*, 644–650.

Manuck, S. B., Corse, C. D., & Winkelman, P. A. Behavioral correlates of individual differences in blood pressure reactivity. *Journal of Psychosomatic Research*, 1979, *23*, 281–288.

Manuck, S. B., Craft, S. A., & Gold, K. J. Coronary-prone behavior pattern and cardiovascular response. *Psychophysiology*, 1978, *15*, 403–411.

Manuck, S. B., & Garland, F. N. Coronary-prone behavior pattern, task incentive and cardiovascular response. *Psychophysiology*, 1979, *16*, 136–147.

Matthews, K. A. Assessment and developmental antecedents of the coronary-prone behavior pattern in children. In T. M. Dembroski, S. W. Weiss, J. L. Shields, S. G. Haynes, & M. Feinleib (Eds.), *Coronary-prone behavior*. New York: Springer-Verlag, 1978.

Matthews, K. A., & Brunson, B. I. The attentional style of Type A coronary-prone individuals: Implications for symptom reporting. *Journal of Personality and Social Psychology*, 1979, *37*, 2081–2090.

Matthews, K. A., Glass, D. C., Rosenman, R. H., & Bortner, R. W. Competitive drive, Pattern A, and coronary heart disease: A further analysis of some data from the Western Collaborative Group Study. *Journal of Chronic Diseases*, 1977, *30*, 489–498.

Matthews, K. A., & Saal, F. E. The relationship of the Type A coronary-prone behavior pattern to achievement, power, and affiliation motives. *Psychosomatic Medicine*, 1978, *40*, 631–636.

Menninger, K. A., & Menninger, W. C. Psychoanalytic observations in cardiac disorders. *American Heart Journal*, 1936, *11*, 10.

Michaels, L. Aetiology of coronary artery disease: A historical approach. *British Heart Journal*, 1966, *28*, 258–264.

MRFIT Collaborating Investigators. *Journal of the American Medical Association*, 1976, *235*,825.

Myers, A., & Dewar, H. A. Circumstances attending 100 sudden deaths from coronary artery disease with coroners' necropsies. *British Heart Journal*, 1975, *37*, 1133–1143.

O'Brien, J. R. Variability in the aggregation of human platelets by adrenaline. *Nature*, 1963, *200*, 763–764.

Osler, W. *Lectures on angina pectoris and allied states*. New York: Appleton, 1892.

Peterson, J. E., Keith, R. A., & Wilcox, A. A. Hourly changes in serum cholesterol concentration: Effects of the anticipation of stress. *Circulation*, 1962, *25*, 798–803.

Pittner, N. S. & Houston, B. K. Response to stress, cognitive coping strategies, and the Type A behavior pattern. *Journal of Personality and Social Psychology*, 1980, *39*, 147–157.

Price, K. P., & Clarke, L. K. Behavioral and psychophysiological correlates of the coronary-prone personality: New data and unanswered questions. *Journal of Psychosomatic Research*, 1978, *40*, 478–486.

Raab, W. Cardiotoxic biochemical effects of emotional-environmental stressors—fundamentals of psychocardiology. In L. Levi (Ed.), *Society, stress, and disease*. New York: Plenum, 1971.

Rose, R. M., Jenkins, C. D., & Hurst, M. W. *Air traffic controller health change study*. Report to the Federal Aviation Administration, June, 1978.

Rosenman, R. H. The interview method of assessment of the coronary-prone behavior pattern. In T. M. Dembroski, S. M. Weiss, J. L. Shields, S. G. Haynes, & M. Feinleib (Eds.), *Coronary-prone behavior*. New York: Springer-Verlag, 1978a.

Rosenman, R. H. The role of the Type A behavior pattern in ischaemic heart disease: Modification of its effects by beta-blocking agents. *British Journal of Clinical Pratice*, 1978b, *32* (Suppl. 1), 58–65.

Rosenman, R. H., & Friedman, M. Association of a specific overt behavior pattern in females with blood and cardiovascular findings. *Circulation*, 1961, *24*, 1173–1184.

Rosenman, R. H., & Friedman, M. Neurogenic factors in pathogenesis of coronary heart disease. *Medical Clinics of North America*, 1974, *58*, 269–279.

Rosenman, R. H., Friedman, M., Straus, R., Wurm, M., Kositchek, R., Hahn, W., & Werthessen, N. T. A predictive study of coronary heart disease: The Western Collaborative Group Study. *Journal of the American Medical Association*, 1964, *189*, 15–22.

Ross, R., & Glomset, J. A. The pathogenesis of atherosclerosis. *New England Journal of Medicine*, 1976, 295, 369–377; 420–425.

Ross, R., & Harker, L. Hyperlipidemia and atherosclerosis. *Science*, 1976, *193*, 1094–1100.

Scherwitz, L., Berton, K., & Leventhal, H. Type A behavior, self-involvement, and cardiovascular response. *Psychosomatic Medicine*, 1978, *40*, 593–609.

Scherwitz, L., Leventhal, H., Cleary, P., & Laman, C. Type A behavior: Consideration for risk modification. *Health Values: Achieving High Level Wellness*, 1978, 6, 291–296.

Schneiderman, N. Animal models relating behavioral stress and cardiovascular pathology. In T. M. Dembroski, S. M. Weiss, J. L. Shields, S. G. Haynes, & M. Feinleib (Eds.), *Coronary-prone behavior*. New York: Springer-Verlag, 1978.

Schwartz, G. E. Psychosomatic disorders and biofeedback: A psychobiological model of disregulation. In J. Maser, & M. Seligman (Eds.), *Psychopathology: Experimental Models*. San Francisco: W. H. Freeman, 1977.

Stokols, D., Novaco, R. W., Stokols, J., & Campbell, J. Traffic congestion, Type A behavior, and stress. *Journal of Applied Psychology*, 1978, *63*, 467–480.

Streufert, S., Streufert, S., Dembroski, T., & MacDougall, J. Complexity, coronary-prone behavior and physiological response. In D. Oborne, M. Grunberg, & J. Eiser (Eds.), *Research in psychology and medicine*, London: Academic Press, 1979.

Taggart, P., Carruthers, M., & Somerville, W. Electrocardiogram, plasma catecholamines and lipids, and their modification by oxprenolol when speaking before an audience. *Lancet*, 1973, Aug., 341–346.

Trousseau, A. *Clinical medicine*. Philadelphia: 1882.

Von Dusch, T. *Lehrbuch der Herzkrankheiten*. Leipzig: Verlag Von Wilhem Engelman, 1868.

Van Egeren, L. F. *Electrocardiographic ST and T changes in Type A (Coronary-prone) subjects in computer-simulated interpersonal situations.* Unpublished manuscript.

Van Egeren, L. F. Social interactions, communications, and the coronary-prone behavior pattern: A psychophysiological study. *Psychosomatic Medicine,* 1979a, 41, 2–18.

Van Egeren, L. F. Cardiovascular changes during social competition in mixed motive game. *Journal of Personality and Social Psychology,* 1979b, 37, 858–864.

Vickers, R. *A short measure of the Type A personality.* Unpublished manuscript, University of Michigan, 1973.

Von Holst, D. Renal failure as the cause of death in *Tupaia belangeri* (tree shrews) exposed to persistent social stress. *Journal of Comparative Physiology,* 1972, 78, 236–273.

Waldron, I., Hickey, A., Butensky, R., Gruss, L., Overall, K., Schmader, A. & Wohlmuth, D. Type A behavior pattern: Relationship to variation in blood pressure, paternal characteristics, and academic and social activities of students. *Journal of Human Stress,* 1980, 6, 16–27.

Wardrop, J. *Diseases of the heart.* London: 1851.

Weidner, G., & Matthews, K. A. Reported physical symptoms elicited by unpredictable events and the Type A coronary-prone behavior pattern. *Journal of Personality and Social Psychology,* 1978, 36, 213–220.

Weiss, J. M. Effects of coping responses on stress. *Journal of Comparative and Physiological Psychology,* 1968, 65, 251–260.

White, P. D. The historical background of angina pectoris. *Modern Concepts of Cardiovascular Disease,* 1974, 43, 109.

Williams, R. B. Psychophysiological processes, the coronary-prone behavior pattern, and coronary heart disease. In T. M. Dembroski, S. M. Weiss, J. L. Shields, S. G. Haynes, & M. Feinleib (Eds.), *Coronary-prone behavior.* New York: Springer-Verlag, 1978.

Williams, R. B., Haney, T. L., Lee, K. L., Kong, Y., Blumenthal, J. A., & Whalen, R. E. Type A behavior, hostility, and coronary atherosclerosis. *Psychosomatic Medicine,* 1980, 42, 539–549.

Zierler, K. L., Maseri, A., Klassen, D., Rabinowitz, D., & Burgess, J. Muscle metabolism during exercise in man. *Transcripts of the Association of American Physicians,* 1968, 81, 266–273.

Zyzanski, S. J. Coronary prone behavior pattern and coronary heart disease: Epidemiological evidence. In T. M. Dembroski, S. M. Weiss, J. L. Shields, S. G. Haynes, & M. Feinleib (Eds.), *Coronary-prone behavior.* New York: Springer-Verlag, 1978.

4 Attention and Coronary Heart Disease

J. Richard Jennings
University of Pittsburgh

INTRODUCTION

In this chapter we will examine evidence indicating that attention may be an influential psychological factor influencing coronary heart disease (CHD).

What is meant by attention? All of us can only perceive and act upon a limited portion of the massive amount of information available from the environment and from ongoing thoughts and actions. Therefore, a limited portion of information must be selected. This process is termed attention, and the limitation defines processing capacity (See Broadbent, 1971; Kahneman, 1973; Norman, 1969). Some individuals allocate full processing capacity to tasks at hand and, thus, ignore distracting information. Others do not allocate full capacity, but maintain spare capacity, tolerate distraction and are willing to take ample time to finish a task. Stated differently, individuals vary in their policies for allocating processing capacity.

To many readers, the "cold", cognitive process of allocation of capacity (attending) may seem an unlikely influence on CHD. Indeed, we have a cultural association between visceral function, disease, and "hot" emotional events (Averill, 1974). Attention as a "higher function" does not fit that association. Cardiovascular changes during extreme excitement are common knowledge. Thus, it is not surprising that our culture and many authors have chosen to emphasize strong emotions and overwhelming stress as psychological factors contributing to heart disease. Students of physiological reaction, on the other hand, have, however, historically been concerned about whether emotion or the cognitive and motoric preparation for action are the primary cause of physiological reactions. This concern has become more critical as we learn that mundane

85

episodes of attending and remembering as well as psychologically intense events produce reliable physiological change. Note also that reactions to intense events include coping efforts that necessarily involve mobilization of resources for problem solving—that is, the allocation of processing capacity (e.g. Lazarus, 1966). Furthermore, individual differences in allocation policy imply differences in what is attended to as well as differences in physiological responses concomitant with allocation. Inattention to some events may influence the perception and treatment of CHD.

CHD seems to develop over years, not days or minutes, thus chronic, everyday processes may reasonably be implicated in the disease process (See Davignon, 1977, 1978). In this chapter, we review recent evidence suggesting that individuals allocating full capacity may neglect subtle but informative cues, that when perceived and acted on, can protect against coronary heart disease. Furthermore, the allocating of processing capacity produces brief changes in cardiovascular function which may have implications for the disease processes involved in CHD.

The discussion of allocation of capacity and CHD will be organized in three sections. The first section describes evidence showing that allocation of capacity leads to cardiovascular change. The second section examines allocation of capacity and the neglect of subtle environmental cues. Finally, the third section relates individual differences in the allocation of capacity to behavioral risk factors for CHD and to CHD itself. The scope of this review will not permit exhaustive reviews of each issue. Therefore, illustrative evidence will be presented with appropriate referencing of review articles germane to specific questions.

CAPACITY ALLOCATION AND CARDIOVASCULAR RESPONSE

Psychological influences on disease processes must be expressed through the actions of the brain and related neuroendocrine apparatus. Peripherally, the sympathetic and parasympathetic branches of the autonomic nervous system innervate the heart and the vasculature. The control of these peripheral afferents and efferents is well represented throughout the brain—including so called "higher centers" such as the frontal cortex (Calaresu, Faiers, & Mogenson, 1975). Peripherally, the endocrine system, particularly the adrenal gland, provides important controls of electolyte and fluid balances critical for the maintenance of blood flow and pressure. Centrally, the pituitary-hypothalamic axis of the brain regulates the activity of the endocrine system. Our increasing understanding of these systems provides a plethora of mechanisms by which psychological events as represented in the brain can act on the cardiovascular system.

Historically, cardiovascular responses to psychological events were considered a component of an "arousal" response. Cannon (1939) first described an arousal response termed the "flight or fight" response. As is widely known, this response is an "en masse" reaction of the sympathetic nervous system leading to adrenalin excretion, heart rate speeding, blood pressure increases, palmar sweating, and enhanced blood flow to the muscles. Overall, this response prepares the body for extreme exertion. The role of the parsympathetic nervous system (vagal effectors) was seen as directly opposite to the sympathetic system—it conserved energy and restored the body after periods of arousal. In the 1950's and 1960's this view was elaborated and related to brain function via the actions of the reticular activity system of the brain stem and midbrain (Duffy, 1957, 1972; Lindsley, 1960). Arousal was seen as an unidimensional continuum from sleep to extreme excitement—a continuum with parallel psychological and physiological expressions.

Current physiological and psychophysiological evidence suggests, however, that a simple arousal notion is not a complete explanation of psychophysiological change (see Cofer & Appley, 1964; Lacey & Lacey, 1974). Arousal is not unidimensional. A relevant line of investigation for example, suggested that arousal could not explain the cardiovascular changes that occurred when a person performed an information processing task. These experiments are important because they suggest that information processing, as well as emotional excitement, could control cardiovascular responding.

Much of the recent work on information processing and cardiovascular change can be traced to the work of John and Bea Lacey in the late 1950's and 1960's. In an early paper (Lacey, Kagan, Lacy, & Moss, 1963), heart rate and skin conductance responses to a number of tasks were examined. Volunteers performed mental arithmetic, made up sentences, solved anagrams, listened to the rules for a novel game, attended to an emotive drama, listened to white noise, and observed light flashes. All of the tasks produced physiological reactions. Most importantly, however, skin conductance increased in all the tasks, while heart rate increased in some and decreased in others. Listening to the rules of the game, the emotive drama, white noise, and observing light flashes elicited a slowing of heart rate (cardiac deceleration). Two important claims were made: first, that arousal, anxiety, or emotion could not account for the results; and second, information processing demands of the tasks could.

What is the basis for these claims? Many factors varied between the tasks—sensory modality, appeal to emotions, requirements for motor responding. For example, the drama task required the volunteer to empathize with an actor verbalizing the thoughts and feelings of a dying man. Yet this presumably emotional task yielded a cardiac deceleration similar to that induced by watching lights flash. The Laceys' argue that the tasks eliciting deceleration shared a requirement to note and detect environmental occurrences. The tasks producing acceleration were seen as requiring mental work rather than sensitivity to environmental input. Heart rate seemed to classify the tasks by information processing requirements rather than by degree of motivational or affective involvement.

A second reason for questioning an emotional or arousal interpretation was the patterning of skin conductance and heart rate responses. This pattern was not consistent with a change in general arousal or a view of emotion that is tied to such arousal. Arousal should produce heart rate acceleration and palmar sweating. The results for half the tasks used by the Laceys', however, showed palmar sweating combined with decreases in heart rate (see also Lazarus, Speisman, & Mordkoff, 1963).

How does the Lacey interpretation relate to our concern with attention and processing capacity? Although some ambiguity exists, (see Hahn, 1973), Lacey and Lacey generally associated heart rate deceleration with an acceptance of environmental input or the intention to note and detect such input. Cardiac acceleration was related to rejection of environmental input or mental elaboration. The Laceys seem to be suggesting that what we commonly call "mental concentration" is related to cardiac acceleration. Their concept can be redefined in terms of a processing capacity view of attention (Jennings, Lawrence, & Kasper, 1978). Such a redefinition states that the direction of cardiac change is determined by whether processing capacity is (a) allocated to monitoring input channels[1] and inhibiting ongoing processing, or (b) allocated to ongoing processing. Cardiac deceleration is associated with (a) and acceleration with (b). The primary virtue of reframing the Lacey hypothesis is to suggest the relevance of previous work using measures of processing capacity. Such measures can then be used to examine precisely the concomitance of heart rate and the allocation of processing capacity. This strategy, for example, has proven successful for the study of pupillary dilation (Kahneman, 1973).

In order to show that allocation of processing capacity is directly related to cardiovascular function, these must be evidence first, that a change in allocation of processing capacity has occurred, and second, that specific cardiovascular changes are induced. These changes should be independent of emotional, motivational, or motoric variation. The demonstration of these points must be considered separately for those situations inducing cardiac deceleration and those inducing cardiac acceleration. A complete review of these issues will not be attempted here and, the interested reader is referred to Bohlin and Kjellberg,

---

[1]This term does not refer only to sensory input, but rather to any information required and not presently available. In this sense, an input channel is identical with Posner's (1980) concept of psychological pathway. In terms of heart rate research, this means anticipated nonenvironmental input, e.g. time estimation or attending to bodily cues, would be expected to lead to cardiac deceleration (see Johnson & May, 1969).

(1979), Carroll and Anastasiades (1978), Elliott (1972), Hahn (1973), and Lacey and Lacey (1974, 1978).

Allocation of Capacity to Anticipation: Cardiac Deceleration and Associated Responses

Cardiac deceleration is commonly observed either just preceding an expected event, e.g. before the respond signal in a fixed foreperiod reaction time task, or just after an unexpected but significant stimulus, such as a loud sound. The unexpected sound elicits an immediate orientation toward the source of the stimulus, heightened alertness and, frequently, subjectively experienced physiological change, e.g. pounding heart or sweaty palms. Similar but less striking experiences may occur during anticipation.

In order to avoid circular reasoning, we must first show that anticipation and orienting induce behavioral responses indicative of a change in the allocation of processing capacity. The most acceptable evidence of this sort is based on the dual task paradigm (see Kerr, 1973). Capacity limitation is defined as the portion of available information that an individual can deal with at any instant. If all capacity is allocated, none should be available to deal with another task. This is the rationale for the dual task paradigm. Two tasks are presented. One task, e.g. anticipating a weak stimulus, is presented to the volunteer as the main task. The other task, e.g. a reaction time task, is presented as secondary and typically occurs less frequently than the main task. When all capacity has not been allocated to anticipating the weak stimulus, reaction speed should be fast. When all capacity is allocated to the anticipation task, reaction speed should be slow. Performance on the secondary task measures the capacity allocated to the main task.

Just prior to an expected event, secondary task performance has been shown to decline (see review in Posner, 1978), and motor activity irrelevant to the primary task disappears (see review in Obrist, Howard, Lawler, Galosy, Meyers, & Gaebelein, 1974). Under some conditions simple reflexes such as the eye blink are also inhibited during anticipation (Bohlin & Graham, 1977; Brunia, 1979; Silverstein & Graham, 1978).

Less behavioral evidence of changes in the allocation of processing capacity is available for periods immediately following an unexpected event because data collection is difficult. Regularly presented events quickly become expected rather than unexpected. We do know, however, that ongoing activity is inhibited during orienting to an unexpected event, and there is some evidence of secondary task decrements during a mildly surprising event (Jennings, Lawrence, & Kasper, 1978). Overall, allocation of significant (if not necessarily full) capacity appears to be a feature of both the anticipation of an expected event or the orientation to an unexpected one.

We can now discuss heart rate changes that occur when processing capacity is allocated *after* a novel event. In an early paper, Graham and Clifton (1966) suggested that heart rate deceleration was a component of the "orienting reflex" examined extensively in Soviet psychophysiology (Kimmel, van Olst, & Or-lebeke, 1979; Sokolov, 1963). The orienting reflex refers to both somatic and autonomic responses to unexpected and significant stimulus change (Bernstein & Taylor, 1979), and can readily be interpreted as analogous to the allocation of processing capacity to expected input. Alerted by the "orienting" stimulus, the organism allocates capacity to the receipt of further environmental information. Intense abrupt change may, however, lead to startle rather than orienting and noxious stimuli may lead to a "defense reaction". Both the startle and defense are associated with heart rate speeding rather than slowing (cf. Graham, 1979). Between extremes of startle and defense, however, heart rate slowing is an invariant feature of orienting.

The heart rate changes that occur when processing capacity is allocated to an anticipated event, that is a change *before* an expected event, have been extensively studied using a preparatory interval paradigm. This paradigm has been used extensively by the Laceys in following up their initial work (e.g. Lacey & Lacey, 1974). Figure 4.1 shows a typical result from this paradigm (Jennings, Averill, Opton, & Lazarus, 1971). Volunteers perform a choice reaction time task with the possibility of electric shock occurring at the same time as the signal to react (the Discriminative-Go signal in the figure). Cardiac deceleration occurs in the 10-second interval between a ready signal and the signal to react. Using Lacey's term, an interval has been created during which the primary task is to note and detect an environmental event. The figure shows that in all cases the heart speeds briefly after the ready signal and then slows up to the time of the signal to react.

How do these results contribute to our demonstration of a specific cardiac response to information processing? The figure illustrates that the threat of certain or probabilistic shock does not eliminate the cardiac deceleration. Many demonstrations are available of such brief cardiac slowing prior to affect generating stimuli (e.g., Hare, Wood, Britian, & Shadman, 1971; Hastings & Obrist, 1967). Related demonstrations have also shown that increasing incentives, e.g. increasing the reward for fast reaction times will, if anything, *increase* the depth of cardiac deceleration (e.g., Lacey, 1972; Jennings, 1981). Indeed, cardiac deceleration does not seem to occur unless the stimulus events have psychological significance for the volunteer (Brown, Morse, Leavitt, & Graham, 1976).

The anticipation paradigm has yielded a number of other relevant results (cf. Bohlin and Kjelberg, 1979). For example, a precise temporal expectancy is a prerequisite for the cardiac deceleration, but, contrary to earlier hypotheses, variables such as stimulus uncertainty do not have a powerful effect on the phenomenon (see Jennings, Averill, Opton, & Lazarus, 1971). The requirement for a response to the expected event also amplifies the deceleration, but is not

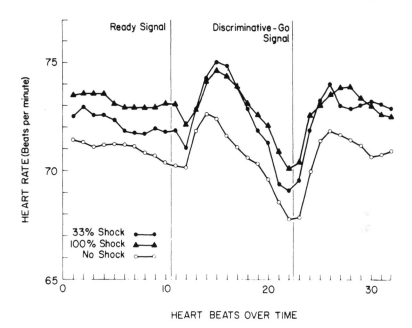

FIG. 4.1. Beat by beat heart rate in a choice reaction time task. At the time of the Ready signal, volunteers saw a light initiating a 10-second anticipatory period. At the end of this time, one of two lights lit indicating the speeded key press required. This Discriminative-Go signal was accompanied by electrical shock 0, 33, or 100% of the time in different experimental conditions. The three beat by beat responses correspond to these conditions. (From Jennings, Averill, Opton, & Lazarus, 1971 with permission of the Society for Psychophysiological Research).

necessary for the emergence of the deceleration. Finally, the association of either significant muscular effort or strongly aversive events with the expected event appear to attenuate but not eliminate the anticipatory deceleration. In sum, the evidence supports the primacy of a temporally focused anticipation over other variables known to alter heart rate responses.

Heart rate is only one aspect of a response pattern that includes changes in the blood vessels and hormonal responses. The slowing of heart rate in fact is a puzzling phenomenon because the individual is expecting action as well as an event. Adequate preparation would seem to call for a speeding of the pumping action of the heart not a slowing. Muscular action requires heightened metabolic support and waste elimination and thus heightened circulatory function. Do the vascular and endocrine responses that occur appear to be more supportive of the anticipated action than the heart rate change? Experiments of Obrist (Obrist, Gaebelein, Teller, Langer, Grignolo, Light, & McCubbin, 1978; Obrist, Langer, Light, Grignolo, & McCubbin, 1979; Obrist, Lawler, Howard, Smithson, Martin, & Manning, 1974) and Williams (Williams, Bittker, Buschsbaum, &

Wynne, 1975; Williams, Poon, & Burdette, 1977) provide information relevant to this question. During periods of anticipation, blood pressure and rate of change of pressure are elevated relative to control periods, but forearm blood flow decreases. Skin blood flow also appears to increase at the time of anticipatory heart rate slowing (Jennings, Schrot, & Wood, 1980). In sum, during anticipation heart rate and blood flow to the muscle seem temporarily inhibited while blood pressure parameters show increases suggestive of sympathetic nervous system activation.

Increases in blood pressure would serve to support forthcoming action but the studies cited, at least, do not suggest any adaptive role for the heart rate and muscle blood flow changes. Concomitant increases in catecholamines (largely noradrenalin and adrenalin) would provide a mobilization of the body for action, but endocrine responses during the allocation of capacity to anticipation have not been widely studied. Increases in adrenalin have been reported with a vigilance task (Williams, 1975) and during a task requiring close observation and selective processing of information (Frankenhauser & Johansson, 1976). In the latter, adrenalin levels were higher in tasks requiring greater selectivity. Although both studies appear to involve attentional processes, our intepretation of the courses of these changes must be tentative as the studies were not designed to relate the allocation of capacity to endocrine response.

Allocation of Capacity to Ongoing Processing: Cardiac Acceleration and Associated Responses

In contrast to situations of anticipation or orienting, a different pattern of cardiovascular response occurs when full capacity is allocated to the processing of ongoing thoughts and actions. Such allocation is likely to occur, for example, during the memorization of a set of items or during mental calculations. Processing capacity is being used as opposed to being held available for impending events and actions. (Most information processing tasks require this form of capacity allocation.)

When full capacity is allocated for immediate use, physiological changes occur similar to those accompanying physical exercise: heart rate, blood pressure, and catecholamines increase and blood is shunted to the muscles and away from the skin (see reviews in Henry & Stephens, 1977; Kahneman, 1973).[2] Such changes have frequently been associated with the general activation of the physiological system (Duffy, 1957; Freeman, 1948; Lindsley, 1960).

---

[2]It should be emphasized that the induced changes are only similar to those associated with exercise. Langer, Obrist, and McCubbin (1979) have demonstrated differences between exercise induced and psychologically induced changes in dogs. The current level of discussion does not permit a detailed discussion of the known differences between physiological arousal responses.

Since physiological activation can occur for many reasons, moment by moment concomitance of physiological change with an index of allocation of capacity must be demonstrated in order to rule out alternative explanations. Although few studies have focused directly on cardiovascular change, the relation of allocation of capacity and heart rate change is generally supported (e.g., Kahneman, Tursky, Shapiro, & Crider, 1969; Tursky, Schwartz, & Crider, 1980). In one study, for example, heart rate during a learning task was shown to relate directly to performance on a secondary reaction time task (Jennings, Lawrence, & Kasper, 1978). In this experiment, items were memorized and tested in a paradigm resembling the classic serial anticipation technique (Millward, 1971). A comparison task had volunteers recite sequential numbers as paced by the serial anticipation method. Both the secondary task measure, reaction time and degree of cardiac acceleration reflected the allocation of greater capacity to the memorization task relative to the recitation task. Similarly, both measures suggested that the recall of items required greater capacity allocation than their initial learning. The parallelism of secondary task and heart rate measures of capacity did, however, disappear late in the experimental session. Heart rate and reaction time appeared to be differentially sensitive to fatigue. This study as well as other work (Jennings, 1975; Jennings & Hall, 1980) failed to find any evidence of an association between heart rate change and specific types of mental work, such as memorizing and performing cognitive transformations. Furthermore, in these studies variations in emotional reactions do not seem to predict the physiological changes. Overall, the available evidence supports the concomitance of heart rate change and capacity allocated to ongoing processing, but warns that physiological variables, (e.g., fatigue) as well as information processing requirements are important.

Heart rate acceleration during information processing is embedded in an overall pattern of cardiovascular and endocrine responses. However, the variety of psychophysiological influences on cardiac acceleration preclude the clear determination that these responses are unique to the allocation of attended capacity. Dual task studies are not available to document that changes in processing capacity have occurred. Typically, systolic and diastolic blood pressure increase during the performance of tasks. Williams (Williams et al., 1975, 1977) has further shown that blood flow to the muscles is increased during tasks, such as mental arithmetic. Similarly, increases in catecholamines and cortisol have been frequently observed in information processing tasks (Frankenhauser, 1971, 1975; Rose, Jenkins, & Hurst, 1978). Thus, allocation of full capacity to current processing may elicit an increase in cardiovascular and endocrine function, but this increase cannot at present be attributed solely to information processing.

The neural basis of the brief heart changes associated with information processing is known to some extent. Pharmacological studies reviewed by Obrist, Langer, Light, Gringnolo, and McCubbin (1979) suggest that vagal (parasympathetic) influences largely control the heart rate responses. The heart rate deceleration during anticipation is blocked by a drug that reduces vagal influences on the heart. Drugs blocking the sympathetic nervous system lessen heart rate acceleration, but acceleration is due to a release of vagal inhibition as well. Associated vascular and endocrine changes may be due to sympathetic nervous system influences, but this has not been as clearly established.

In summary, allocation of processing capacity appears to elicit consistent physiological responses. Strong evidence for this position require that secondary task measures of capacity allocation be related to physiological responses. Difficulties with the concept of arousal and available evidence led us, however, to suggest that cardiovascular changes during two forms of capacity allocation must be considered separately. Direction of heart rate change, muscle blood flow, and relative amount of parasympathetic influence on the heart depend on whether capacity is allocated to ongoing or anticipated cognitive processing. Blood pressure and hormonal responses at least tentatively, appear responsive to amount of capacity allocated irrespective of whether allocated to ongoing or anticipated processing.

Alternative Positions

Early challenges to the association of information processing and heart rate change were from suggestions that deceleration reflected an absence of physiological or affective arousal (e.g. Johnson & Campos, 1967). Hopefully, the research just reviewed has answered this objection. Heart rate deceleration has been shown to, if anything, be enhanced in relatively "arousing" situations such as performing a difficult discrimination with high incentive.

A significant and challenging objective to the Lacey's interpretation has been consistently voiced by Paul Obrist. In a number of experiments (reviewed in Obrist, 1981), he found a decrease in electromyographic (EMG) activity simultaneous with cardiac deceleration. This suggested a cardiac-somatic coupling, i.e. heart rate decelerated only when the EMG was inhibited. This formulation can be separated in a weak and strong form (Jennings et al., 1971). The strong form states that the EMG changes are primary and heart rate necessarily follows EMG. The weak form suggests that a "central attentional state" occurs that frequently leads to concomitant cardiac and EMG changes. Empirically, the frequent concomitance of cardiac and EMG changes cannot be questioned. Available evidence, however, suggests that the weak form of the cardiac-somatic hypothesis is more defensible than the strong form. An experiment by Coles and Duncan-Johnson (1975) is most relevant in this regard. Sequential stimuli were arranged to provide a variation in information processing requirements. Heart rate change reflected these variations but EMG change did not. Other instances can be cited in which the amplitude of motor reflexes increased rather than decreased concomitantly with heart rate deceleration (Brunia, 1979; Graham, 1979). Thus, heart rate change during information processing does not seem to be an artifact of motor changes.

Obrist's (1981) point of view does raise an important caution about the interpretation of heart rate change and physiological change in general. The cardiovascular system serves to maintain the supply of necessary nutrients to the cells of the body. The nervous system has adapted to this need with a number of control systems related to respiration and local metabolic needs. These control systems would seem to necessarily take precedence over many psychologically induced changes. For example, the heart rate responses we have described are related to respiratory variables (Jennings & Wood, 1977). A complete understanding of heart rate responses must consider the relationship of physiological and psychological responses and thus, the limiting conditions of both types of control.

Implications of Allocation Capacity for Disease Processes

Thus far, we have shown that the allocation of processing capacity induces physiological change. On the other hand, many activities, e.g., exercise, alter physiology and may have no effect on disease or may even enhance health. Indeed, physiological changes during information processing may be adaptive in the sense that both endocrine (Frankenhauser, 1975) and cardiovascular (e.g. Jennings & Hall, 1980) responses have been positively related to performance.

We can only speculate at present that an exacerbation of intensity or chronicity of these responses may be related to CHD. Frankenhauser (1971) has, for example, developed the concept of physiological cost. Each neuroendocrine or pressor response may cause a certain amount of wear and tear on the blood vessel (see below). The cost can be balanced by reparative processes, but only if the costs are not too high or too frequent.

A brief digression on CHD is necessary to establish the relative importance and possible sites of action of psychological factors. Currently, atherosclerosis is viewed as a multifactorial disease (Stammler, 1978), which has an initial phase of injury to the wall of the blood vessel and a subsequent phase of development of atherosclerotic plaque. Psychological factors are one of the multiple factors contributing to atherosclerosis. For example, the catecholamines adrenalin and noradrenalin, which increase during psychological stress (see Levi, 1971), are thought to be among several factors which influence the initial phase of injury to the wall of the blood vessel. Clearly, the multifactorial model suggests that if psychological factors influence atherosclerosis, they do so interactively with a large number of physical, biochemical, and physiological factors.

Atherosclerotic plaque contributes to the decreased blood flow heart tissue but myocardial infarction appears to be an acute event related either to material lodging in already narrowed vessels or disturbances of the normal pumping rhythm of the heart, arrhythmia. Thus, psychological factors may relate differently to the various clinical manifestations of CHD such as myocardial infarction, sudden death, and angina pectoris.

Much of the speculation about the mechanisms by which psychological factors influence CHD has focused on individual differences because not everyone suffers from CHD. A number of authors have reviewed possible mechanisms of psychological influence on CHD (Dembroski, MacDougall, Herd, & Shields, this volume; Krantz, Glass, Schaeffer, & Davia, 1982; Schneiderman, 1978; Verrier & Lown, this volume, Williams, 1977). Two broad categories of causation are cited. First an acute event may induce neural discharges in a diseased individual that disturb cardiac rhythm and cause sudden death (see Verrier & Lown, this volume). Second, chronic events may influence factors implicated in atherosclerosis such as catecholamine responses and blood pressure changes (see Schneiderman; Dembroski et al., this volume). Frequently, "repeated and excessive activation of sympathetic autonomic and neuroendocrine mechanisms" are viewed as the primary source of pathophysiological change (Dembroski et al., this volume).

Vagal, as well as sympathetic, influences on the heart may also play a role in cardiac arrhythmia and possibly in sudden death (see Jennings, in press). Allocation of capacity to anticipation is rather uniquely linked to cardiac deceleration (a vagal effect) occurring in a behavioral active state. Levy and Martin (1979) have reviewed in detail the influence of vagal and combined sympathetic vagal stimulation on heart rate and stroke volume. Under a variety of conditions, vagal input can lead to arrhythmia. Behavioral work by Brener, Phillips, and Connally (1977) found an association between learned heart rate slowing and arrhythmia. This animal work may be supplemented by our recent observation of the occurrence of arrhythmia in four of the 31 executives participating in an experiment involving cardiac deceleration (Jennings & Choi, 1981). Another suggestive piece of evidence is the induction of arrhythmia in ischemic animals by stimulation of brain regions known to also regulate the cardiac decelerative response (Skinner, 1982; Skinner, Lie, & Entman, 1975; Skinner & Yingling, 1977). Thus, available results would argue that we should not ignore the potential CHD risk of repeated or intense elicitors of combined vagal-sympathetic activation— particularly in the diseased individual.

Any convincing relation to CHD must, however, be based on studies directly relating the allocation of processing capacity to either CHD itself or established risk factors for CHD. Evidence of this sort, although still meager, will be reviewed after discussing the psychological implications of capacity allocation.

SELECTIVE ATTENTION, CAPACITY OVERLOAD, AND AROUSAL

Recent developments in social psychology have linked the overload of processing capacity with stress and often with arousal—one component of which is cardiovascular change. This section briefly reviews this work. Although the social psychological work has not been directly integrated with the psychophysiological work just reviewed, cardiovascular indices of increased capacity allocation should be concomitant with the "overloading" of processing capacity. Such overload has also been related to selective attention. In particular, we will review the ignoring of health and social cues as a function of full capacity allocation. The review will conclude again by asking the relevance of the effects to CHD.

Social psychologists became interested in the overloading of capacity through a concern with urban stress (Glass & Singer, 1972; Milgram, 1970). The increased complexity and industrialization of our society has led to an increase in urban noise, crowding, and time pressures. These may generally be viewed as creating a chronic state of overstimulation. A substantial literature exists showing the detrimental effects of such overstimulation (e.g. Glass & Singer, 1972; Cohen, Evans, Krantz, & Stokols, 1980; Baum & Valins, 1977). The mechanisms translating urban stress into psychological deficits and physiological anomalies are a focus of current interest. A number of proposals have invoked attentional mechanisms, such as capacity overload, salience, and attributions initiated by arousal states (e.g. Gochman, 1979; Stokols, 1975; Suedfeld, 1975; Taylor & Fiske, 1978).

The conceptual roots of these applications of processing capacity concepts derive from early work on arousal and performance (Cofer & Appley, 1964; Hebb, 1955). Animal studies typically varied rewards or punishments and observed their effects upon the performance of learning tasks that varied in complexity. In 1959, Broadhurst summarized the studies relating high arousal and decreased efficiency in complex tasks. Easterbrook (1959) extended this argument by suggesting specifically that arousal narrowed the span of attention leading to the ignoring of incidental cues. Once again, the term arousal must be discussed. Early work equated the concepts of arousal, motivation, and drive. Furthermore certain manipulations, such as the addition of noxious noise or threat of electric shock, have also been equated with arousal. Such manipulations are, however, complex and even the subjective report of increased arousal does not guarantee that the manipulation had the sole effect intended by the experimenter (see Poulton, 1977). These definitional problems are not easily solved by moving to a physiological index of arousal. As we saw in the previous section, psychologically induced variation in a physiological measure is complex and not easily separated from biological variation.

Despite these definitional problems, manipulations defined by the experimenter to increase either arousal or demands on processing capacity appear to decrease sensitivity to low salience cues. Reviews by Broadbent (1971), Tecce and Cole (1976) and Hockey (1979) provide a balanced view of the strengths and weaknesses of the arousal-attention relationship. An experiment by Hockey (1973) and subsequent follow-up work will illustrate the nature of the evidence available. Volunteers were given a primary pursuit tracking task but also asked to note the occasional lighting of one of a set of lamps arranged in a semi-circle around the volunteer. The lamps were arranged so that the task could be performed without head turning; with an easy tracking task, performance on the light detection task is perfect. Increases in pursuit tracking difficulty or the addition of noise cues, however, lead to failure to detect some of the visual signals from the lamps. In such cases, pursuit tracking performance is maintained, but the detection deteriorates on the less perceptually salient lamps. Hockey (1979) reports that the opposite effect occurs when low arousal is induced by sleep loss—tracking performance declines more than detection. Increased "arousal" is associated with increased attentional selectivity. Hockey's (1973) experiment produced an orderly result in which the lamps most peripheral to the volunteer showed the greatest decrement during the noise condition. In two experiments, however, Forster and Grierson (1978a, b) failed to replicate this result. Noise altered the performance on the lamps but the exact result of Hockey could not be replicated. Discussion of this failure (Hockey, 1978) emphasized the complexity of dual task techniques and possible differences between the experiments in the tracking tasks. Thus, it may not always be possible to predict exactly what the volunteer will deem "peripheral", but manipulations deemed "arousing" do generally seem to enhance attention to central events at the expense of peripheral events. Knowledge of the specific "arousal" states induced and the specific cognitive processes required by the tasks may ultimately allow us to predict selectivity more exactly. For now, however, we can return to the social psychological work relating significant social cues to stress conceptualized as capacity overload.

A discussion of social and health cues obviously moves us away from cues such as experimenter provided lights and sounds which are very well defined but socially insignificant. As we deal with less well defined cues we also move into research areas in which the dual task paradigm has not been widely applied. Therefore, capacity allocation must usually be inferred from environmental conditions or task complexity without the benefit of measures of capacity allocated. In these designs general decrements in performances may be difficult to separate from maintained performance on a central task with decreased performance on a peripheral task. With these caveats in mind, let us see if situations eliciting full capacity also encourage disregard of social and health cues.

Taylor and Fiske (1978), Suedfeld (1975), and Cohen (1978) have provided useful reviews of the application of attention to socially relevant cues. Cohen's (1978) review is particularly relevant. In addition to the usual assumptions of a processing capacity model, Cohen suggests that capacity is required by the selection process itself. Furthermore, when selectivity is chronically required capacity is used up or depleted. Literature is reviewed suggesting that the variables relevant to urban stress, noise, unpredictability, and crowding, do adversely effect secondary task performance on a dual task paradigm. These same variables can also be shown to hasten cognitive fatigue as indicated by performance over time and performance in subsequent tasks, i.e. after effects. How does this relate to cues of possible relevance to CHD?

Awareness of Social and Health Cues

The final step in Cohen's (1978) argument is that subtle, but important, social cues may be ignored as a result of capacity overload. Social cues are observed events, such as facial expressions, which are noted and interpreted in terms of social relationships. Awareness of social cues provides us with information about the impact of our behavior on others, and thus, with information necessary for the maintenance of adequate relationships. The susceptibility of social cues to selective ignoring has been demonstrated by Cohen and Lezak (1977). Volunteers were asked to memorize a list of items with a secondary task of noting slides showing persons. When noise was added to this task, memory for the slides showing persons was decreased; the person slides acted as low salience cues. Similar effects on personality judgments were reported by Siegal and Steele (1979, 1980); distracting stimuli reduced the amount of information volunteers used in forming judgments. While these studies show a reduction in attention to social cues, some evidence goes beyond this by showing that social behavior is influenced by full capacity allocation. For example, helping behavior appears to be decreased in situations that would appear to elicit full allocation of capacity (e.g., Korte, Ypma, & Toppen, 1975; Matthews & Canon, 1975). For helping, the chain of reasoning between allocation of full capacity and social relations is completed by studies showing that interpersonal relations suffer when one individual fails to act on another's cues indicating help seeking (Berkowitz, 1972).

Awareness of physical symptoms that signal disease is a second type of information that may be lost due to the allocation of all or nearly all capacity to central events. Many physical symptoms appear as the aches and pains of everyday life rather than as overwhelming pain. Awareness of physical symptoms is required if low intensity but consistent and significant disease symptoms are to be discriminated from transient aches and pains. An interesting experimental analog of this effect is presented by Matthews, Scheier, Brunson, and Carducci (1980). The influence of predictable and unpredictable noise on symptom reporting was compared. Unpredictable noise was first shown to require greater allocation of capacity than predictable noise using a secondary reaction time task. Symptom reporting was then shown to be markedly less during unpredictable as compared to predictable noise. Presumably, individuals allocating full capacity fail to act on symptoms since they are not perceived; however, direct evidence on this point seems unavailable.

Implication for Disease

Selective attending to social and health cues is of itself a normal response just as the cardiovascular responses discussed earlier were normal. Relationships to disease must again depend on the exacerbation of a normal response via intensity or chronicity. Individuals who react to overload with extreme selectivity may miss even important social cues of, for example, a spouse's dissatisfaction. A more likely impact, however, may be a relationship between chronic overload and chronic inattentiveness to social and health cues. Such a chronic condition may, at least conceptually, be related to the breaking down of important health maintaining buffers against disease. For example, the chronic failure to notice social cues and thus maintain social relations may impoverish a person's social network. Social support appears to buffer individuals against the initiation and consequences of disease and aid recovery from disease (see Cobb, 1976; Pinneau, 1976). Longitudinal evidence for this position has been presented by Gore (1978) in a study of the health consequences of unemployment. Among men who remained unemployed after factory closing, men with strong social support reported fewer illness symptoms than those who were unsupported. Physical health cues as well as social cues can be related to disease buffers. A chronic failure to notice and act on physical symptoms would necessarily seem to eliminate the person's own health maintaining behavior (see Gillum, Feinleib, Margolis, Fabsitz, & Brasch, 1976; Insull, 1973). Needed rest, vacations, and alterations in eating and smoking will not be initiated because the person has not perceived the need for change. In addition, early medical treatment will not be sought and prophylactic medications and health maintaining regimes will obviously be unavailable.

Although plausible, such arguments must be supported by relating them directly to CHD. Individuals who develop CHD, relative to those who do not, should chronically allocate full processing capacity and thus ignore social and health cues. The remainder of the chapter will focus on such evidence as well as evidence that the same individuals show cardiovascular responses consistent with the allocation of full capacity.

ALLOCATION OF CAPACITY AND RISK FOR CHD

The literature reviewed to this point suggests that allocation of a significant amount of processing capacity to a primary task will (a) produce well defined cardiovascular responses and (b) reduce awareness of secondary events. We have suggested possible ways in which both of these consequences could influence the course and outcome of CHD. These speculations centered on individual differences in intensity, chronicity, and temporal patterning between those of risk and not at risk for CHD. What evidence can be cited that such individual differences exist?

Two basic approaches can be taken: First, looking at those with clearly diagnosed CHD versus comparable controls and second, looking at those who possess characteristics placing them at risk for the disease versus those who don't. The advantage of looking at those with CHD is that the disease state is clearly present. The disadvantage is that the disease itself will alter physiological and psychological functioning. The advantages of examining groups at risk is that normal functioning can be examined in the absence of disease; conversely, only a small portion of those examined will actually develop the disease. In this chapter, we will take both approaches and examine studies of the risk factors of work overload and the Type A behavior pattern as well as studies comparing CHD patients with controls.

Work Overload

For many individuals the workplace presents an environment requiring significant allocation of processing capacity. Demands for efficiency and productivity may presumably lead many individuals to allocate significant amounts of capacity, and thus, show cardiovascular responses and changes in selective attention. If these changes are important for CHD, we might expect epidemiological surveys of certain on the job factors such as work overload, to show correlations with CHD. These correlations should be stronger than correlations with other factors, such as global job satisfaction, which only indirectly tap the amount of processing capacity habitually allocated to job activities. Although not without contradictions, the literature generally supports a significant and relatively specific correlation between work overload and CHD (Caplan, Cobb, French, Harrison, & Pinneau, 1975; Sales & House, 1971; House, 1974; Haynes, Feinleib, & Kannel, 1980).

Sales (1969) wrote an influential review of the area which also clearly conceptualized work overload. Overload was defined as a ''condition in which the individual is faced with a set of obligations which, taken as a set, requires him to do more than he is able in the time available.'' This formulation does not demand that the demands be considered illegitimate. Studies are reviewed (e.g. Friedman, Rosenman, & Carrol, 1958) suggesting that during periods of high work demand or in individuals reporting work overload, serum cholesterol is elevated. In addition, Sales related the Type A behavior pattern to work overload.

A more recent review by Kasl (1978) details the current status of the work overload concept. He notes that work overload, simply conceived, has not been consistently related to CHD. Various facets of work overload, quantitative but not qualitative work overload, job dissatisfaction, and fatigue on awakening have been found correlated to CHD. On the other hand, a number of studies have shown that workers with a considerable amount of administrative responsibility or numerous time deadlines fail to show increased CHD risk. In addition, a number of the studies reporting positive results only show such results for subgroups of their sample, e.g. blue collar workers or younger workers. The results of Haynes et al. (1980) are typical of evidence in this area. In this study, the Framingham epidemiological data were examined for psychosocial relations to CHD incidence in the age ranges, 45-54 years, 55-64, and over 65. Five categories of variables were examined: behavior type, reactions to anger, situational stress, sociocultural mobility, and somatic strain. None of the variables predicted CHD incidence in the 45-54-year-old cohort. In the 55-64-year cohort, positive relations were found for work overload, a modified Type A scale, anger directed at others, and times promoted in the past 10 years. In the 65 and over cohort, only anxiety symptoms correlated with CHD incidence. These relations held for men but not women. In brief, work overload cannot be ignored as a potential predictor of CHD, but we are far from understanding its contribution with any precision. Thus, the work overload literature provides only a modicum of support for our notion that the physiological and psychological sequelae of the allocation of processing capacity may be related to CHD.

Type A Behavior

Recent interest in Type A behavior permits a relatively fine grained analysis of the potential role of capacity allocation. Epidemiological evidence shows that Type A individuals are approximately twice as likely to develop CHD as individuals with the opposite pattern termed B (Rosenman, Brand, Jenkins, Friedman, Straus, & Wurm, 1975; Rosenman, Brand, Sholtz, & Friedman, 1976). Do Type A individuals show the physiological responses and selective focusing that we have associated with the allocation of full capacity? The Type A individual, identified initially by Friedman and Rosenman (1974), is usually described as somewhat hostile and impatient with a strong sense of competitiveness and time urgency. This description seems intuitively to accord well with a policy of the chronic allocation of all or nearly all processing capacity. Examples from the work of Glass (1977) illustrate the similarity between the characteristics of Type A individuals and those that might arise from the chronic allocation of full capacity. In the absence of clear goals, Type A but not Type B students work hard on a simple task (Burnam, Pennebaker, & Glass, 1973). After being challenged by a small number of difficult problems, the performance efforts of Type A students are even further intensified relative to Type B's (Glass, 1977; Matthews, 1981). A more specific analysis of the allocation of capacity is required, however, to make a convincing case for allocation of capacity. Do As and Bs differ in how they allocate capacity and in how they react physiologically to changes in capacity allocation?

Allocation of Capacity in As and Bs.   Dembroski et al. (this volume) describe Type A as a complex of behaviors. All of these behaviors may not relate to CHD, (e.g. Matthews, Glass, Rosenman, & Bortner, 1977), and, of course, not all of these behaviors relate to allocation of processing capacity. Two superficially contradictory behaviors relevant to the allocation of capacity were noted in the initial definitions of Type A behavior. First, Type As were observed to be "very alert but inattentive to details extraneous to the task" (Bortner & Rosenman, 1967, p. 577). Second, Type As were observed to "schedule more and more in less and less time" and thus, "indulge in polyphasic thought or performance, frequently striving to think or do two things simultaneously" (Friedman & Rosenman, 1974, pp. 82–83). These styles are said by Friedman and Rosenman (1974) to be among the "most common" in Type As and a "core component". The two styles are superficially contradictory in that alertness to a primary task to the disregard of extraneous events would seem to preclude thinking or doing two or more things at once.

A resolution of this contradiction provides a hypothesis concerning the allocation of capacity in Type A individuals (or at least in some Type A individuals, see Dembroski et al. [this volume]). Faced with a primary ongoing task, Type A individuals might be expected to allocate maximal capacity to the task only when absolutely necessary; between these critical seconds the Type A individual would be expected to allocate capacity to motivationally relevant events (independent of the task). In short, the Type A individual allocates most of his capacity most of the time, but, in the view of the experimenter, Type A individuals may appear distractible. The findings of Glass (1977) and his colleagues are relevant here. They report that their theoretical predictions about Type As' behavior are only verified when the experimental cues are extremely salient to the participants. For example, uncontrollable noise bursts of 80 dBA do not elicit enhanced responding by Type As; whereas bursts of 108 dBA do (Glass, 1977). Apparently Type As don't attend to the information provided by the noise bursts until they reach a certain level of prominence. Stated differently, Type As do not appear to be allocating processing capacity to events that are deemed peripheral.

While these observations can be interpreted as consistent with the allocation of full processing capacity by Type As, this interpretation is post hoc. A more explicit test is provided in three experiments conducted by Matthews and Brunson (1979). These experiments used the Stroop Color Word task which requires the identification of the color of the ink in which a stimulus word is printed. The task is challenging because the stimulus words are the names of colors. Thus, in most cases the meaning of the word and the ink color of the word will be conflicting cues. In one experiment, a secondary light detection task was combined with the color-word task. In the other two, distracting noise was combined with the color-word task. Noise has been previously shown to improve performance on the color-word task presumably by inducing an inhibitory set toward both noise and word meaning (Hartley & Adams, 1974; Houston, 1968, 1969, Houston & Jones, 1967, cf. discussion above of arousal and selectivity). If Type As show heightened attention to central events, they should perform well on a primary but not a secondary task (Experiment 1) and be minimally disrupted by the addition of distracting noise (Experiment 2 & 3). Furthermore, distracting noise should compete with the polyphasic thought of Type As. These expectations were confirmed. In both Experiments 2 and 3 the performance of Type A individuals actually improved in the presence of distracting noise. These results indicated that Type As attend to their environment in a manner consistent with that of individuals whose processing capacity is fully allocated. Type As focused their attention to central environmental information; consequently, they attended less to peripheral events than did Bs. Moreover, distracting noise may have inhibited the Type As attention to self-generated distractors (i.e., polyphasic thought).

Four recent experiments support the findings of Matthews and Brunson (1979). Stern, Harris, and Elverum (1981) compared the performance of As and Bs on arithmetic tasks with an embedded recall task and vice versa (arithmetic embedded in a recall task). In both cases, the performance of As was superior to Bs on the task defined as primary. Humphries, Neumann, and Carver (1981) compared As and Bs on a memory task with both frequently and infrequently occurring items. With moderate and high but not low incentive for performances, As recalled more frequently occurring items than Bs. Gastorf, Suls, and Sanders (1980) examined the distractibility of As in the context of a study of social facilitation. The distractor, a coactor performing the task, was designed to elicit the competitive aspect of Type As. Thus, the design provides a relevant focus for the polymodal activity of Type As—a focus not provided by the incidental cues used in the other studies. The presence of the Type A-relevant distractor was shown to impair the performance of Type As in a complex form of the task—which presumably required more capacity allocation than a less complex form. Thus, a reasonable amount of evidence seems to support our hypothesis concerning capacity allocation in Type As.

According to our argument, a chronic allocation of full processing capacity in Type As should alter the likelihood of their noting and acting upon social and health cues. Type A individuals do appear to be less likely to report health relevant signs than Pattern B individuals. The work of Carver and colleagues (Carver, Coleman, & Glass, 1976) is illustrative. A treadmill was used to induce exertion and measures of experienced fatigue and maximum exercise capacity were obtained. The results revealed that while Type As reached a higher proportion of their maximum oxygen absorption rate during the walking test then did Bs, they also reported less subjective fatigue than did Bs. More direct evidence is provided by Weidner and Matthews (1978). If As actively ignore fatigue during allocation of full capacity, they should fail to report symptoms during a task, but not at the end of a task. In this experiment, Type As and Bs performed a demanding task for 4 minutes and then completed a symptom checklist. Half of each Type believed that they were to continue for an additional 4 minutes on the task, half believed they had completed the task. Results indicated that although As and Bs were equally fatigued at the end of the task, As reported less fatigue than did Bs during the task. These results are supported by Stern et al. (1981). When As were engaged in an arithmetic task, they reported less fatigue than Bs. Interestingly, if fatigue ratings were made a primary focus, this effect disappeared.

These laboratory findings were supported and extended to significant medical symptoms in an observational study (Carver, DeGregorio, & Gillis, 1980). Coaches of a University team were asked to make subjective ratings of football players who were injured by midseason. As relative to Bs were rated as having pushed themselves closer to their limits, disregarded their injuries to a greater extent during games, and performed better. Thus, systematic observations and experimentation concur that the tendency of Type As to allocate full capacity to the task at hand may lead to their ignoring health cues. In doing so, Type As may ignore the early symptoms of CHD and not seek medical attention. Indeed, this notion is consistent with the observations of Greene, Moss, and Goldstein (1974) who reported that infarction victims, who were predominantly Type As, were likely to delay seeking care.

The second health implication of heightened selectivity is the ignoring of social cues. Do Type As chronically ignore social cues and thus tend to have impoverished social networks? Available evidence suggests that this may be true. College male Type As have been found to have low scores on an index of social support and report some difficulties in interpersonal relations (Waldron, Hickey, McPherson, Butensky, Gruss, Overall, Schmader, & Wohlmuth, 1980). Although Type As show high participation in social activities and are elected to office, they do not necessarily develop strong social networks (Burke & Weir, 1980). Quality of relationship may well be the important factor—the difference between a nodding acquaintance and a confidant with whom highly personal thoughts can be shared. Burke, Weir, and DuWors (1979) for example, report low levels of marital satisfaction among the wives of Type A administrators. Other correlations suggested that Type A husbands may be less likely than Type B husbands to confide in their wives. This interpretation is supported by data we recently collected from a sample of business executives. Half of the Type A individuals reported no confidant or only a single confidant; while the non-A executives all reported two or more (Jennings & Pilkonis, 1980). The groups did not vary on other dimensions of social network, e.g. number of acquaintances. Thus the available evidence indicates that Type As have impoverished social networks but the role of insensitivity to social cues as a mediator has not been established.

The evidence reviewed suggests that Type As and Bs may allocate processing capacity differently and do so in ways that may potentially influence CHD. Type As seem to chronically allocate full capacity and distribute that capacity in time differently than Type Bs. Do psychophysiological studies suggest that this A-B difference in the allocation of processing capacity has physiological con-comitants.

Physiological Response during the Allocation of Capacity in As and Bs. Psychophysiological responses to appropriate experimental conditions should reflect differences in the allocation of capacity of As and Bs. As might be expected to allocate full capacity to tasks and show enhanced physiological changes. Whenever full capacity is not required by the task, however, As may engage in extra experimental activities and thus show less task linked physiological reactivity than Bs. As previously reviewed, however, the cardiovascular change elicited by a task will depend on whether capacity is allocated to anticipated or ongoing use.

Our review will focus on studies of Type A in which the allocation of processing capacity can be directly related to a physiological response. General reviews of the psychophysiological responsivity of Type As can be found in Dembroski et al. (this volume), Krantz, Glass, Schaeffer, and Davia (1982), Matthews (1982), and Rosenman and Chesney (1980). These reviews suggest that Type As show greater blood pressure and catecholamine responses to tasks that exceed some threshold level of challenge. We do not believe it is adequate to glibly suggest that high challenge is equivalent to significant allocation of capacity. Thus, we shall focus on psychophysiological studies that can reasonably be interpreted as relevant to the allocation of capacity to ongoing or anticipated use.

Allocation of Capacity to Ongoing Use.   Do Type A's show heightened heart rate and blood pressure when they allocate capacity to ongoing information processing? Williams (1977) has previously argued that the Laceys' concepts of sensory intake and rejection may be important mediators of cardiovascular response to events and, thus, mediators of the pathophysiology of CHD. Clearly, this approach is quite consistent with that taken in this chapter, e.g., "sensory rejection" is directly comparable to the allocation of capacity to ongoing use. Williams (Williams, Lane, White, Kuhn, & Schanberg, 1981) has recently reported initial results from a large study designed to test the importance of sensory intake and rejection. Type A and B students performed mental arithmetic and cardiovascular and catecholamine responses were measured. Volunteers were not harassed or "stressed". Thus, an attempt was made only to examine "sensory rejection" as opposed to a hostile challenge, although independent measures of sensory rejection, i.e. dual task measures, were not obtained. The task produced the expected changes in forearm blood flow, adrenalin and noradrenalin. More significantly, Type A students responded significantly more than B students. Heart rate and blood pressure differences were, presumably, not obtained. Williams' results, although preliminary, do provide important support for heightened vascular and endocrine changes in Type As being associated with the allocation of capacity to ongoing use.

Somewhat similar results were obtained by Glass, Krakoff, Finkelman, Snow, Contrada, Kehoe, Mannucci, Isecke, Collins, Hilton, and Elting (1980). This experiment was directed at work overload and combined two tasks: one requiring allocation of capacity to ongoing use and the other to anticipated use. More concretely a perceptual tracking task was combined with a memorization task. Although, the overall cardiovascular responses to such a task are difficult to predict, the experiment does provide a clear requirement for the allocation of significant capacity. Furthermore, the instructions emphasized task performance rather than attempting to induce motivational or affective states. For these reasons, the experiment provides a reasonable response to our query of whether significant allocation of processing has a direct effect on physiological responding. Type As relative to Bs did, in fact, show greater blood pressure and adrenalin responses during task performance. Heart rate change did not separate the groups; however, average heart rate was analyzed as opposed to heart rate change in response to specific task events. A trend was observed toward higher error scores on the secondary but not primary task in Type As over Bs. This would indicate greater allocation of capacity to the primary task in Type A volunteers, and thus account for their greater physiological reactivity (given that the physiological response was largely to the primary task). The Glass results support a heightened physiological response of Type As during the allocation of capacity but only weakly. Learning effects and a surprisingly ineffective white noise manipulation complicate the interpretation of the Glass experiment.

A relevant, but inconclusive, experiment by Diamond and Carver (1980) must also be mentioned. Following Williams (1977), the effects of sensory intake and rejection in student As and Bs were examined. As and Bs did not differ in heart rate, blood pressure, or pulse volume responses. We have noted earlier, however, that cardiovascular changes occur reliably only with significant allocations of capacity. Diamond and Carver's (1980) tasks were minimally effective in inducing the expected heart rate changes—the average heart rate change induced by the sensory intake task was less than a one beat per minute deceleration. Furthermore, no indices of task performance are offered to verify the involvement of the volunteers. Thus, Diamond and Carver's (1980) data are unconvincing. This work should be repeated with tasks requiring significant allocations of capacity and more intensive training of volunteers. All and all heightened physiological reactivity to the allocation of capacity to ongoing use in Type As is supported in two studies, but truly convincing evidence is not yet available.

Allocation of Capacity to Anticipated Use.   Type As may also allocate capacity to anticipation differently than Bs and thus show distinctive changes in cardiac deceleration and related responses. Our review of performance data showing allocation of processing capacity differences between As and Bs did not explicitly examine anticipation tasks. We will do so here in order to point up the parallelism of performance and physiological data.

Both the performance and psychophysiology of As and Bs seem to differ in tasks requiring anticipation. Fortunately, a similar performance paradigm has been used by a number of investigators although the detail of the analysis of physiological change has varied widely. Focusing first on the performance results, Abrahams and Birren (1973) and Glass and coworkers (1977) examined simple and choice reaction time (RT) with fixed and variable foreperiods. Abrahams and Birren (1973) found the RT's of As slowed relative to Bs in both simple and choice fixed foreperiod RT paradigms. They interpreted their results as showing a subclinical precursor of the psychomotor slowing sometimes reported for CHD patients. Glass and coworkers (1977) viewed their work as a behavioral test of the impatience characteristic imputed to Type As by Friedman and Rosenman. They argued that relatively long times (4 to 9 sec.) between RT trials would create impatience and attendent distractibility, thus interfering with performance. Similar effects were not expected with short (i.e., 2 sec.) intervals between RT trials. Their results for long intervals replicated those of Abrahams and Birren (1973)—Type As were slower than Type Bs. As predicted, however, RT differences were not found with short intervals between RT trials. Subsequent work (also in Glass, 1977) showed that the Type A deficit at long intervals could be reversed by a failure pretreatment. Glass' (1977) and Abraham and Birren's (1973) work validate impatience as a feature of Type A, and show that impatience is sensitive to experimental manipulations. In our view, it supports the contention that allocation of capacity in Type As is controlled by their time urgency—full capacity is allocated at critical times for task performance but polymodal thought and activity intervenes whenever possible. Later experiments using similar techniques, however, failed to replicate the slowing of RT's in Type As (Dembroski, MacDougall, & Shields, 1977; Goldband, 1979).

Two experiments in this laboratory (Jennings, 1981) reexamined the RT of A and B volunteers under conditions of a long interval between trials. These experiments were designed to yield trials with slow, accurate choice RT's as well as trials with rapid, inaccurate RT's (see Jennings, Wood, & Lawrence, 1976; Wood & Jennings, 1976). Two samples were used: a student sample classified by the student form of the Jenkins Activity Survey (JAS) employed by Glass (1977) and a business executive sample classified on the Speed-Impatience component of the Structured Interview (see Dembroski, 1978). Overall, As and Bs did not differ on average RT's or accuracy. RT's constrained by instructions to range from 350-500 msec., however, showed an interesting effect replicating earlier work. Type A students and executives working for minimal incentives responded more slowly and less accurately than Type B volunteers. Furthermore, this difference reversed when incentives were increased. Unfortunately, this high incentive condition was only available for the student sample. In addition, both students and executive Type As in the low incentive condition reported the slow RT condition as being more attention demanding or frustrating. These results support the Glass (1977) contention that the impatience of Type As interferes with the maximum allocation of processing capacity. Temporal delays combined with low incentive permit distracting thoughts or actions. Extensions of this work should obviously probe the degree of task focus maintained by As during relatively long intervals between RT's. As we shall see below, however, physiological evidence supports this interpretation.

Does cardiovascular data from RT tasks with long intertrial intervals show that Type As allocate maximal capacity to anticipation only when absolutely necessary? Initial work (Dembroski et al., 1977) on *average* as opposed to event related second-by-second, heart rate and blood pressure supported a relation between impatience and capacity allocation to anticipation. Heart rate and blood pressure were found to increase during the task for As as opposed to Bs; and the variability of the heart rate of As was greater than Bs prior to the task and to a lesser extent during the task. A follow-up report (Dembroski et al., 1978) indicated that the heart rate results were particularly correlated with the Impatience component of the Structured Interview. These changes in heart rate and blood pressure were replicated in a separate experiment (Dembroski, MacDougall, Herd, & Shields, 1979), however, the heart rate variability result and the specific relationship of the Speed-Impatience component were not replicated.

Two studies which explicitly measured the heart rate deceleration occurring just prior to the RT stimulus (second by second rather than average heart rate change) also failed to find differences between As and Bs (Abrahams, 1974; Goldband, 1979). In one, however, (Goldband, 1979) an index of vascular reactivity distinguished between behavior types. These reports suggest that As and Bs may allocate different amounts of capacity to the task, inducing differences in relatively sustained cardiovascular change suggestive of sympathetic nervous system activation, e.g. increases in mean heart rate and blood pressure. (See Obrist et al., 1978). Specific episodes of anticipated use of capacity do not, however, induce differing amounts of cardiac deceleration in As and Bs.

Detailed observations of cardiac deceleration by Jennings (Jennings & Choi, 1981; Jennings, submitted a), however, suggest that As and Bs may differ in how they allocate capacity to anticipation. Cardiovascular variables were measured in the experiments with student and executive samples mentioned previously. We found as had Dembroski et al. (1978) that heart rate variability was higher in As than in Bs—particularly just before and after RT performance. Changes in average vascular and cardiac responses and depth of deceleration parameters during the task did not significantly differ between As and Bs. The results for cardiac deceleration were complex and not completely consistent between the student and executive samples. The evidence showed, however, that Type As (especially those high in the Speed-Impatience component, see Dembroski, 1978) might show anticipatory cardiac deceleration in response to events of less significance than those responded to by Type Bs—i.e. during the initial warm-up trials of the experiment and during trials with relatively low incentives. Furthermore, among Type As high in the Speed-Impatience components the cardiac deceleration response developed rapidly and terminated quickly. Executive As showed a response that was not initiated until the last instant prior to the RT, while student As terminated their response immediately at the occurrence of the RT stimulus. Despite their brevity, the amplitude of cardiac deceleration was either equal in A and B executives or in the case of rapid RT's, larger in Type A students.

These beat by beat heart rate results suggest a tentative picture of an "impatient" form of capacity allocation in the Type A. Heart rate variability has been rather consistently associated with degree of task involvement (see Mulder, Mulder-Hajonides, van der Meulen, 1973; Walter & Porges, 1976; Wierville, 1979). The high between trial heart rate variability of Type As may indicate a lack of task involvement and presence of polymodal thoughts and actions. This allocation of capacity to multiple events is suspended for the minimum amount of time necessary to achieve task performance—as indexed by the brief, intense cardiac deceleration responses. This interpretation is consistent with the performance results received in the previous sections. Some important ambiguities remain, however. Most importantly the performance results for students were based on the JAS but only Structured Interview variables were related significantly to the physiological changes. The failure of student and executive samples to show identical A-B differences is also of concern. In general, however, impatient Type As seem to show a distinctive cardiovascular reaction during the allocation of capacity to anticipated use.

In summary, both performance and physiological data suggest that Type As allocate processing capacity differently than Bs. Given the risk status of Type As, this supports our contention that differences in chronic policies of allocating processing capacity may be important to CHD. The review also showed that Type As were not simply hyperreactive in their performance and physiology. The Type A concern with time translates into a particular policy for the allocation of processing capacity: maximal capacity is allocated to a task but only for the minimum necessary time. Thus, performance and physiology results suggest that although Type As frequently allocate more capacity than Bs, they do not consistently maintain allocation to anticipated events. In multiple task settings the Type A focuses attention on central rather than peripheral events and is aided by the presence of nominal distractors. Extraneous "distraction" seems to focus the polymodal thought and activity of the Type A on the task at hand. The central focus of Type As may contribute to a disregard of health and social cues. Increased blood pressure and catecholamine responses in Type A's were observed during the allocation of capacity to both ongoing and anticipated processing. Differences between As and Bs were also noted in the timing of the cardiospecific vagal responses during the allocation of processing capacity to anticipated use. Such A-B psychophysiological differences may be relevant to the pathophysiology of CHD.

Allocation of Capacity and CHD

Patients with CHD obviously provide a direct test of hypotheses about CHD. Unfortunately, differences contributing to the disease are difficult to dissociate from differences induced by the disease process. For example, a reduced oxygen supply to the heart due to CHD may reduce responsivity to neural stimulation. Thus, advanced stage CHD patients may respond *less* than controls to a psychological stimulus; while early stage patients might respond more. Such problems are important for interpreting the small amount of literature on psychological and psychophysiological differences between CHD patients and controls. For purposes of discussion we shall separate cardiac sudden death from atherosclerotic heart disease.

A significant proportion of sudden cardiac deaths occur in persons with minimal pathological evidence of heart disease (see Jennings, in press). Can sudden death be related to physiological changes during the allocation of processing capacity? Disturbances of cardiac rhythm leading to ventricular fibrillation are usually presumed to be the cause of death. For a number of years the psychosomatic literature suggested that vagal effects, such as we have related to cardiac deceleration contributed to such fatal arrhythmia (e.g. Wolf, 1978). Continuing evidence for this position is reviewed in Jennings (in press). A particularly intriguing report (Schneider, 1957), found that post heart attack patients who produced large cardiac decelerations following a surprising stimuli were more likely than other patients to suffer sudden death. If replicated and shown to be specific to novel stimuli, evidence of this sort would provide a strong link between CHD and the allocation of capacity to anticipated use. At present, however, a rapidly growing literature suggests that sympathetic nervous system influences are more potent inducers of arrhythmia than vagal influences (see Lown & Verrier, this volume; Lown, DeSilva, & Lenson, 1978; Lown, Verrier, & Corbalan, 1973; Lown, DeSilva, Reich, Murawski, 1980; Krantz et al., 1982). Post heart attack patients when exposed to stressful interviews and complicated tasks have been reported to show increased incidence of arrhythmia. This induction of arrhythmia may be relevant to the sympathetic-like changes observed during the allocation of capacity to ongoing use. Such a specific interpretation cannot, however, be proven without measures directly related to the current interpretation. The multifactorial nature of the pathogenesis of CHD is emphasized nicely in this work showing that both psychological events and a physiological state are required to induce increased arrhythmia.

Most studies of CHD patients have involved the comparison of patients with clinical symptoms of ischemic heart disease with matched controls. Thus, these studies focus on atherosclerosis as opposed to sudden death. The presence of disease has sometimes been positively related to the amount of physiological reactivity during a general challenge, e.g. an interview (see review in Krantz et al., 1982; Sime, Buell, & Eliot, 1980). In one report (Dembroski, MacDougall, & Lushene, 1979), Type A patients with a history of myocardial infarction increased their blood pressure more than Type B patients and case controls during an interview and quiz challenge. The Impatience, Competitive, and Hostile component of the interview predicted the degree of physiological response in Type A patients and Type A controls. Such individual difference relations are important, but less direct than specific manipulations of the allocation of capacity. Van Doornen, Orlebeke, and Somsen (1980) reported the beat by beat heart rate of patients and controls while anticipating a noxious tone. During a fixed anticipation period heart rate initially slowed after a warning stimulus, then accelerated, and finally decelerated in anticipation of a noxious tone. Patients with a recent history of myocardial infarction (including subsamples receiving and not receiving β blockers) were compared to age appropriate control groups who either were high or low in risk factors for CHD. Patients and those high in CHD risk responded similarly. The low risk controls, however, showed both a greater initial acceleration and a greater anticipatory deceleration. Our work (Jennings & Choi, 1981) suggested an examination of the timing of deceleration. Mean response of low risk patients showed decelerative changes during about 7 of the 12 seconds of the anticipation intervals; while the patients and high risk controls showed similar changes for only about 4 of the 12 seconds. Behavior types were not, however, assessed by Van Doornen et al. (1980) so we can only suggest a similarity of deceleration between Type As, patients, and high risk controls. We must also be aware of the probability that the control of heart rate is physiologically impaired in CHD patients (Coghlan, Phares, Cowley, Copley, & James, 1979; Eckberg, Drabinsky, & Braunwald, 1971; Goldstein, Beisar, Stampfer, & Epstein, 1975).

Does the behavioral performance of CHD patients suggest that they allocate processing capacity differently from controls? Patients generally perform less well than controls (see review in Spieth, 1965; Welford, 1977). One source of these deficits might be a failure to allocate as much capacity to tasks as control. Studies which have compared tasks that vary in information processing requirements have generally reported that performance deficits in CHD patients occur when task complexity increases and particularly when dual tasks are performed. These results are *not* consistent with studies of risk groups, such as Matthews and Brunson (1979) in which the groups at risk for CHD perform better than the control. Such discrepancies must, however, be viewed cautiously until patients and controls at risk are classified by the same instruments and receive the same performance tasks.

In summary, the relation of capacity allocation to CHD has not been strengthened by examining the patient data. Allocation of capacity to ongoing use may be related to sympathetic activity in patients and thus to cardiac arrhythmia and chronic influences on atherosclerosis. At present, however, no evidence has been gathered that explicitly supports this hypothesis. Scattered studies suggest that depth of cardiac deceleration during the allocation of capacity to anticipation might be related positively to sudden death and negatively to presence of CHD. Finally, performance decrements have been found in CHD patients performing complex tasks. Such decrements may be due to a general decline in health, but are not predicted by views relating CHD to the chronic allocation of full processing capacity.

SUMMARY, IMPLICATIONS AND PROBLEMS

This chapter attempts to show that individual differences in one psychological construct, attention, may influence CHD. As a psychological contruct, attention integrates results associating CHD with overt behaviors, dispositions, and environmental conditions. The concept of allocation of processing capacity was introduced in order (1) to define attention operationally with paradigms that assess capacity, and (2) to relate physiological and psychological results to concepts such as work overload. The cardiovascular and neuroendocrine changes which occur during changes in allocating processing capacity were then reviewed. Broadening our focus to social and health cues, we then examined the selective awareness of cues resulting from the allocation of significant amounts of processing capacity to a central task. Finally, individual differences in the policies of allocating processing capacity were related to buffers against disease, behavioral risk factors, and CHD. A necessarily simplified schemata of the flow of ideas in the chapter is presented in Figure 4.2.

Figure 4.2 schematically presents the possible steps between the allocation of processing capacity and factors relevant to coronary heart disease (CHD). Allocation of all or nearly all processing capacity routinely causes two concomitant changes: characteristic physiological responses and a focus on central events. The physiological responses are normal but if chronically elicited may contribute to CHD through wear and tear on blood vessels and vulnerability to arrhythmia. Similarly, a sustained focus on central events should lead to reduced awareness of health and social cues. This unawareness may directly influence buffers against disease—social networks and health maintenance behavior.

The schematic nature of Figure 4.2 must be emphasized. Each of the relations portrayed is complex. Hopefully, the global outline of steps will have a heuristic purpose in focusing research questions. Once these questions are posed, the answers will necessarily render Figure 4.2 obsolete. Figure 4.2 does portray some important cautionary statements. First, cardiovascular health is viewed as a function of both the presence of CHD pathophysiology and the strength of buffers against disease. Secondly, psychological influences are shown as only contributing to CHD rather than being its sole cause. Finally, for the sake of simplicity the figure ignores the very real probability that a policy of chronic allocation of full processing capacity is not the sole psychological factor acting against disease buffers or contributing to pathophysiology.

What have we learned from our review? First, the allocation of a high proportion of processing capacity does appear to induce a focus of attention and have a physiological impact. The physiological impact and the exact nature of the focusing of attention may be a function of individual differences, such as Type A, and of the environmental conditions. Very little information is available on the everyday chronicity of these allocation processes although characteristics, such as Type A, physiological reactivity, and allocation of processing capacity

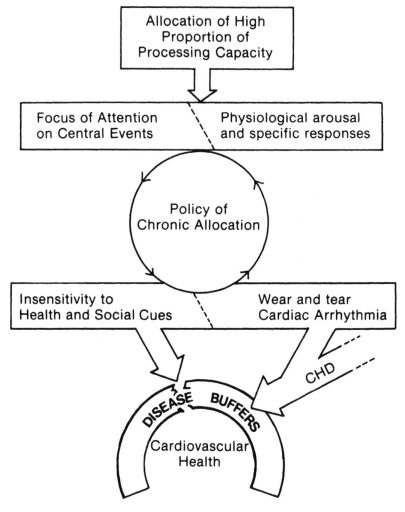

FIG. 4.2.   A schematic presentation of ways in which attention defined as the allocation of processing capacity might be related to coronary heart disease.

can be related to behavioral risk factors. Very little information is available relating the allocation of capacity directly to CHD. The need for further research is self-evident.

Problems

As indicated above, the major current problem is the scarcity of data which specifically relates a measure of the allocation of processing capacity to CHD and related risk factors. Specific and general problems also are present. A specific problem is the complexity of measuring of processing capacity. The dual task methodology is complex, and it's becoming clear that a single concept of processing capacity may be an oversimplification (see Navon & Gopher; 1979, Wickens, 1980). Hopefully, continuing developments in experimental psychology will provide a robust dual task paradigm suitable for our applications. Results to date furthermore suggest that behavioral risk groups may differ in specific responses to specific situations rather than in global responses that may be tapped with any type of global challenge (cf. Dembroski et al., this volume). Considerable experimental efforts will be required to address only relatively narrow questions. CHD is a complex, long-term disease and no single marker for CHD is available prior to overt physiological impairments. Thus, studies must rely on fallible criteria such as psychological and physiological risk factors. This problem is acute when a multifaceted risk factor such as Type A is used. Examining components of Type A provides some conceptual clarity but at the cost of losing the empirical link to CHD provided by prospective epidemiological studies.

Implications

If the allocation of processing capacity is related to CHD, individuals at risk can be identified on the basis of environmental conditions as well as individual characteristics. In short, existing knowledge about the allocation of capacity permits reasoned generalizations to conditions of CHD risk. Allocation of capacity provides an alternative, and in some ways simpler, explanation of data usually interpreted in terms of affective or motivational states. For example, Glass (1977) has suggested that a proneness to "learned helplessness" is related to the pathophysiology of CHD. The evidence which prompted Glass' suggestion can be conceptualized in terms of capacity allocation if the concept of capacity depletion introduced by Cohen (1978) is applied. Individuals working in a noisy environment after leaving that environment appear to experience a decrease in efficiency of performance (Glass & Singer, 1972). As noted earlier, Cohen (1978) suggested that ignoring the noise required processing capacity and that the after-effect on performance was due to capacity depletion. The allocation policy of Type As should make them particularly prone to such after-effects. Glass (1977) reports two experiments showing such an effect. In one, Type A and B volunteers were initially challenged by a long session of either insoluble or soluble tasks. Performance on a subsequent soluble set of problems was then observed. Type A, but not B, individuals showed a performance decrement after the insoluble problems. If we presume that the challenge of the insoluble task elicited sustained allocation of full capacity in the Type As, depletion of capacity may explain the performance decrement on the second task. Glass (1977) interprets the results in terms of the "learned helplessness" concept—that is, clear failure on the initially challenging task induced a generalized perception of helplessness yielding the observed performance decrement. Although any choice between interpretations would be premature, a capacity allocation interpretation seems more consistent with other aspects of Type A behavior than the learned helplessness concept. Note also that a personality concept such as control may be expressed through the differences in allocation policy between As and Bs. A variety of psychosocial factors may conceivably be integrated through their common effects on the chronicity and intensity of allocations of processing capacity.

In conclusion, we have reviewed evidence which establishes the possibility that attention, defined in processing capacity terms here, is related to CHD. Although further research is clearly required, existing evidence suggests that this will be fruitful. Hopefully, attending to attention will allow us to better understand the role of psychological factors in heart disease.

ACKNOWLEDGMENTS

I would like to thank Dr. Karen A. Matthews for her substantial contribution to this chapter. Dr. Matthews is largely responsible for developing the relationship between attention and buffers against disease which is discussed in the chapter. Dr. Kay A. Jennings and Dr. Matthews are both thanked for helpful critiques of various drafts of the chapter.

REFERENCES

Abrahams, J. P. Psychomotor performance and change in cardiac rate in subjects behaviorally predisposed to coronary heart disease (Doctoral dissertation, University of Southern California, 1974). *Dissertation Abstracts International*, 1974, *35/04B*, 1931.

Abrahams, J. P., & Birren, J. E. Reaction time as a function of age and behavioral predisposition to coronary heart disease. *Journal of Gerontology*, 1973, *28*, 471–478.

Averill, J. R. An analysis of psychophysiological symbolism and its influence on theories of emotion. *Journal for the Theory of Social Behavior*, 1974, *4*, 147–190.

Baum, A., & Valins, S. (Eds.). *The social psychology of crowding: Studies of the effects of residential group size*. Hillsdale, N.J.: Lawrence Erlbaum Associates, 1977.

Berkowitz, L. Social norms, feelings, and other factors affecting helping and altruism. In L. Berkowitz (Ed.), *Advances in experimental social psychology*, 1972, *6*, 63–108.

Bernstein, A. S., & Taylor, K. W. The interaction of stimulus information with potential stimulus significance in eliciting the skin conductance orienting response. In H. D. Kimmel, E. H. van Olst, & J. H. Orlebeke (Eds.), *The orienting reflex in humans*. Hillsdale, N.J.: Lawrence Erlbaum Associates, 1979, pp. 499–452.

Bohlin, G., & Graham, F. K. Cardiac deceleration and reflex blink facilitation. *Psychophysiology*, 1977, *14*, 423–430.

Bohlin, G., & Kjellberg, A. Orienting activity in two-stimulus paradigms as reflected in heart rate. In H. D. Kimmel, E. van Olst, & J. F. Orlebeke (Eds.), *The orienting reflex in humans*. Hillsdale, NJ: Lawrence Erlbaum Associates, 1979, pp. 169–189.

Bortner, R. W., & Rosenman, R. H. The measurement of Pattern A behavior. *Journal of Chronic Diseases*, 1967, *20*, 525–533.

Broadbent, D. E. *Decision and stress*. London: Academic Press, 1971.

Broadhurst, P. L. The interaction of task difficulty and motivation: The Yerkes-Dodson law revisited. *Acta Psychologica*, 1959, *16*, 321–338.

Brener, J., Phillips, K., & Connally, S. R. Oxygen consumption and ambulation during operant conditioning of heart rate increases and decreases in rats. *Psychophysiology*, 1977, *14*, 483–491.

Brown, J., Morse, P., Leavitt, L., & Graham, F. Specific attentional effects reflected in the cardiac orienting response. *Bulletin of the Psychonomic Society*, 1976, *7*, 1–4.

Brunia, C. H. M. Some questions about the motor inhibition hypothesis. In H. D. Kimmel, E. H. van Olst, & J. H. Orlebeke (Eds.), *The orienting reflex in humans*. Hillsdale, NJ: Lawrence Erlbaum Associates, 1979. pp. 241–258.

Burke, R. J., & Weir, T. A. Personality, value and behavioral correlates of the Type A individual. *Psychological Reports*, 1980, *46*, 171–181.

Burke, R. J., Weir, T., & DuWors, R. E., Jr. Type A behavior of administrators and wives' reports of marital satisfaction. *Journal of Applied Psychology*, 1979, *64*, 57–65.

Burnam, M. A., Pennebaker, J. W., & Glass, D. C. Time consciousness, achievement striving, and the Type A coronary-prone behavior pattern. *Journal of Abnormal Psychology*, 1973, *84*, 76–79.

Calaresu, F. R., Faiers, A. A., & Mogensen, G. J. Central neural regulation of heart and blood vessels in mammals. *Progress in Neurobiology*, 1975, *5*, 1–35.

Cannon, W. B. *The wisdom of the body* (2nd Ed.). New York: Norton, 1939.

Caplan, R. D., Cobb, S., French, J. R. P., Jr., Harrison, R. V., & Pinneau, S. R. J. *Job demands and worker health*. Washington, DC: HEW Publication No. (NIOSH) 75-160, 1975.

Carroll, D., & Anastasiades, Z. The behavioral significance of heart rate: The Lacey's hypothesis. *Biological Psychology*, 1978, *1*, 249–275.

Carver, C. S., Coleman, A. E., & Glass, D. C. The coronary-prone behavior pattern and the suppression of fatigue on a treadmill test. *Journal of Personality and Social Psychology*, 1976, *33*, 460–466.

Carver, C. S., DeGregorio, E., & Gillis, R. *Challenge and Type B behavior among intercollegiate football players*. Unpublished manuscript, 1980.

Cobb, S. Social support as a moderator of life stress. *Psychosomatic Medicine*, 1976, *38*, 300–314.

Cofer, C. N., & Appley, M. H. *Motivation: Theory and research*. New York: Wiley, 1964.

Coghlan, H. C., Phares, P., Cowley, M., Copley, D., & James, T. N. Dysautonomia in initial valve prolapse. *American Journal of Medicine*, 1979, *67*, 236–244.

Cohen, S. Environmental load and the allocation of attention. In A. Baum, J. E. Singer, & S. Valins (Eds.), *Advances in environmental psychology*. Hillsdale, NJ: Lawrence Erlbaum Associates, 1978.

Cohen, S., Evans, G. W., Krantz, D. S., & Stokols, D. Physiological, motivational, and cognitive effects of aircraft noise on children: Moving from the laboratory to the field. *American Psychologist*, 1980, *35*, 231–243.

Cohen, S., & Lezak, A. Noise and inattentiveness to social cues. *Environment and Behavior*, 1977, *9*, 559–572.

Coles, M. G. H., & Duncan-Johnson, C. C. Cardiac activity and information processing: The effects of stimulus significance and detection and response requirements. *Journal of Experimental Psychology: Human Perception and Performance*, 1975, *1*, 418–428.

Davignon, J. Current views on the etiology and pathogenesis of atherosclerosis. In J. Gerest, E. Koiw, & O. Kuchel (Eds.), *Hypertension: Physiopathology and treatment*. New York: McGraw Hill, 1977, pp. 961–989.

Davignon, J. The lipid hypothesis: Pathophysiological basis. *Archives of Surgery*, 1978, *113*, 28–34.

Dembroski, T. M. Reliability and validity of procedures used to assess coronary-prone behavior. In T. Dembroski, S. M. Weiss, J. L. Shields, S. G. Haynes, & M. Feinleib (Eds.), *Coronary-prone behavior*. New York: Springer-Verlag, 1978, pp. 95–106.

Dembroski, T. M., MacDougall, J. M., Herd, J. A., & Shields, J. L. Perspectives on coronary-prone behavior pattern. In A. Baum, D. S. Krantz, & J. E. Singer (Eds.), *Handbook of medical psychology*, in press.

Dembroski, T. M., MacDougall, J. M., Herd, J. A., & Shields, J. L. Effects of level of challenge on pressor and heart rate responses in Type A and B subjects. *Journal of Applied Social Psychology*, 1979, *9*, 209–228.

Dembroski, T. M., MacDougall, J. M., & Lushene, R. Interpersonal interaction and cardiovascular response in Type A subjects and coronary patients. *Journal of Human Stress*, 1979, *5*, 28–36.

Dembroski, T. M., MacDougall, J. M., & Shields, J. L. Physiologic reactions to social challenge in persons evidencing the Type A coronary prone behavior pattern. *Journal of Human Stress*, 1977, *3*, 2–10.

Dembroski, T. M., MacDougall, J. M., Shields, J. L., Petitto, J., & Lushene, R. Components of the Type A coronary-prone behavior pattern and cardiovascular responses to psychomotor performance challenge. *Journal of Behavioral Medicine*, 1978, *1*, 159–176.

Diamond, E. L., & Carver, C. S. Sensory processing, cardiovascular reactivity, and the Type A coronary-prone behavior pattern. *Biological Psychology*, 1980, *10*, 265–275.

Duffy, E. The psychological significance of the concept of "arousal" or "activation". *Psychological Review*, 1957, *64*, 265–275.

Duffy, E. Activation. In N. S. Greenfield & R. A. Sternbach (Eds.), *Handbook of psychophysiology*. New York: Holt, 1972. pp. 577–622.

Easterbrook, J. A. The effect of emotion on cue utilization and the organization of behavior. *Psychological Review*, 1959, *66*, 183–201.

Eckberg, D. L., Drabinsky, M., & Braunwald, E. Defective cardiac parasympathetic control in patients with heart disease. *New England Journal of Medicine*, 1971, *285*, 877–883.

Elliott, R. The significance of heart rate for behavior: A critique of Lacey's hypothesis. *Journal of Personality and Social Psychology*, 1972, *22*, 398–409.

Forster, P. M., & Grierson, A. T. Noise and attentional selectivity: A reproducible phenomenon? *British Journal of Psychology*, 1978, *69*, 489–498. (a)

Forster, P. M., & Grierson, A. T. Attentional selectivity: A rejoinder to Hockey. *British Journal of Psychology*, 1978, *69*, 505–506. (b)

Frankenhauser, M. Experimental approaches to the study of human behavior as related to neuroendocrine functions. In L. Levi (Ed.), *Society, stress, and disease* (Vol. I). London: Oxford University, 1971. pp. 22–35.

Frankenhauser, M. Sympathetic-adrenomedullary activity, behavior and the psychosocial environment. In P. H. Venable & M. J. Christie (Eds.), *Research in psychophysiology*. London: Wiley, 1975. pp. 71–94.

Frankenhauser, M., & Johansson, G. Task demand as reflected in catecholamine excretion and heart rate. *Journal of Human Stress*, 1976, *2*, 15–23.

Freeman, G. L. *The energetics of human behavior*. Ithaca, NY: Cornell University Press, 1948.

Friedman, M., & Rosenman, R. H. *Type A behavior and your heart*. New York: Knopf, 1974.

Friedman, M., Rosenman, R. H., & Carrol, V. Changes in the serum cholesterol and blood clotting time in men subjected to cyclic variation of occupational stress. *Circulation*, 1958, *17*, 852–861.

Gastorf, J. W., Suls, J., & Sanders, G. S. Type A coronary-prone behavior pattern and social facilitation. *Journal of Personality and Social Psychology*, 1980, *38*, 773–780.

Gillum, R. F., Feinleib, M., Margolis, J. R., Fabsitz, R. R., & Brasch, R. D. Delay in the prehospital phase of acute myocardial infarction. *Archives of Internal Medicine*, 1976, *136*, 649–654.

Glass, D. C. *Behavior patterns, stress, and coronary disease.* Hillsdale, NJ: Lawrence Erlbaum Associates, 1977.

Glass, D. C., & Singer, J. E. *Urban stress: Experiments on noise and social stressors.* New York: Academic Press, 1972.

Glass, D. C., Krakoff, L. R., Contrada, R., Hilton, W. F., Kehoe, K., Mannucci, E. C., Collins, C., Snow, B., & Elting, E. Effect of harassment and competition upon cardiovascular and plasma catecholamine response in Type A and Type B individuals. *Psychophysiology,* 1980, *17,* 453–463.

Glass, D. C., Krakoff, L. R., Finkelman, J., Snow, B., Contrada, R., Kehoe, K., Mannucci, E. G., Isecke, W., Collins, C., Hilton, W. F., & Elting, E. Effect of task overload upon cardiovascular and plasma catecholamine response in Type A and Type B individuals. *Basic and Applied Social Psychology,* 1980, *1,* 199–218.

Gochman, I. R. Arousal, attribution, and environmental stress. In I. G. Sarason, & C. D. Spielberger (Eds.), *Stress and anxiety* (Vol. 6). Washington, D.C.: Hemisphere, 1979, pp. 27–54.

Goldband, S. *Environmental specificity of physiological response to stress in coronary-prone subjects.* Unpublished doctoral dissertation, State University of New York at Buffalo, 1979.

Goldstein, R. E., Beiser, G. D., Stampfer, M., & Epstein, S. E. Impairment of autonomically mediated heart rate control in patients with cardiac dysfunction. *Circulation Research,* 1975, *36,* 571–578.

Gore, S. The effect of social support in moderating the health consequences of unemployment. *Journal of Health and Social Behavior,* 1978, *19,* 157–165.

Graham, F. K. Distinguishing among orienting, defense, and startle reflexes. In H. D. Kimmel, E. H. van Olst, & J. H. Orlebeke (Eds.), *The orienting reflex in humans.* Hillsdale, N.J.: Lawrence Erlbaum Associates, 1979, pp. 137–168.

Graham, F. K., & Clifton, R. K. Heart rate change as a component of the orienting response. *Psychological Bulletin,* 1966, *65,* 305–320.

Greene, W. A., Moss, A. J., & Goldstein, S. Delay, denial, and death in coronary heart disease. In R. S. Eliot (Ed.), *Stress and the heart.* Mount Kisco, NY: Futura, 1974, pp. 123–142.

Hartley, L. R., & Adams, R. G. Effect of noise on the Stroop test. *Journal of Experimental Psychology,* 1974, *102,* 62–66.

Hahn, W. W. Attention and heart rate: A critical appraisal of the hypothesis of Lacey and Lacey. *Psychological Bulletin,* 1973, *79,* 59–70.

Hare, R., Wood, K., Britian, S., & Shadman, J. Autonomic responses to affective visual stimulation. *Psychophysiology,* 1971, *7,* 408–417.

Hastings, S., & Obrist, P. Heart rate during conditioning in humans: Effects of varying the interstimulus (CS-UCS) interval. *Journal of Experimental Psychology,* 1967, *74,* 431–442.

Haynes, S. G., Feinleib, M., & Kannel, W. B. The relationship of psychosocial factors to coronary heart disease in the Framingham Study: III. Eight-year incidence of coronary heart disease. *American Journal of Epidemiology,* 1980, *14,* 37–58.

Hebb, D. O. Drives and the C. N. S. (Conceptual Nervous System). *Psychological Review,* 1955, *62,* 243–253.

Henry, J. P., & Stephens, P. M. *Stress, health, and the social environment.* New York: Springer-Verlag, 1977.

Hockey, G. R. J. Changes in information-selection patterns in multisource monitoring as a function of induced arousal shifts. *Journal of Experimental Psychology,* 1973, *101,* 35–42.

Hockey, G. R. J. Attentional selectivity and the problems of replication: A reply to Forster and Grierson. *British Journal of Psychology,* 1978, *69,* 499–503.

Hockey, G. R. J. Stress and the cognitive components of skilled performance. In V. Hamilton & D. M. Warburton (Eds.), *Human stress and cognition.* Chichester: Wiley, 1979. pp. 141–178.

House, J. S. Occupational stress and coronary heart disease: A review and theoretical integration. *Journal of Health and Social Behavior*, 1974, *15*, 12–27.

Houston, B. K. Inhibition and the facilitating effect of noise on interference tasks. *Perceptual and Motor Skills*, 1968, *27*, 947–950.

Houston, B. K. Noise, task difficulty, and Stroop color-word performance. *Journal of Experimental Psychology*, 1969, *82*, 403–404.

Houston, B. K., & Jones, T. M. Distraction and Stroop color-word performance. *Journal of Experimental Psychology*, 1967, *74*, 54–56.

Humphries, C., Neumann, P. G., & Carver, C. S. *Cognitive characteristics of the Type A coronary-prone behavior pattern*. Unpublished manuscript, 1981.

Insull, W. (Ed.) *Coronary risk handbook*. New York: American Heart Association, 1973.

Jennings, J. R. Information processing and concomitant heart rate changes in the overweight and underweight. *Physiological Psychology*, 1975, *3*, 290–296.

Jennings, J. R. Could the vagal responses during information processing be related to clinically significant arrhythmia? In C. Twentyman, L. Epstein, E. Blanchard, & J. V. Brady (Eds.), *Progress in Behavioral Medicine*, New York: Springer-Verlag, in press.

Jennings, J.R. *Anticipatory cardiac deceleration, variability, and components of the Type A pattern*. Manuscript submitted for publication, 1981.

Jennings, J. R., Averill, J. R., Opton, E. M., & Lazarus, R. S. Some parameters of heart rate change: Perceptual versus motor task requirements, noxiousness, and uncertainty. *Psychophysiology*, 1971, *7*, 194–212.

Jennings, J. R., & Choi, S. Type A components and the psychophysiological responses to an attention demanding performance task. *Psychosomatic Medicine*, 1981, *43*, 475–487.

Jennings, J. R., & Hall, S. W., Jr. Recall, recognition, and rate: Memory and the heart. *Psychophysiology*, 1980, *17*, 37–46.

Jennings, J. R., Lawrence, B. E., & Kasper, P. Changes in alertness and processing capacity in a serial learning task. *Memory and Cognition*, 1978, *6*, 45–53.

Jennings, J. R., & Pilkonis, P. Unpublished data, University of Pittsburgh, October 1980.

Jennings, J. R., Schrot, J., & Wood, C. C. Cardiovascular response patterns during choice reaction time. *Physiological Psychology*, 1980, *8*, 130–136.

Jennings, J. R., Wood, C. C., & Lawrence, B. E. Effects of graded doses of alcohol on speed-accuracy tradeoff in choice reaction time. *Perception and Psychophysics*, 1976, *19*, 85–91.

Jennings, J. R., & Wood, C. C. Cardiac cycle time effects on performance phasic cardiac responses, and their intercorrelation in choice reaction time. *Psychophysiology*, 1977, *14*, 297–307.

Johnson, H. J., & Campos, J. J. The effect of cognitive tasks and verbalization instructions on heart rate and skin conductance. *Psychophysiology*, 1967, *4*, 143–150.

Johnson, H. J., & May, J. R. Phasic heart rate changes in reaction time and time estimation. *Psychophysiology*, 1969, *6*, 351–357.

Johnston, W. A., & Heinz, S. P. Flexibility and capacity demands of attention. *Journal of Experimental Psychology: General*, 1978, *107*, 420–435.

Kahneman, D. *Attention and effort*. Englewood Cliffs, NJ: Prentice-Hall, 1973. pp. 1–49.

Kahneman, D., Tursky, B., Shapiro, D., & Crider, A. Pupilary, heart rate, and skin resistance changes during a mental task. *Journal of Experimental Psychology*, 1969, *79*, 164–167.

Kasl, S. V. Epidemiological contributions to the study of work stress. In C. L. Cooper & R. Payne (Eds.), *Stress at work*. New York: Wiley, 1978. Pp. 3–50.

Kerr, B. Processing demands during mental operations. *Memory and Cognition*, 1973, *1*, 401–412.

Kimmel, H., van Olst, E., & Orlebeke, J. F. *The orienting reflex in humans*. Hillsdale, NJ: Lawrence Erlbaum Associates, 1979.

Korte, C., Ypma, A., & Toppen, C. Helpfulness in Dutch society as a function of urbanization and environmental input level. *Journal of Personality and Social Behavior*, 1975, *32*, 996–1003.

Krantz, D. S., Glass, D. C., Schaeffer, M. A., & Davia, J. E. Behavior patterns and coronary disease: A critical evaluation. In J. T. Cacioppo & R. E. Petty (Eds.), *Perspectives on cardiovascular psychophysiology*. New York: Guilford Press, 1982.

Lacey, J. I. Some cardiovascular correlates of sensorimotor behavior: Example of visceral afferent feedback? In C. H. Hockman (Ed.), *Limbic system mechanisms and autonomic function*. Springfield, IL: Thomas, 1972, Pp. 175–201.

Lacey, J. I., Kagan, J., Lacey, B. C., & Moss, H. A. The visceral level: Situational determinants and behavioral correlates of autonomic response patterns. In P. H. Knapp (Ed.), *Expression of the emotions in man*. New York: International Universities Press, 1963, pp. 161–196.

Lacey, B. C., & Lacey, J. I. Studies of heart rate and other bodily processes in sensorimotor behavior. In P. A. Obrist, A. H. Black, J. Brener, & L. V. DiCara (Eds.), *Cardiovascular psychophysiology-current issues in response mechanisms, biofeedback and methodology*. Chicago, IL: Aldine-Atherton, 1974. pp. 538–564.

Lacey, B. C., & Lacey, J. I. Two way communication between the heart and the brain. *American Psychologist*, 1978, *33*, 99–113.

Langer, A. W., Obrist, P. A., & McCubbin, J. A. Hemodynamic and metabolic adjustments during exercise and shock avoidance in dogs. *American Journal of Physiology*, 1979, *236*, H225–H230.

Lazarus, R. S. *Psychological stress and the coping process*. New York: McGraw Hill, 1966.

Lazarus, R. S., Speisman, J. C., & Mordkoff, A. M. The relationship between autonomic indicators of psychological stress: Heart rate in conductions. *Psychosomatic Medicine*, 1963, *25*, 19–30.

Levi, L. (Ed.). *Society, stress, and disease* (Vol. 1). London: Oxford University Press, 1971.

Levy, M. N., & Martin, P. J. Neural control of the heart. In R. M. Berne, N. Sperelakis, & S. R. Geiger, (Eds.), *Handbook of physiology: Section 2: The cardiovascular system*. Bethesda, MD: American Physiological Society, 1979, pp. 581–620.

Lindsley, D. B. Attention, consciousness, sleep, and wakefulness. In H. W. Magoun (Ed.), *Handbook of physiology* Section I: *Neurophysiology*. (Vol. 3). Bethesda, MD: American Physiological Society, 1960. pp. 1553–1593.

Lown, B., DiSilva, R. A., & Lenson, R. Roles of psychologic stress and autonomic nervous system changes in the provocation of ventricular premature complexes. *The American Journal of Cardiology*, 1978, *41*, 979–985.

Lown, B., DiSilva, R. A., Reich, P., & Murawski, B. J. Psychophysiologic factors in sudden cardiac death. *American Journal of Psychiatry*, 1980, *137*, 1325–1335.

Lown, B., Verrier, R., & Corbalan, R. Psychologic stress and threshold for repetitive ventricular response. *Science*, 1973, *182*, 834–836.

Matthews, K. A. Psychological perspectives on the Type A behavior pattern. *Psychological Bulletin*, 1982, *91*, 293–323.

Matthews, K., & Brunson, B. Allocation of attention and Type A coronary prone behavior. *Journal of Personality and Social Psychology*, 1979, *37*, 2081–2090.

Matthews, K. A., Glass, D. C., Rosenman, R. H., & Bortner, R. W. Competitive drive, pattern A, and coronary heart disease: A further analysis of some data from the Western Collaborative Group Study. *Journal of Chronic Diseases*, 1977, *30*, 489–498.

Matthews, K. A., Scheier, M. F., Brunson, B. I., & Carducci, B. Attention, unpredictability, and reports of physical symptoms: Eliminating the benefits of predictability. *Journal of Personality and Social Psychology*, 1980, *38*, 525–537.

Matthews, K. E., Jr., & Canon, L. K. Environmental noise level as a determinant of helping behavior. *Journal of Personality and Social Psychology*, 1975, *32*, 571–577.

McCullagh, K. G. Revised concepts of atherogenesis: A review. *Cleveland Clinic Quarterly*, 1976, *43*, 247–266.

Milgram, S. The experience of living in cities: A psychological analysis. *Science*, 1970, *167*, 1461–1468.

Mulder, G., Mulder, H., & van der Meulen, W. R. E. H. Mental load and the measurement of heart rate variability. *Ergonomics*, 1973, *16*, 69–84.

Millward, R. B. Theoretical and experimental approaches to human learning. In J. W. Kling, & L. A. Riggs (Eds.), *Experimental psychology*. New York: Holt, Rinehart, & Winston, 1971, pp. 905–1017.

Navon, D., & Gopher, D. On the economy of the human processing system. *Psychological Review*, 1979, *86*, 214–255.

Norman, D. A. *Memory and attention*. New York: Wiley, 1969.

Obrist, P. A. *Cardiovascular psycophysiology: A perspective*. New York: Plenum, 1981.

Obrist, P. A., Gaebelein, C. J., Teller, E. S., Langer, A. W., Grignolo, A., Light, K. C., & McCubbin, J. A. The relationship among heart rate, carotid dP/dt and blood pressure in humans as a function of the type of stress. *Psychophysiology*, 1978, *15*, 102–115.

Obrist, P. A., Howard, J. L., Lawler, J. E., Galosy, R. A., Meyers, K. A., & Gaebelein, C. J. The cardiac-somatic interaction. In P. A. Obrist, A. H. Black, J. Brener, & L. V. DiCara (Eds.), *Cardiovascular psychophysiology-Current issues in response mechanisms, biofeedback, and methodology*. Chicago, IL: Aldine, 1974. pp. 136–162.

Obrist, P. A., Langer, A. W., Light, K. C., Grignolo, A., & McCubbin, J. A. Myocardial performance and stress: Implications for basic and clinical research. In H. D. Kimmel, E. H. van Olst, & J. H. Orlebeke (Eds.), *The orienting reflex in humans*. Hillsdale, NJ: Lawrence Erlbaum Associates, 1979. pp. 199–218.

Obrist, P. A., Lawler, J. E., Howard, J. L., Smithson, K. W., Martin, P. L., & Manning, J. Sympathetic influences on cardiac rate and contractility during acute stress in humans. *Psychophysiology*, 1974, *11*, 405–427.

Pinneau, S. R. *Effects of social support on occupational stresses and strains*. Presented at a symposium on job demands and worker health. Held at the 84th annual convention of the American Psychological Association, Washington, DC, September, 1976.

Posner, M. I. *Chronometric explorations of mind*. Hillsdale, NJ: Lawrence Erlbaum Associates, 1978.

Poulton, E. C. Arousing stresses increase vigilance. In R. R. Mackie (Ed.), *Vigilance: Theory, operational performance, and physiological correlates*. New York: Plenum, 1977, pp. 423–459.

Rose, R. M., Jenkins, C. D., & Hurst, M. W. Air traffic controller health change study. Report to Federal Aviation Administration (Contract No. DOT-FA73WA-3211) August, 1978.

Rosenman, R. H., Brand, R. J., Jenkins, C. D., Friedman, M., Straus, R., & Wurm, M. Coronary heart disease in the Western Collaborative Group Study. *Journal of American Medical Association*, 1975, *233*, 872–877.

Rosenman, R. H., Brand, R. J., Sholtz, R. I., & Friedman, M. Multivariate prediction of coronary heart disease during 8.5 year follow-up in the Western Collaborative Group Study. *American Journal of Cardiology*, 1976, *37*, 903–910.

Rosenman, R. H., & Chesney, M. A. The relationship of Type A behavior to coronary heart disease. *Activitas Nervosa Superior*, 1980, *22*, 1–45.

Sales, S. M. Organizational role as a risk factor in coronary disease. *Administrative Sciences Quarterly*, 1969, *14*, 325–336.

Sales, S. M., & House, J. Job dissatisfaction as a possible risk factor in coronary heart disease. *Journal of Chronic Diseases*, 1971, *23*, 861–873.

Schneider, R. A. Patterns of autonomic response to startle in subjects with and without coronary artery disease. *Clinical Research*, 1957, *15*, 59. (Abstract)

Schneiderman, N. Animal models relating behavioral stress and cardiovascular pathology: A position paper on mechanisms. In T. M. Dembroski, S. Weiss, J. Shields, S. Haynes, & M. Feinleib (Eds.), *Proceedings of the forum on coronary-prone behavior*. Bethesda, MD: DHEW Publication No. (NIH) 78-1451, 202–233.

Siegal, J. M., & Steele, C. M. Noise level and social discrimination. *Personality and Social Psychology Bulletin*, 1979, *5*, 95–99.

Siegal, J. M., & Steele, C. M. Environmental distraction and interpersonal judgments. *British Journal of Social and Clinical Psychology*, 1980, *19*, 23–32.

Silverstein, L. D., & Graham, F. K. *Selective attention effects on reflex activity*. Paper presented at the 18th annual meeting of the Society for Psychophysiological Research, September, 1978.

Sime, W. E., Buell, J. C., & Eliot, R. S. Cardiovascular responses to emotional stress (Quiz Interview) in post-myocardial infarction patients and matched control subjects. *Journal of Human Stress*, 1980, *6*(3), 39–46.

Skinner, J. E. The role of the frontal cortex in the regulation of cardiac vulnerability to ventricular fibrillation: A new concept of Cannon's cerebral defense mechanism to appear in E. Donchin, G. Galbraith, & M. Kietzman (Eds.), *Neurophysiology and psychology: Basic mechanisms and clinical applications*. New York: Academic Press, 1982.

Skinner, J. E., Lie, J. T., & Entman, M. L. Modification of ventricular fibrillation latency following coronary artery occlusion in the conscious pig: The effects of psychological stress and beta-adrenergic blockade. *Circulation*, 1975, *51*, 656–667.

Skinner, J. E., & Yingling, C. D. Central gating mechanisms that regulate event-related potentials and behavior: A neural model for attention. In J. E. Desmedt (Ed.), *Attention, voluntary contraction and event-related cerebral potentials*. Basel: Karger, 1977. pp. 30–69.

Sokolov, E. N. *Perception and the conditioned reflex*. Oxford: Pergamon Press, 1963.

Spieth, W. Slowness of task performance and cardiovascular disease. In A. T. Welford & J. E. Birren (Eds.), *Behavior, aging, and the nervous system*. Springfield, IL: Charles C. Thomas, 1965, pp. 366–400.

Stammler, J. Dietary and serum lipids in the multifactorial etiology of atherosclerosis. *Archives of Surgery*, 1978, *113*, 21–25.

Stern, G. S., Harris, J. R., & Elverum, J. Attention to important versus trivial tasks and salience of fatigue-related symptoms for coronary prone individuals. *Journal of Research in Personality*, 1981, *15*, 467–474.

Stokols, D. A congruence analysis of human stress. In I. G. Sarason, & C. D. Spielberger (Eds.), *Stress and anxiety* (Vol. 6). Washington, D.C.: Hemisphere, 1975, pp. 27–53.

Suedfeld, P. Stressful levels of environmental stimulation. In I. G. Sarason, & C. D. Spielberger, (Eds.), *Stress and anxiety* (Vol. 6). Washington, D.C.: Hemisphere, 1975, pp. 109–127.

Taylor, S. E., & Fiske, S. T. Salience, attention, and attribution: Top of the head phenomena. In L. Berkowitz (Ed.), *Advances in experimental social psychology* (Vol. 2). New York: Academic Press, 1978.

Tecce, J. J., & Cole, J. O. The distraction-arousal hypothesis, CNV, and schizophrenia. In D. I. Mostofsky (Ed.), *Behavior control and modification of physiological activity*. Englewood Cliffs, NJ: Prentice-Hall, 1976. pp. 162–219.

Tursky, B., Schwartz, G. E. & Crider, A. Differential patterns of heart rate and skin resistance during a digit-transformation task. *Journal of Experimental Psychology*, 1980, *83*, 451–457.

Van Doornen, L. J. P., Orlebeke, J. F., & Somsen, R. J. M. Coronary risk and coping with aversive stimuli. *Psychophysiology*, 1980, *17*, 598–603.

Verrier, R., & Lown, B. Sudden death. In A. Baum, D. S. Krantz, & J. E. Singer (Eds.), *Handbook of medical psychology*, in press.

Waldron, I., Hickey, A., McPherson, C., Butensky, A., Gruss, L., Overall, K., Schmader, A., & Wohlmuth, D. Type A behavior pattern: Relationship to variation in blood pressure, parental characteristics, and academic and social activities of students. *Journal of Human Stress*, 1980, *6*, 16–27.

Walter, G. F., & Porges, S. W. Heart rate and respiratory responses as a function of task difficulty: The use of discriminant analysis in the selection of psychologically sensitive physiological responses. *Psychophysiology*, 1976, *13*, 563–571.

Walton, K. W. Pathogenetic mechanisms in atherosclerosis. *American Journal of Cardiology*, 1975, *35*, 542–558.

Weidner, G., & Matthews, K. A. Reported physical symptoms elicited by unpredictable events, and the Type A coronary-prone behavior pattern. *Journal of Personality and Social Psychology,* 1978, *36,* 1213–1220.

Welford, A. T. Motor performance. In J. E. Birren & K. W. Schaie (Eds.), *Handbook of the psychology of aging.* New York: Van Nostrand, 1977, pp. 450–496.

Wickens, C. D. The structure of attentional resources. In R. S. Nickerson (Ed.), *Attention and performance* (Vol. 8). Hillsdale, N.J.: Lawrence Erlbaum Associates 1980, pp. 239–258.

Wierville, W. W. Physiological measures of aircrew mental workload. *Human Factors,* 1979, *21,* 573–593.

Williams, R. B., Jr. Physiological mechanisms underlying the association between psychosocial factors and coronary disease. In W. D. Gentry & R. B. Williams, Jr. (Eds.), *Psychologic aspects of myocardial infarction and coronary care.* St. Louis, MO: C. V. Mosby, 1975. pp. 37–50.

Williams, R. B., Jr. Psychophysiological differences between the Type A and Type B individuals that may lead to CHD. In T. M. Dembroski, S. Weiss, J. Shields, S. Haynes, & M. Feinleib (Eds.), *Proceedings of the forum on coronary-prone behavior.* Bethesda: DHEW Publication No. (NIH) 78-1451, 1977.

Williams, R. B., Jr., Bittker, T. E., Buchsbaum, M. S., & Wynne, L. C. Cardiovascular and neurophysiologic correlates of sensory intake and rejection. I. Effect of cognitive tasks. *Psychophysiology,* 1975, *12,* 427–433.

Williams, R. B., Jr., Lane, J. D., White, A. D., Kuhn, C. M., & Schanberg, S. M. Type A behavior pattern and neuroendocrine response during mental work. *Psychosomatic Medicine,* 1981, *43,* 92–93.

Williams, R. B., Jr., Poon, L. W., & Burdette, L. J. Locus of control and vasomotor response to sensory processing. *Psychosomatic Medicine,* 1977, *39,* 127–133.

Wolf, S. Psychophysiological influences on the dive reflex in man. In P. J. Schwartz, A. N. Brown, A. Mallaiani, & A. Zanchetti (Eds.), *Neural mechanisms in cardiac arrhythmia.* New York: Raven Press, 1978, pp. 237–250.

Wood, C. C., & Jennings, J. R. Speed-accuracy tradeoff functions in choice reaction time: Experimental designs and computation procedures. *Perception and Psychophysics,* 1976, *19,* 92–102.

5 Psychological Factors in Cardiac Arrhythmias and Sudden Death

Richard L. Verrier
Regis A. DeSilva
Bernard Lown

Cardiovascular Division, Department of Medicine of the Brigham and Woman's Hospital, Harvard Medical School and Cardiovascular Laboratories, Department of Nutrition, Harvard School of Public Health, Boston, Massachusetts

The main objective of this chapter is to give an overview of contemporary issues related to the role of psychologic factors in the precipitation of sudden cardiac death. Accordingly, we will discuss the scope of the problem, the clinical evidence implicating psychologic factors, and the insights derived from animal studies of psychophysiologic factors in sudden cardiac death. It should be stated at the onset that this review is not intended to cover the entire waterfront of this rapidly growing discipline. Rather, we will attempt to be selective and highlight current investigations which, in our opinion, will set the trajectory for future research.

SCOPE OF THE PROBLEM

Sudden death is the leading cause of fatality in the industrially developed world (Lown 1979). In the United States alone, 450,000 victims are claimed annually, accounting for nearly 25% of all deaths. It is the prime cause of mortality for individuals aged 20 to 64. Almost two-thirds of coronary heart disease (CHD) deaths occur within less than 24 hours after onset of symptoms. In the majority of those dying suddenly, death is unexpected, occurs instantaneously and strikes outside of the hospital. The median age of sudden death is 59 years. Indeed in nearly 25% of these victims, the presence of clinical heart disease is first indicated by sudden death (Kuller, 1966).

While victims have a high prevalence of risk factors for CHD, they are not distinguishable from other patients with CHD (Chiang, Perlman, Fulton, Ostrander, & Epstein, 1970, Doyle, Kannel, McNamara, Quickenton & Gordon, 1976). The victim of sudden death does not differ from other coronary-prone individuals in the occurrence of hypercholesterolemia, prevalence of cigarette smoking, hypertension, obesity, diabetes, and a positive family history. Sudden death occurs far more frequently in men than in women (Kuller 1966, Wikland 1968). Although the total number of cases increases with age, the fraction of all coronary deaths that are sudden and unanticipated is higher in the young adult male than in the older male (Croce 1960). Prospective, cross-sectional, and retrospective studies indicate that the incidence of sudden death from CHD per 1000 subjects aged 50 to 60 is approximately 2 per year for white males, 1.3 for black males, 1.1 for black females, and 0.5 for white females (Kannel, Dawber, & McNamara, 1966, Kuller, Lilienfeld, & Fisher, 1967, Weinblatt, Shapiro, Frank, and Sager 1968).

Although witnessing someone die suddenly during exercise leaves an indelible impression, this is a most unusual sequence. To date there have been no persuasive reports linking sudden death with strenous physical exertion or work. Nearly 75% of all sudden deaths occur at home, 8 to 12% at work (Kuller 1966, 1967; Wikland 1968), and only 2 to 5% have been preceded by vigorous physical effort (Spain, 1964).

Pathologic Features

Of the CHD sudden deaths, 61% have been reported to have three or all four major coronary vessels showing greater than 75% luminal stenosis, while only 24% had one vessel or no vessel with that degree of involvement (Peper, Kuller, & Cooper, 1975). In the majority, the coronary arteriosclerotic process is diffuse, severe, and multivascular and is frequently associated with chronic myocardial damage. Acute coronary artery occlusion or thrombosis is the exception, and its occurrence is related to the duration of the terminal episode (Spain & Bradess 1970, Schwartz & Walsh 1971). In only a minority of patients is myocardial infarction the underlying mechanism. Electrocardiographic confirmation of acute transmural myocardial infarction was present in 39 of 239 patients (16%) (Cobb, Baum, Alvarez, & Schaffer 1975). In fact, two distinct syndromes can be distinguished in sudden death: a minority of patients experiencing myocardial infarction and a majority having cardiac electrical failure. Thus, in most subjects dying suddenly, acute pathologic lesions either in the coronary arteries or in the myocardium are inadequate to account for the fatal event (Lown 1979). How then is the lethal episode precipitated? Lown and coworkers (Lown & Wolf 1971, Lown, Verrier, & Rabinowitz, 1977, Lown & Verrier 1982) have promulgated three main hypotheses to account for the occurrence of sudden cardiac death. The first is that sudden death is primarily due to electrical disorder of the heart beat in the form of ventricular fibrillation (VF). This arrhythmia has been characterized as chaotic electrical depolarization of the heart resulting in disorganized and ineffective mechanical activity with cessation of blood flow. Death occurs within minutes if cardiopulmonary resuscitation and defibrillation are not promptly instituted. Coronary care unit experience (Lown & Wolf 1971) and out of hospital experience (Cobb et al. 1975) have provided ample evidence that ventricular fibrillation is indeed the mechanism of sudden death and thus the first tenet is on firm grounds.

The second hypothesis is that electrical instability of the myocardium may long precede the onset of the malignant arrhythmias. It has been suggested that certain types of premature beats may reflect the presence of electrical instability (Lown & Wolf 1971). The existence of such instability in patients with ischemic heart disease is demonstrable by administration of programmed electrical impulses to the ventricular myocardium (Greene, Reid, & Schaeffer 1978, Mason & Winkle 1978, Podrid, Schoeneberger, Lown, Matos, Porterfield, & Corrigan 1981). The occurrence of repetitive electrical responses to electrical stimuli has predictive value with respect to the subsequent occurrence of malignant arrhythmias and sudden cardiac death (Mason & Winkle 1978, Podrid et al. 1981). Some investigators have claimed that in fact the repetitive ventricular response may be a useful index in the management of patients prone to life-threatening arrhythmias (Mason & Winkle 1978, Podrid et al. 1981). The third hypothesis proposed by Lown and coworkers (Lown et al. 1977, Lown & Verrier 1982) is that transient risk factors, primarily of neural origin, can trigger ventricular fibrillation in the electrically unstable heart. This suggestion is of considerable contemporary medical significance and thus observes careful evaluation. The remainder of the review will focus on the central issue. Specifically, what evidence is available to support the view that neural and psychologic factors constitute a major risk factor for sudden cardiac death?

ANIMAL STUDIES

Early evidence of a link between higher nervous activity and cardiac arrhythmias was derived mainly from anesthetized animal experiments. Levy (1913–1914) demonstrated over 60 years ago that injection of drugs such as nicotine, barium chloride or epinephrine into certain areas of the brain in chloroform-anesthetized cats provoked major ventricular arrhythmias even when the coronary circulation was intact (1913–1914). The neural pathways involved in arrhythmogenesis were subsequently defined by means of stereotaxically positioned electrodes (Lown & Verrier 1976). Despite reasonable progress in anesthetized animal experimentation, advances in the psychologic dimension were few and far between.

The classic studies of Cannon (1942) suggested that the biologically active amine adrenaline was secreted in response to stimuli that produced fear and rage reactions in animals, and he considered these biogenic amines to play a role in Voodoo death. Subsequently, the experiments of Richter (1957) exerted a profound influence in shifting the attention of psychologic investigators from the sympatho-adrenal system to the vagus as a precipitating element of sudden death. Richter demonstrated that rats forced to swim in water tanks died in bradycardia and asystole rather than from VF, presumably as a result of intense vagal discharge. While the simple faint in humans is caused by this means, this is unlikely to be the mechanism for sudden cardiac death for two main reasons. First, whereas enhanced vagal activity is capable of permanently arresting the small rat heart, it is incapable of doing so in the larger mammalian hearts of the dog and human (McWilliam 1887). Second, VF, not asystole, is the primary mechanism for sudden cardiac death (Lown 1973).

Subsequent studies were directed toward exposing normal animals to severe behavioral stress until the animals either died or exhibited signs of extensive cardiac damage. These stresses involved interference of animals' access to food (Raab, Chaplin, & Bajusz 1964; Raab 1966), exposing rats to tape recordings of noisy rat-cat fights (Raab et al. 1964; Raab 1966), "yoked chair" aversive avoidance experiments in monkeys (Corley, Mauck, & Shiel 1975) and animal crowding (Raab 1966). Subjecting normal pigs to unavoidable small electrical shocks while they were paralyzed by muscle relaxants likewise induced cardiac myofibrillar damage within 24 hours (Johannsson, Jonsson, Lannek, Blomgren, Lindberg, & Poupa 1974).

Thus, until recently (Table 5.1), psychophysiologic studies in the area of sudden death research were oriented largely toward the provocation of myocardial injury and asystole in normal animals. This was an unfortuante trend because

TABLE 5.1
Historical Perspective of Experimental Modelling of
Bio-Behavioral Factors in Sudden Cardiac Death

Investigators	Period	Biological Model	Proposed Mechanism of Death
Cannon	1942	"Voodoo Death"	Sympatho-adrenal activation
Richter	1957	Swimming Rats	Vagally-induced asystole
Raab	1964	Sensory and emotional stress in rats	Cardiac myofibrillar damage
Corley	1974	Shock avoidance in squirrel monkeys	Myocardial degeneration leading to asystole
Johansson	1974	Restraint stress in pigs	Myocardial necrosis

TABLE 5.2
Characteristics of Sudden
Cardiac Death Syndrome

Mechanism	Electrical Failure (VF)
Duration of final event	Seconds to minutes
Coronary artery disease	Present
Acute coronary occlusion	Absent
Myocardial damage (ECG, enzymes, etc.)	Absent

major features of the clinical syndrome which already were evident from coronary care unit experience in the 1960's (Lown, Kosowsky, & Klein 1969) were ignored in designing biological models. For example, sudden death usually occurs in the presence of underlying coronary disease, not in normal individuals. The fatal event is usually abrupt in onset (symptoms lasting seconds to minutes) and is due primarily to VF not asystole. And finally, significant myocardial damage is rarely present, suggesting that sudden death is due to a derangement in cardiac electrical function rather than to an anatomical lesion (Table 5.2).

Thus, it was necessary to shift the research focus toward defining the influence of psychologic factors on ventricular electrical stability. This, however, presented difficult methodologic problems. In particular, how can we assess vulnerability to VF in the free-moving conscious animal? Such assessment requires the use of painful test stimuli, induction of VF, and use of traumatic resuscitation procedures that preclude meaningful investigation of psychologic variables.

Assessment of Cardiac Vulnerability in Conscious Animals

To circumvent these difficulties, we utilized a different marker of ventricular vulnerability (Matta, Verrier, and Lown 1976, Lown & Verrier 1982). Classically, the threshold for ventricular fibrillation has been assessed by delivering small electric currents to the heart during the narrow zone of the so-called vulnerable period of the ventricle, coinciding with the apex of the T wave in the surface electrocardiogram. By stepwise increases of current intensity, ventricular fibrillation can be provoked and the electrical threshold for this measured. Since ventricular fibrillation is preceded by repetitive extrasystoles, the threshold for the later endpoint may be utilized, since it is not detected by the animal (Figure 5.1). This marker, which reliably tracks the threshold current required to provoke ventricular fibrillation, acts as a substitute for the ventricular fibrillation threshold and obviates the need for cardiac resuscitation.

Stimulus
Intensity
(ma)

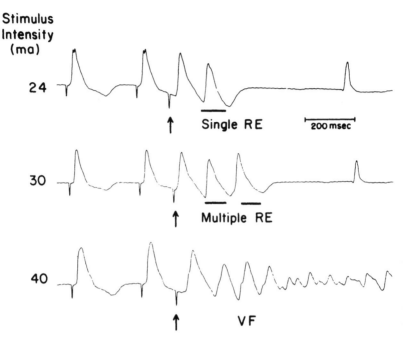

FIG. 5.1.   Repetitive responses preceding ventricular fibrillation (VF). At a stimulus intensity of 24*mA* (arrow), a repetitive extrasystole (RE) is elicited (upper panel). At 30 *mA*, multiple RE ensue (middle panel) that degenerated into VF when stimulus intensity was raised to 40 *mA* (lower panel). Heart rate was maintained constant at 214 beats/min by pacing. Tracings are intracavitary ECGs recorded at 125 mm/sec (From Matta, Verrier & Lown, 1976)

Psychologic Influences on Ventricular Vulnerability

The repetitive extrasystole therefore served as our essential electrophysiologic endpoint for examining the effects of diverse psychologic states on cardiac vulnerability. In our initial studies, a simple classical aversive conditioning protocol was utilized (Lown, Verrier & Corbalan 1973). Dogs were exposed to two different environments: a cage in which the animal was left largely undisturbed, and a Pavlovian sling in which the animal received a single 5 joule transthoracic shock at the end of each experimental period for 3 successive days. The two environments were compared on days 4 and 5. At these times, dogs in the sling were restless, frequently salivated excessively, exhibited somatic tremor, demonstrated sinus tachycardia, and had increased mean arterial blood pressure. In the cage, the animals appeared relaxed as evidenced by behavioral signs and hemodynamic variables. Transferring the animals from the nonaversive to the aversive environment resulted in a substantial 40% reduction in vulnerable period threshold (DeSilva, Verrier, & Lown, 1979, Liang, Verrier, Melman, &

Lown 1979) (Figure 5.2). These findings indicate that psychologic stress profoundly lowers the threshold for ventricular fibrillation.

It was pertinent to determine whether the type of stress was crucial to the changes in ventricular vulnerability. We therefore examined an entirely different psychologic stress model in which dogs were subjected to programmed signaled shock avoidance (Matta, Lawler, & Lown 1976). Exposure to such an aversive conditioning program resulted in a 50% reduction in the repetitive extrasystole threshold, a change comparable to that observed in the cage-sling paradigm

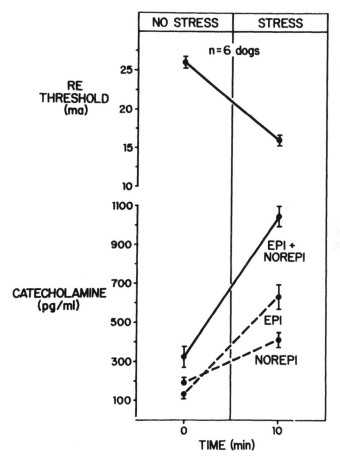

FIG. 5.2 Effect of aversive sling environment on repetitive extrasystole (RE) threshold and circulating plasma catecholamine level. After removal from the cage the RE threshold decreased by 41% within 10 min of placing the animals in the sling, accompanied by substantial increases in both norepinephrine and epinephrine. (Values are means ± SEM) (From Liang, Verrier, Melman & Lown, 1979)

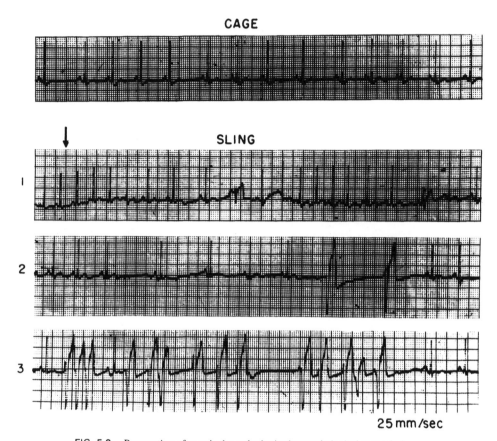

CAGE

SLING

1

2

3

25 mm/sec

FIG. 5.3.   Provocation of ventricular arrhythmias by psychological stress during myocardial infarction. In the nonstressful environment (cage, upper tracing), the animal exhibited normal sinus rhythm at a rate of 90 beats/min. In comparison, when the animal was placed in the stressful environment (sling, lower three continuous tracings), ventricular arrhythmias were evoked. 1, upon presentation of stressful stimuli (arrow) a brief period of sinus tachycardia (160 beats/min) was followed by (2) sinus bradycardia (72 beats/min). 3, normal rhythm was interrupted by ventricular premature beats, culminating in ventricular tachycardia with bouts of R-on-T phenomena. The observations were made 48 hours after myocardial infarction. (From Corbalan, Verrier, Lown, 1974)

described above. Recently, we have also found that still a different stress involving the induction of an anger-like state by food-access-denial in dogs lowered the vulnerable period threshold by 30 to 40% (Verrier, Lombardi, & Lown 1982). Though the vulnerable period threshold was similarly altered in three different psychologic stress models, it by no means proves that the specificity of the stress is immaterial. The problem invites much more comprehensive investigation.

An important issue to be resolved was whether these moderate aversive psychologic states were sufficient in magnitude to provoke ventricular arrhythmias in the predisposed animal without the need to subject the heart to external electrical stimulation.

This question was examined in dogs subjected to coronary artery occlusion (Corbalan, Verrier, & Lown 1974). The animals were conditioned according to the cage-sling paradigm. After 5 consecutive days in which they spent 1 hour in the cage and 1 hour in the sling, a balloon occluder previously implanted around the left anterior descending coronary artery was inflated. Once the animals had recovered fully from the occlusion and were entirely free of arrhythmia, they were reexposed to the two environments. The sling environment consistently resulted in diverse ventricular arrhythmias including ventricular tachycardia and R-on-T extrasystoles; these effects disappeared when the animals were returned to the nonaversive cage (Figure 5.3). In these dogs recovering from myocardial infarction, despite the consistent induction of serious arrhythmias, ventricular fibrillation was not precipitated. This was the case even when the animals were exposed to the aversive environment within only a few hours following occlusion of a major coronary vessel. It remained uncertain whether these psychologic stresses were of sufficient magnitude to trigger ventricular fibrillation.

To shed light on the question, we examined whether imposition of psychologic stress during the very inception of acute myocardial ischemia would predispose to ventricular fibrillation. Our experimental model involved a 10-minute period of left anterior descending coronary artery occlusion followed by abrupt release. This model was chosen because it exhibits a consistent time course of changes in ventricular vulnerability. Specifically, within 1 to 2 minutes of coronary occlusion, the vulnerable period threshold falls to extremely low levels. This period of enhanced vulnerability persists for 6 to 7 minutes after which time the vulnerable period threshold recovers despite continued occlusion. Upon release of the occlusion after an ischemic period of 10 minutes, a brief period of vulnerability reappears within 20 to 30 seconds and lasts for less than 1 minute (Figure 5.4) (Verrier & Lown, 1979).

An additional reason for choosing an occlusion-release model is that it is unclear whether the provocation of ventricular fibrillation in man results from an ischemic lesion caused by infringement of arterial flow or from the release of obstruction with ensuing reperfusion such as might be observed with transient coronary artery spasm. The effects of the cage and the sling environments were therefore evaluated in the occlusion-release model. When acute myocardial

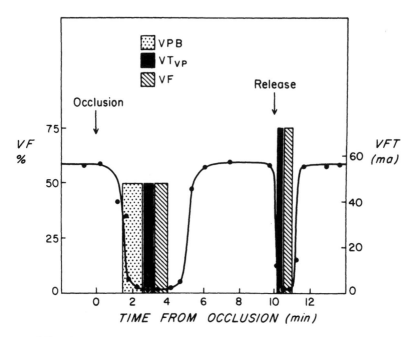

FIG. 5.4. Changes in ventricular fibrillation (VF) threshold induced by a 10-min period of left anterior descending coronary artery occlusion and by release. Note relation between the occurrence of ventricular arrhythmia and the reduction in threshold (solid line). VPB, ventricular premature beats; VT_{vp}, ventricular tachycardia of the vulnerable period. (From Lown & Verrier, 1976)

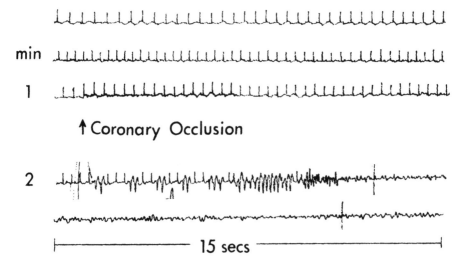

FIG. 5.5. While the animal was in a sling environment, coronary occlusion resulted within 2 minutes in ventricular fibrillation. Note the instability of the baseline due to restlessness when the animal was merely standing quietly. When coronary occlusion was carried out the animal was in the nonaversive cage environment, ventricular fibrillation did not occur.

ischemia was induced in the aversive sling setting, the incidence of ventricular fibrillation was more than three times greater (46% vs. 14%, p < 0.01) than that observed in the nonaversive environment (Verrier and Lown 1979). The episode of ventricular fibrillation occurred within 3 to 5 minutes of coronary artery occlusion or within 20 to 30 seconds of release of obstruction (Figure 5.5). These intervals correspond closely with the periods of maximum ventricular vulnerability exposed by electrical testing of the heart.

Skinner and coworkers (1975) have also reported a significant influence of psychologic stimuli on susceptibility to ventricular fibrillation during acute coro-

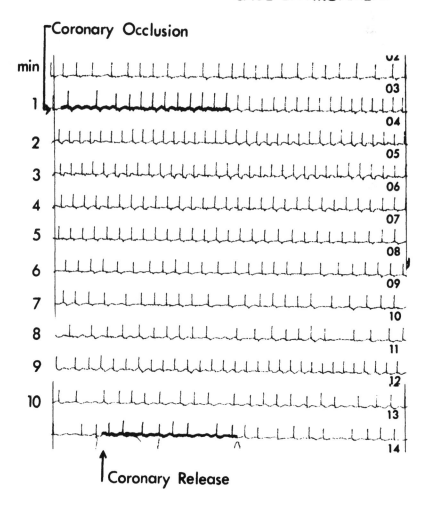

CAGE ENVIRONMENT

nary artery occlusion in pigs. Myocardial ischemia was induced in either a familiar or unfamiliar environment. In the unfamiliar setting, following coronary artery occlusion, fibrillation occurred within a few minutes; however, onset of fibrillation was greatly delayed and even entirely prevented in some animals in an environment to which the pigs had been previously adapted.

The precise pathways mediating psychophysiologic activity to the heart which · affect vulnerability to ventricular fibrillation in the conscious animal are as yet undefined. Recently, Skinner and Reed (1981) shed some light on this question by means of sophisticated cryogenic techniques. They adapted farm pigs to a laboratory environment during a 4 to 8-day period and noted significant retardation or even prevention in the onset of ventricular fibrillation associated with coronary occlusion. These effects of stress on susceptibility to fibrillation appeared to be mediated via the thalamic gating mechanism. This conclusion was based on the findings that cryogenic blockade of this system or its output from the frontal cortex to the brainstem delays or prevents the occurrence of ventricular fibrillation.

These results indicate that diverse biobehavioral stresses are capable of lowering the vulnerable period threshold in the normal heart and predisposing the acutely ischemic heart to ventricular fibrillation during both occlusion and reperfusion. How then does higher nervous system activity conduce the ventricular myocardium to fibrillation?

Adrenergic Factors and Vulnerability During Psychologic Stress

Do adrenergic factors play a substantial role in mediating ventricular vulnerability during biobehavioral stress in conscious animals? This appears to be the case with respect to effects of aversive conditioning on ventricular electrical stability and is supported by several observations. First, the levels of circulating catecholamines vary directly with the changes in ventricular vulnerability during psychologic stress. When dogs were transferred from a nonaversive cage to an aversive sling environment, there was a substantial rise in blood epinephrine and norepinephrine concentrations indicative of enhanced sympathetic neural activity as well as adrenal medullary discharge. The observed reductions in vulnerable period threshold corresponded with the concomitant elevations in circulating catecholamine levels (Liang, Verrier, Melman & Lown 1979).

An essential involvement of adrenergic mechanisms is also suggested by the effects of pharmacologic (Matta, Lawler, Lown 1976, Verrier & Lown 1977) and surgical sympathectomy (Verrier & Lown 1977) on stress-induced changes in ventricular vulnerability. Indeed, it has shown that beta-adrenergic blockade with propranolol (Verrier & Lown 1977) or the cardioselective agent tolamolol (Matta, Lawler, & Lown 1976) completely prevents the effects of aversive conditioning on the vulnerable period threshold. This is the case whether the

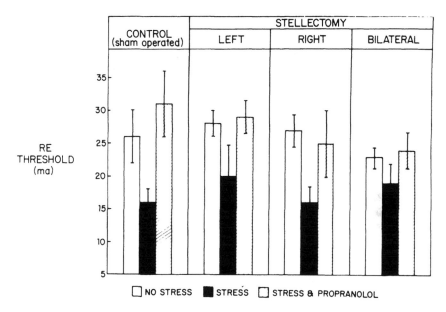

FIG. 5.6.   Effect of beta-adrenergic blockade with propranolol (0.25 mg/kg) and stellectomy on ventricular vulnerability during psychologic stress. Stress induced a significant decrease in vulnerable period threshold which decrease is prevented by propranolol. Unilateral stellectomy did not prevent the decrease in threshold and only partial protection was afforded by bilateral stellectomy. (From Verrier & Lown, 1977)

conditioning is classical or instrumental. It is of interest that stellectomy, whether of the left or right ganglion, did not prevent the reduction in repetitive extrasystole threshold associated with aversive conditioning. Only partial protection was conferred by bilateral stellectomy (Verrier & Lown 1977) (Figure 5.6). Thus, adrenergic inputs in addition to those derived from stellate ganglia impinge upon the myocardium during psychologic stress to alter ventricular vulnerability. Most probably these additional inputs derive from other thoracic ganglia and from adrenal medullary catecholamines.

Psychophysiologic Mechanisms During Myocardial Ischemia

The precise neural mechanisms involved in the biobehavioral provocation of ventricular arrhythmias during myocardial ischemia and infarction are only partially understood. For example, whereas farm pigs adapted to a laboratory environment have a reduced and delayed onset of ventricular fibrillation during coronary artery obstruction, surprisingly, beta-adrenergic blockade with propranolol did not afford any protection against the development of ventricular fibrillation in unadapted animals (Skinner, Lie, Entman 1975). Pharmacologic blockade of adrenergic inputs to the heart and environment adaptation did not yield equivalent results. It remains to be determined whether the failure of propranolol to protect against ventricular fibrillation resulted from inadequate blockade of adrenergic inputs to the heart or from the involvement of extra-adrenergic factors in the antifibrillatory effect of psychologic adaptation.

By contrast, Rosenfeld, Rosen, and Hoffman (1978) found a significant pro-tective effect of beta-adrenergic blockade against malignant ventricular ar-rhythmias associated with acute coronary artery occlusion in dogs exposed to behavioral stresses. The animals were chronically instrumented to record elec-trocardiograms and electrograms for ischemic and nonischemic ventricular epi-cardium during either left anterior descending or circumflex coronary artery occlusion. The dogs were exposed to several forms of behavioral stress experi-mentation in an unfamiliar environment, or were presented with stressful stimuli which were either a light followed by a sudden noise, or a noise followed by subcutaneous electrical shock. Shock significantly decreased latency and in-creased the grade of ventricular arrhythmias. Beta-adrenergic blockade with the cardioselective agent tolamolol substantially reduced the adverse effects of stress on cardiac rhythm. Moreover, they found that the quaternary analog of pro-pranolol, UM 272, which causes no beta-adrenergic blockade but exerts direct local anesthetic effects on the heart, did not confer a protective action. Thus, the beneficial effect of tolamolol appears to result from its antiadrenergic action rather than from a nonspecific effect on myocardial tissue. These workers also demonstrated an antiarrhythmic effect of the antianxiety drug, diazepam.

Cholinergic Influences and Vulnerability During Stress

Do cholinergic factors also modulate ventricular electrical properties in response to environmental stimuli? Two sets of observations suggest an affirmative an-swer to this question. First, it has been shown that administration of morphine sulfate to dogs in the aversive sling environment increased the vulnerable period threshold to the value observed in the nonaversive cage setting (DeSilva et al. 1978). When vagal efferent activity was blocked by atropine, a major component of morphine's protective effect was annulled. When morphine was given in the nonaversive environment, where adrenergic activity was reduced as indicated by low circulating catecholamine levels (DeSilva et al. 1978, Liang et al. 1979), drug-induced vagotonia did not affect the vulnerable period threshold. Thus, the beneficial effect of morphine during psychologic stress appeared to result partly from vagal antagonism of the fibrillatory influence of enhanced adrenergic input to the heart and partly from the drug's sedative action.

It remained uncertain, however, whether intrinsic vagal tone in the stressed animal was sufficient to exert a stabilizing influence on ventricular vulnerability. To study this question, relatively small doses of atropine (0.05 mg/kg) were given to block selectively vagal efferent activity to the heart. In the aversive sling

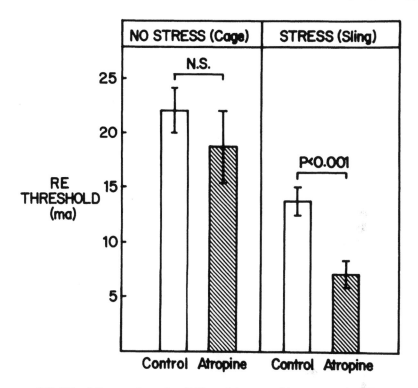

FIG. 5.7.   Influence of atropine (0.05 mg/kg) on repetitive extrasystole (RE) threshold in conscious dogs exposed to nonaversive and aversive environments. In the aversive setting, blockade of vagal efferent activity with atropine substantially reduced the vulnerable period threshold, indicating an enhanced propensity for ventricular fibrillation. In the nonstressful setting, where adrenergic activity was low, atropine was without effect. During cardiac electrical testing heart rate was maintained constant by ventricular pacing (From Verrier & Lown, 1980)

setting, vagal efferent blockade resulted in a substantial 50% reduction in the vulnerable period threshold. The implication is that in the stressed animal, a considerable level of vagal tone is present which partly offsets the profibrillatory influence of aversive psychophysiologic stimuli. In the cage, where adrenergic input was low, vagal blockade was without effect on the threshold (Verrier & Lown 1980) (Figure 5.7).

Sympathetic-Parasympathetic Interactions

What then is the basis for the protective effect of the vagus on ventricular vulnerability? Our thesis has been that the effect of the vagus on ventricular vulnerability is contingent on the level of preexisting cardiac sympathetic tone (Lown & Verrier 1982). At a low level of sympathetic tone, no vagus effect is demonstrated (Kolman, Verrier, & Lown 1975). By contrast, when sympathetic tone to the heart is augmented by thoracotomy (Kolman, Verrier, & Lown, 1975), sympathetic nerve stimulation (Kolman et al. 1975), or catecholamine infusion (Rabinowitz et al. 1976), simultaneous vagal activation exerts a protective effect on ventricular vulnerability. Vagus nerve stimulation is without effect on vulnerability when adrenergic input to the heart is ablated by beta-adrenergic blockade (Figure 5.8) (Kolman et al. 1975, Rabinowitz, Verrier, & Lown 1976).

The influence of the vagus on ventricular vulnerability appears to result from activation of muscarinic receptors, since these changes in vulnerability are prevented by atropine administration (Lown & Verrier 1981). The diminution of adrenergic effects by muscarinic activation has a physiologic and cellular basis. Muscarinic agents inhibit the release of norepinephrine from sympathetic nerve endings (Levy & Blattberg 1976) and attenuate the response to norepinephrine at receptor sites by cyclic nucleotide interactions (Watanabe & Besch 1975).

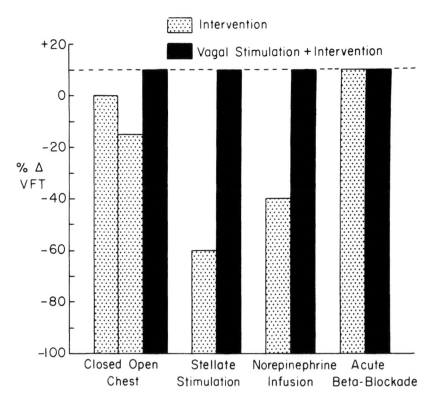

FIG. 5.8. Influence of vagal stimulation in the presence of various levels of adrenergic tone. The vagal effect on ventricular fibrillation (VF) threshold is demonstrable only when neural or humoral activity is increased (From Lown & Verrier, 1976)

Thus, results from both anesthetized and conscious animal experiments indicate that enhanced cardiac vagal tone, whether occurring spontaneously or induced pharmacologically, decreases susceptibility to ventricular fibrillation. This beneficial action is primarily caused by antagonism of adrenergic inputs to the heart.

Vagal Influences in the Ischemic and Infarcted Heart

The role of vagus nerve activity in altering predisposition to VF during acute coronary artery occlusion is a subject of current reappraisal. Kent, Smith, Redwood, & Epstein (1973) found that vagus nerve stimulation significantly increased the VF threshold and decreased susceptibility to fibrillation in the ischemic canine heart. Subsequently, Corr, Gillis, and coworkers (1974, 1976) observed that the presence of intact vagi protected against VF in chloralose-anesthetized cats during left anterior descending but not right coronary artery ligation. Yoon, Han, Tse, and Rogers (1977) and James, Arnold, Allen, Pantridge, and Shanks (1977) were unable to demonstrate any effect of vagus nerve stimulation on VF threshold during left anterior descending coronary artery occlusion in the canine heart. Corr and coworkers (1974) have found that cholinergic stimulation may actually exacerbate rather than ameliorate the arrhythmias which ensue upon release of occlusion, with attendant reperfusion of the ischemic myocardium.

Our own investigations indicate that intense cholinergic stimulation by electrical stimulation of the decentralized vagi or by direct muscarinic enhancement with methacholine affords only partial protection during myocardial ischemia in dogs in which heart rate was maintained constant by pacing. No salutary influence of cholinergic stimulation, however, was noted during reperfusion (Verrier & Lown, 1978). However, additional countervailing factors come into play when myocardial perfusion is impaired. Thus, vagal stimulation does not completely suppress the arrhythmias which result from myocardial infarction (Kerzner, Wolf, Kosowsky, & Lown 1973). In fact, it has been demonstrated that enhanced vagus activity or acetylcholine infusion consistently elicited ventricular tachycardia during the quiescent arrhythmia-free phase of myocardial infarction in dogs. This effect was completely rate-dependent since preventing the vagally induced bradycardia abolished the arrhythmias. Thus, the antiarrhythmic effects of the vagus may be augmented or reversed by its profound influence on heart rate in the setting of acute myocardial infarction.

Effect of Sleep on Ventricular Arrhythmias

Kleitman's (1963) pioneering work made evident that prolonged sleep deprivation in animals led to disorganized aggressive behavior, and eventually, sudden death. Post-mortem examination demonstrated no anatomic lesions or chemical imbalance to account for death. Cardiac arrhythmia was considered as a possible cause. This is not an unreasonable surmise. Sleep, as a neural event, probably influences cardiac behavior predominantly through autonomic nervous system mediation. Much evidence suggests that diencephalic areas in the central nervous system serve as focal points of cardiac control (Rushmer, Smith & Lasher, 1960; Smith, 1960) and that this control is transmitted through peripheral autonomic pathways (Bond 1942, Cohen & Pitts 1968). The same catecholamine neurotransmitters which subserve myocardial function are also associated with specific sleep stages (Reite et al., 1969, Jouvet 1969, Koella, Feldstein, & Czicman 1968), while other specific neurochemical subsystems govern the deep sleep stages which are associated with cardiac arrhythmic activity (Rosenblatt, Zwilling, & Hartmann, 1969). Baust and coworkers (1969) have shown that denervation of the heart prevents the usual cardiac response to various arousal states.

To date, there are no reports defining the precise relationship between altered sleep stages and heart rhythm. As a matter of fact, barring a single report by Skinner, Mohr & Kellaway (1975), there is a paucity of meaningful observations in the literature. This study explores the influence of sleep stage on the occurrence of ventricular arrhythmias during left anterior descending coronary artery occlusion in conscious pure-bred farm pigs. Skinner, Mohr & Kellaway (1975) found that the period during the early sleep cycle wherein transitional and slow wave sleep alternate was accompanied by an increase in arrhythmias compared to the awake state. This was true both in the acutely infarcted (2 hours) as well as the recently infarcted (2 days) pig heart. The maximum increase in ventricular arrhythmias was observed during sustained periods of slow wave sleep. Later when rapid eye movement (REM) sleep predominated, the overall arrhythmia incidence suddenly diminished. Acute coronary artery occlusion performed after the inception of slow wave sleep reduced the latency in onset of ventricular fibrillation compared with that observed during the awake state. Coronary occlusion during REM sleep was associated with the very opposite, namely, a delay in the development of ventricular fibrillation.

These investigators reached some unexpected conclusions: (1) slow wave sleep, but not REM sleep, has a deleterious influence on the ischemic heart; (2) REM sleep may be beneficial since it delays the development of ventricular fibrillation during coronary artery occlusion; and (3), the heart rate changes during sleep do not correlate with the effects of slow wave or REM sleep on cardiac rhythm.

The explanation for the above cited changes remains unclear. It is curious that in the pigs with coronary artery occlusion, arrhythmia was reduced not only during REM sleep but also during wakefulness. These investigators cite Baust and Bohnert (1969) who found in cats that reduction in sympathetic tone accounts for the slow tonic heart rates during REM sleep, while during slow wave sleep, bradycardia was due to increased parasympathetic tone. However, increased sympathetic tone is certainly an attribute of the awake state. During wakefulness, Snyder Hobson and Goldfrank (1963) and others (Baccelli et al.

1969; Coccagna et al. 1971) have demonstrated that heart rate and arterial blood pressure are markedly elevated compared to the levels measured during sleep. There may indeed be hemodynamic concomitants, as well as coronary artery flow changes, linked to neural alterations during sleep stages which influence the electrically unstable ischemic heart. These await further investigation.

HUMAN STUDIES

While it is possible to design animal models to simulate biologic problems in humans, the ultimate validation of a causal relationship requires direct investigation of the human condition. Such modelling, however, is difficult if not impossible for a number of ethical and conceptual reasons. Among the major considerations are the difficulty in replicating and quantifying behavioral stresses in human subjects and the problems inherent with the clinical endpoint, namely, ventricular fibrillation and death. Notwithstanding these obstacles, notable progress has been made which sheds light on the relationship between psychophysiologic factors and the occurrence of cardiac arrhythmias and sudden death in humans.

Epidemiologic Studies

Greene, Goldstein, & Moss (1972) interviewed the next-of-kin of 25 men who died suddenly and estimated that "at least 50%" of these individuals had ongoing psychological and social stresses at the time of death. Many of the stresses described were acute in nature and frequently involved the intercept of two or more situations deemed to be psychologically significant. These workers surmised that a combination of depressive and arousal states coexisted at the time of death in the victims. Myers and Dewar (1975) found among 100 men dying suddenly from coronary disease that the most significant factor associated with death was acute psychological stress. Of the 100 cases studied, 23 experienced acute or moderately acute stress in the preceding 30 minutes. If the preceding 24 hours were considered, 40 of the 100 individuals experienced such stress. These stresses were as varied as first attendance at a surgical clinic, attack by dogs, fights over games, involvement in a nontraumatic motor accident and notification of divorce. Moderate physical activity, a recent meal, especially with alcohol, the time of day and day of the week were also significantly related to death. In comparison, chronic psychologic stress, very strenuous exercise, season of year and environmental temperature were not related. It was presumed in this study that abrupt death was due to VF.

Rissanen, Romo, & Siltanen (1978) evaluated the circumstances surrounding sudden death in Helsinki by interviewing next-of-kin. The prevalence of acute and chronic stress, chest pain, heaviness of the arms, dyspnea, fatigue, sweating and nervousness were considered. Unusual fatigue which occurred in 32% of cases was the most common antecedent. Prodromal symptoms were common in individuals who had attacks lasting longer than 2 hours. "Chronic" stress occured in 25%, "acute" stress in 19% of individuals. In all patients with "acute" stress, death was rapid and resulted within 2 hours; myocardial infarction was unusual in this group of 23 patients, and 14 (16%) died instantaneously. Acute myocardial infarction was more common in patients with long-standing stress than in patients with acute stresses. These results suggest that in patients with coronary artery disease, acute psychological stress is more likely to result in instantaneous or rapid death from VF without the evolution of acute myocardial infarction. In patients with chronic stress, or with no evident stress factors, symptoms were of prolonged duration and death was delayed to several hours.

Our own studies in this area consisted of evaluating 117 patients who had malignant ventricular arrhythmia defined as symptomatic ventricular tachycardia (VT) or VF (Reich, DeSilva, Lown, & Murawski, 1981). Of these patients, 53% had been resuscitated from VF. Clinical interviews are conducted by a psychiatrist and a cardiologist in each case, and the possible emotional precipitants in the preceding 24 hours were identified. In 21% of patients, such acute events had occurred and intense emotions such as anger, fear, and excitement were provoked by situations including acute marital and job-related difficulties and bereavement. It was noted that while 66% of the overall study population had coronary heart disease, only 48% of these patients with putative psychophysiologic "triggers" for VT or VF had this condition. A large fraction (44%) of the patients without demonstrable structural heart disease had such triggers for VT or VF.

Psychological Stress and Ventricular Arrhythmias

Ventricular premature beats (VPBs) occurring in patients with coronary heart disease have been shown to be associated with the occurrence of SCD later in life (Lown 1979). Such an endpoint which provides an index of risk for SCD, can be utilized to evaluate prospectively the effects of both psychosocial factors and psychological stress on the heart.

Small numbers of patients have been studied clinically to determine whether induction of stress can evoke ventricular arrhythmias. For example, stresses as disparate as public speaking, motor car racing or driving, loud sounds, and clinical interviews relating to earlier or ongoing emotional trauma have evoked VPBs in patients with and without heart disease (Lown, 1976; Taggart, et al. 1969, 1973, Wellens, Vermeulen, & Durrer, 1972). We have shown in a controlled study in 19 patients, several of whom had been resuscitated from VF, that a three-part psychological stress test resulted in a twofold increase in VPBs; in one patient malignant ventricular tachycardia was induced (Figure 5.9) (Lown & DeSilva 1978).

Control

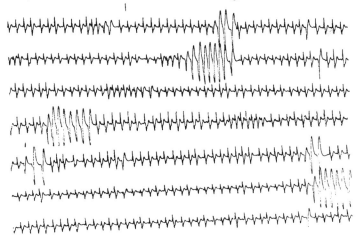

Psychologic Stress Testing

FIG. 5.9. In patient with oft recurring ventricular fibrillation, peripheral autonomic neural manipulation was without effect on arrhythmia. However, psychologic stress testing involving recall of painful past experiences provoked paroxysms of ventricular tachycardia (note concomitant acceleration in rate and development of bundle branch block in trendscription record). (From Lown & DeSilva, 1978)

Educational level has an important psychosocial significance because lack of education is socially handicapping and prevents upward mobility in a technological society. Kitagawa and Hauser (1973) have already shown an inverse relationship between cardiovascular mortality and educational level. Recognizing that the level of education has an important psychosocial impact, Weinblatt et al. (1978) stratified 1739 survivors into categories distinguished by years of schooling. When these men were electrocardiographically monitored for one hour, men with 8 years or less of schooling, exhibited 3 times the risk of SCD if complex ventricular arrhythmias were present. In contrast, better educated men with the same type of arrhythmia had a significantly lower mortality. The cumulative mortality rates were 33% and 9%, respectively for the two groups. Neither standard risk factors nor a variety of clinical characteristics accounted for these differences.

The mechanisms whereby induced or naturally-occurring stresses cause ventricular arrhythmias have been inadequately studied. Taggart et al. (1969) have shown that catecholamine levels are elevated when VPBs occur during psychological stress resulting from car-racing. They were able to abolish stress-induced VPBs with the beta-adrenergic antagonist, oxprenolol. These observations suggest the involvement of the sympatho-adrenal system in stress-induced arrhythmias.

Behavioral Studies

If we assume that certain individuals have a proclivity for psychophysiologically induced arrhythmias, it is logical to examine whether certain behavioral or psychological characteristics predispose to the development of ventricular arrhythmias and SCD. Such studies are lacking for SCD but a similar approach has already been applied to a variety of diseases. Thomas (1976), for example, prospectively evaluated healthy medical students and found that certain features such as nervous tension, anxiety, anger under stress, insomnia, smoking, and alcohol intake were associated with a higher rate of premature death and disease. These precursors were evaluated in relation to the development of suicide, cancer, hypertension, myocardial infarction and mental illness. Thomas (1976) noted that mean depression scores were twice as high in those developing myocardial infarction as in controls.

Depression has been ascribed some importance in relation to sudden death by some investigators. Physicians attending cardiac patients have often noted depression as a precursor to sudden death. Greene et al. (1972) reported in a study where the next-of-kin were interviewed that victims of SCD had a high prevalence of depression and agitation prior to death. A prospective study by Bruhn, Paredes, Adsett, and Wolf (1974) in patients with myocardial infarction indicated that elevated depression scores, a pattern of "joyless striving" at work and Type A behavior characteristics correlated with the occurrence of SCD.

We found, using a variety of psychometric tests, that 25 of 117 patients had identifiable psychophysiologic triggers for VT and VF (Reich et al. 1981). No specific psychological characteristics were apparent except for an exceptionally high depression score. It must be noted, however, that such patients were studied after referral for life-threatening arrhythmias and the presence of depression may have been the consequence rather than a precipitating factor in their illness.

Sleep Studies

Clinical investigations of the effects of sleep on ventricular arrhythmias have yielded conflicting results. Some observers have noted that during sleep VPBs are not affected, while others have observed VPB suppression during sleep (Brodksy et al. 1977, DeSilva, Regestein, & Lown, unpublished observations, Lown, Tykocinski, Garfein, & Brooks 1973, Monti et al. 1975, Pickering, Goulding, & Cobern, 1977; Pickering, Johnston, & Honour, 1978, Rosenblatt et al. 1969, Smith et al. 1972, Winkle et al. 1975). It is of interest that in studies showing little effect of sleep on VPBs or an actual increase in arrhythmia, only small numbers of subjects were used. The patients were also studied in the medicated state or while in the coronary care unit. In studies involving larger numbers of subjects, the results indicate that sleep suppresses VPBs (Brodsky et al. 1977, DeSilva et al. unpublished observations, Lown et al. 1973, Monti et al. 1975, Pickering et al 1977, 1978, Rosenblatt et al. 1969, Smith et al. 1972, Winkle et al. 1975). Lown et al. (1973) observed during Holter monitoring of 54 subjects in their own homes, that VPBs in 22 subjects were reduced at least 50% during sleep, while 13 showed 25–50% decrease. The grade of VPBs was also lowered from a mean of 2.75 while awake to 1.78 during sleep. In several of these patients, antiarrhythmic drugs were less effective than sleep in reducing the grade and frequency of VPBs.

Further investigation in 30 patients indicated that amelioration of VPBs occurred during all sleep stages except REM sleep (DeSilva et al. unpublished observations). Slow wave sleep (Stages 3 & 4) had the most significant effect on VPB suppression. These results differ from those of Rosenblatt et al. (1969) who found an augmentation of arrhythmias during these stages. Frequency of VPBs during awake and REM periods were similar, suggesting that the electrical properties of the heart during these two periods may also be similar. Pickering et al. (1977) reported that in 26% of 31 patients, VPBs were suppressed almost completely during sleep, while in 71% the reduction in VPBs was partial. Multiform and repetitive VPBs were also decreased during sleep. Available evidence in man indicates that non-REM sleep decreases ventricular ectopic activity whereas REM sleep exerts the opposite effect.

Biofeedback, Relaxation Techniques, and Ventricular Arrhythmias

Conscious modulation of sympathetic neural input to the heart may be accomplished by a variety of biofeedback and relaxation techniques. Weiss and Engel (1971) and Pickering and Miller (1977) have shown that VPBs can be suppressed by increasing heart rate with biofeedback. Abolition of VPBs is probably secondary to overdrive suppression of an ectopic focus as a result of acceleration in heart rate. Meditation and relaxation techniques have also been utilized to suppress VPBs. The essential cardiovascular effect of cultic and non-cultic forms of meditation is reduction in heart rate and blood pressure, effects which are probably secondary to decreased sympathetic neural outflow.

Eleven patients with CHD were taught by Benson et al. (1975) to elicit the relaxation response over a period of four weeks. Though VPBs were moderately suppressed during both awake and sleep periods, this effect was significant only during the latter period. Heart rate was not significantly affected by the procedure. Voukydis and Forwand (1977) found that VPBs were reduced by a similar technique in some patients whereas in others, arrhythmia was unaffected or actually increased. Davidson et al. (1979) correlated heart rate decreases with changes in plasma norepinephrine during relaxation therapy. In this study, group means for heart rate did not change significantly between control and relaxation periods.

FINAL COMMENTS

Studies in experimental animals have provided cogent evidence of the potent influence of psychophysiologic factors in altering the stability of cardiac rhythm (Figure 5.10). Psychological stresses of diverse types have been shown to lower the vulnerable period threshold and in the presence of acute myocardial ischemia they can trigger ventricular fibrillation. While the precise neural pathways and neurohumoral mechanisms which alter ventricular vulnerability remain to be defined, the prominent role of the sympathetic nervous system is already firmly established.

While definitive studies establishing a link between behavioral factors and the occurrence of malignant arrhythmias in man are yet lacking, the available data are consonant with the view emerging from the experimental laboratory. Specifically, there is growing epidemiologic data and biobehavioral studies in human subjects suggesting a relationship between psychophysiologic inputs and life-threatening arrhythmias. Current estimates indicate acute psychophysiologic events to be antecedent of sudden cardiac death in about 20 to 40% of cases. Since 450,000 Americans die suddenly every year, the toll of death potentially

INTERACTIONS BETWEEN PSYCOLOGIC VARIABLES
AND MYOCARDIAL ELECTRICAL INSTABILITY

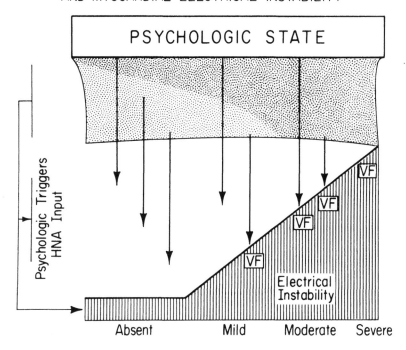

FIG. 5.10.   At least three factors are implicated in the genesis of psychologically provoked ventricular fibrillation; namely, electrical instability of the myocardium, presence of a predisposing psychologic state, and operation of psychologic trigger factors. When electrical instability is absent, as shown at left of figure, neither psychologic state nor trigger can induce ventricular fibrillation. At the opposite and of the spectrum, wherein electrical instability is marked, as shown at right, psychologic inputs are unnecessary. In the intermediate zone an interplay of these three factors determines occurrence of the lethal arrhythmia. (From Lown et al., 1982)

related directly or indirectly to stress is thus of an imposing magnitude. These observations lead naturally to the suggestion that it is not too early to turn to protective interventions, rather than to continue to reiterate the interesting but potentially self-limiting theme that certain psychologic factors may trigger ventricular fibrillation. How can we protect the heart by neurobiologic intervention? What is the appropriate therapeutic role of pharmacologic or surgical blockade of the autonomic nervous system? Can sedative medications be employed effectively? Would dietary intervention alter central neuroendocrine function sufficiently to afford any beneficial effects? These avenues of research seem highly promising and merit vigorous pursuit.

ACKNOWLEDGMENTS

Supported in part by Grants No. HL-07776 and HL-28387 from the National Heart, Lung and Blood Institute, National Institutes of Health, Bethesda, Maryland 20205

REFERENCES

Baccelli, G., Guazzi, M., Mancia, G., and Zanchetti, A. Neural and non-neural mechanisms influencing circulation during sleep. *Nature*, 1969, *223*, 184–185.

Baust, W., Bohnert, B., & Riemann, O. The regulation of the heart rate during sleep. *Electroencephalography and Clinical Neurophysiology*, 1969, 27:626.

Baust, W., Bohnert, B. The regulation of heart rate during sleep. *Experimental Brain Research*, 1969, *7*, 169–180.

Benson, H., Alexander, S., and Feldman, C. L. Decreased premature ventricular contractions through the use of the relaxation response in patients with stable ischemic heart disease. *Lancet*, 1975, *2*, 380.

Bond, D. D. Sympathetic and vagal interaction in emotional responses of the heart rate. *American Journal of Physiology*, 1942, *138*, 468–478.

Brodsky, M., Wu, D., Denes, P., Kanakiz, C., and Rosen, K. M. Arrhythmias documented by 24 hour continuous electrocardiographic monitoring in 50 male medical students without apparent heart disease. *American Journal of Cardiology*, 1977, *39*, 390–395.

Bruhn, J. G., Paredes, A., Adsett, C. A., Wolf, S. Psychological predictors of sudden death in myocardial infarction. *Journal of Psychosomatic Research*, 1974, *18*, 187–191.

Cannon, W. B. Voodoo death. *American Anthropologist*, 1942, *44*, 169–181.

Chiang, B. N., Perlman, L. V., Fulton, M., Ostrander, L. D., Jr., and Epstein, F. H. Predisposing factors in sudden cardiac death in Tecumseh, Michigan: A prospective study. *Circulation*, 1970, *41*, 31–38.

Cobb, L. A., Baum, R. S., Alvarez, H. A, III, and Schaffer, W. A. Resuscitation from out-of-hospital ventricular fibrillation: Four years follow-up. *Circulation*, 1975, 51–52 (suppl 3):223–235.

Coccagna, G., Mantovani, M., Brignani, F., Manzini, A., and Lugaresi, E. Arterial pressure changes during spontaneous sleep in man. *Electroencephalography and Clinical Neurophysiology*, 1971, *31*, 277–281.

Cohen, D. H., & Pitts, L. H. Vagal and sympathetic components of conditioned cardioacceleration in the pigeon. *Brain Research*, 1968, *9*, 15–31.

Corbalan, R., Verrier, R., & Lown, B. Psychological stress and ventricular arrhythmias during myocardial infarction in the conscious dog. *American Journal of Cardiology*, 1974, *34*, 692–696.

Corley, K. C., Mauck, H. P., & Shiel, F. O. M. Cardiac responses associated with "Yoked-Chair" shock avoidance in squirrel monkeys. *Psychophysiology*, 1975, *12*, 439–444.

Corr, P. B., & Gillis, R. A. Role of the vagus nerves in the cardiovascular changes induced by coronary occlusion. *Circulation*, 1974, *49*, 86–97.

Corr, P. B., Pearle, D. L., & Gillis, R. A. Coronary occlusion site as a determinant of the cardiac rhythm effects of atropine and vagotomy. *American Heart Journal*, 1976, *92*, 741–749.

Croce, L., Noseda, V., Bertelli, A., and Bossi, E. Sudden and unexpected death from heart disease. *Cardiologia*, 1960, *37*, 331–360.

Davidson, D. M., Winchester, M. A., Taylor, C. B., Alderman, E. A., and Ingels, N. B., Jr. Effects of relaxation therapy on cardiac performance and sympathetic activity in patients with organic heart disease. *Psychosomatic Medicine*, 1979, *41*, 303–309.

DeSilva, R. A., Regestein, Q. R., & Lown, B. Unpublished observations.

DeSilva, R. A., Verrier, R. L., & Lown, B. The effects of psychological stress and vagal stimulation with morphine on vulnerability to ventricular fibrillation (VF) in the conscious dog. *American Heart Journal*, 1978, *95*, 197–203.

Doyle, J. T., Kannel, W. B., McNamara, P. M., Quickenton, P., and Gordon, T. Factors related to suddenness of death from coronary disease: combined Albany-Framingham studies. *American Journal of Cardiology*, 1976, *37*, 1073–1078.

Greene, H. L., Reid, P. R., & Schaeffer, A. H. The repetitive ventricular response in man: A predictor of sudden death. *New England Journal of Medicine*, 1978, *299*, 729–734.

Greene, W. A., Goldstein, S., & Moss, A. J. Psychosocial aspects of sudden death. *Archives of Internal Medicine*, 1972, *129*, 725–731.

James, R. G. G., Arnold, J. M. O., Allen, J. D., Pantridge, J. F., & Shanks, R. G. The effects of heart rate, myocardial ischemia and vagal stimulation on the threshold for ventricular fibrillation. *Circulation*, 1977, *55*, 311–317.

Johansson, G., Jonsson, L., Lannek, N., Blomgren, L., Lindberg, P., & Poupa, O. Severe stress-cardiopathy in pigs. *American Heart Journal*, 1974, *87*, 451–457.

Jouvet, M. Biogenic amines and the states of sleep. *Science*, 1969, *163*, 32–41.

Kannel, W. B., Dawber, T. R., & McNamara, P. M. Detection of the coronary-prone adult: the Framingham study. *Journal of the Iowa Medical Society*, 1966, *56*, 26–34.

Kent, K. M., Smith, E. R., Redwood, D. R., & Epstein, S. E. Electrical stability of acutely ischemic myocardium: Influences of heart rate and vagal stimulation. *Circulation*, 1973, *47*, 291–298.

Kerzner, J., Wolf, M., Kosowsky, B. D., & Lown, B. Ventricular ectopic rhythms following vagal stimulation in dogs with acute myocardial infarction. *Circulation*, 1973, *47*, 44–50.

Kitagawa, E. M., & Hauser, P. M. *Differential mortality in the United States. A study in socioeconomic epidemiology.* Cambridge, Mass, Harvard University Press, 1973, 11–33, 78–79.

Kleitman, N. *Sleep and Wakefulness.* Chicago, University of Chicago Press, 1963.

Koella, W. P., Feldstein, A., and Czicman, J. S. The effect of parachlorophenylalanine on the sleep of cats. *Electroencephalography and Clinical Neurophysiology*, 1968, *25*, 481–490.

Kolman, B. S., Verrier, R. L., & Lown, B. The effect of vagus nerve stimulation upon vulnerability of the canine ventricle: Role of sympathetic-parasympathetic interactions. *Circulation*, 1975, *52*, 578–585.

Kuller, L., Lilienfeld, A., & Fisher, R. An epidemiological study of sudden and unexpected deaths in adults. *Medicine*, 1967, *46*, 341–361.

Kuller, L. Sudden and unexpected nontraumatic deaths in adults: a review of epidemiological and clinical studies. *Journal of Chronic Diseases*, 1966, *19*, 1165–1192.

Levy, A. G. The genesis of ventricular extrasystoles under chloroform; with special reference to consecutive ventricular fibrillation. *Heart*, 1913–1914, *5*, 299–334.

Levy, M. N., & Blattberg, B. Effect of vagal stimulation on the overflow of norepinephrine into the coronary sinus during cardiac sympathetic nerve stimulation in the dog. *Circulation Research*, 1976, *38*, 81–85.

Liang, B., Verrier, R. L., Melman, J., and Lown, B. Correlation between circulating catecholamine levels and ventricular vulnerability during psychological stress in conscious dogs. *Proceedings of the Society for Experimental Biology and Medicine*, 1979, *161*, 266–269.

Lown, B., & DeSilva, R. A. Roles of psychologic stress and autonomic nervous system changes in provocation of ventricular premature complexes. *American Journal of Cardiology*, 1978, *41*, 979–985.

Lown, B., Kosowsky, B. D., & Klein, M. D. Pathogenesis, prevention and treatment of arrhythmias in myocardial infarction. *Circulation*, 1969, *39–40* (Suppl 4), 261–270.

Lown, B., Temte, J. V., Reich, P., Gaughan, C., Regestein, Q., & Hai, H. Basis for recurring ventricular fibrillation in the absence of coronary heart disease and its management. *New England Journal of Medicine*, 1976, *294*, 623–629.

Lown, B., Tykocinski, M., Garfein, A., and Brooks, P. Sleep and ventricular premature beats. *Circulation*, 1973, *48*, 691–701.

Lown, B., Verrier, R., & Corbalan, R. Psychologic stress and threshold for repetitive ventricular response. *Science*, 1973, *182*, 834–836.

Lown, B., Verrier, R. L., & Rabinowitz, S. H. Neural and psychologic mechanisms and the problem of sudden cardiac death. *American Journal of Cardiology*, 1977, *39*, 890–902.

Lown, B., & Verrier, R. L. Neural activity and ventricular fibrillation. *New England Journal of Medicine*, 1976, *294*, 1165–1170.

Lown, B., & Verrier, R. L. Neural and psychologic factors and the occurrence of ventricular fibrillation. In Riemersma, R., & Oliver, M. F. (Eds.), *Catecholamines in the Non-Ischaemic and Ischaemic myocardium*. Elsevier Biomedical Press, 1982.

Lown, B., & Wolf, M. Approaches to sudden death from coronary heart disease. *Circulation*, 1971, *44*, 130–142.

Lown, B. Sudden cardiac death: the major challenge confronting contemporary cardiology. *American Journal of Cardiology*, 1979, *43*, 313–328.

Lown, B. Sudden death from coronary artery disease. In Waldenstrom, J., Larsson, T., & Ljungstedt, N. (Eds.), *Early Phases of Coronary Heart Disease*. Stockholm: Nordiska Bokhandelns Forlag, 1973:255–277.

McWilliam, J. A. Fibrillar contraction of the heart. *Journal of Physiology* (London) 1887, *8*, 296–310.

Mason, J. W., Winkle, R. A. Electrode-catheter arrhythmia induction in the selection and assessment of antiarrhythmic drug therapy for recurrent ventricular tachycardia. *Circulation*, 1978, *58*, 971–985.

Matta, R. J., Lawler, J., & Lown, B. Ventricular electrical instability in the conscious dog: Effects of psychologic stress and beta-adrenergic blockade. *American Journal of Cardiology*, 1976, *38*, 594–598.

Matta, R. J., Verrier, R. L., Lown, B. Repetitive extrasystole as an index of vulnerability to ventricular fibrillation. *American Journal of Physiology*, 1976, *230*, 1469–1473.

Monti, J. M., Folle, L. E., Peluffo, C., Artuchio, R., Ortiz, A., Sevrini, O., and Dighiero, J. The incidence of premature contractions in coronary patients during the sleep-awake cycle. *Cardiology*, 1975, *60*, 257–264.

Myers, A., & Dewar, H. A. Circumstances attending 100 sudden deaths from coronary artery disease with coroner's necropsies. *British Heart Journal*, 1975, *37*, 1133–1143.

Perper, J. A., Kuller, L. H., & Cooper, M. Arteriosclerosis of coronary arteries in sudden, unexpected deaths. *Circulation*, 1975, 51–52 (suppl 3), 27–33.

Pickering, T. G., Goulding, L., & Cobern, B. A. Diurnal variations in ventricular ectopic beats and heart rate. *Cardiovascular Medicine*, 1977, *2*, 1013–1022.

Pickering, T. G., Johnston, J., & Honour, A. J. Comparison of the effects of sleep, exercise and autonomic drugs on ventricular extrasystoles, using ambulatory monitoring of electrocardiogram and electroencephalogram. *American Journal of Medicine* 1978, *65*, 575–583.

Pickering, T. G., & Miller, N. E. Learned voluntary control of heart rate and rhythm in two subjects with premature ventricular contractions. *British Heart Journal*, 1977, *39*, 152–159.

Podrid, P. J., Schoeneberger, A., Lown, B., Matos, J., Porterfield, J., & Corrigan, E. Programmed premature stimulation as a guide to antiarrhythmic therapy for malignant ventricular arrhythmia in the absence of ambient ectopy. *American Journal of Cardiology*, 1981, *47*, 497.

Raab, W., Chaplin, J. P., & Bajusz, E. Myocardial necroses produced in domesticated rats and in wild rats by sensory and emotional stresses. *Proceedings of the Society for Experimental Biology and Medicine*, 1964, *116*, 665–669.

Raab, W. Emotional and sensory stress factors in myocardial pathology: neurogenic and humoral mechanisms in pathogenesis, therapy and prevention. *American Heart Journal,* 1966, *72,* 538–564.

Rabinowitz, S. H., Verrier, R. L., Lown, B. Muscarinic effects of vagosympathetic trunk stimulation on the repetitive extrasystole (RE) threshold. *Circulation,* 1976, *53,* 622–627.

Reich, P., DeSilva, R. A., Lown, B., & Murawski, B. J. Acute psychological disturbances preceding life-threatening ventricular arrhythmias. *Journal of the American Medical Association,* 1981, *246,* 233–235.

Reite, M. L., Pegram, G. V., Stephens, L. M., Bixler, E. C., & Lewis, O. L. The effect of reserpine and monoamine oxidase inhibitors on paradoxical sleep in the monkey. *Psychopharmacologia* (Berl.) 14, 12–17 (1969).

Richter, C. P. On the phenomenon of sudden death in animals and man. *Psychosomatic Medicine,* 1957, *19,* 191–198.

Rissanen, V., Romo, M., & Siltanen, P. Premonitory symptoms and stress factors preceding sudden death from ischaemic heart disease. *Acta Medica Scandinavica,* 1978, *204,* 389–396.

Rosenblatt, G., Zwilling, G., Hartmann, E. Electrocardiographic changes during sleep in patients with cardiac abnormalities. *Psychophysiology,* 1969, *6,* 233.

Rosenfeld, J., Rosen, M. R., Hoffman, B. F. Pharmacologic and behavioral effects on arrhythmias that immediately follow abrupt coronary occlusion: A canine model of sudden coronary death. *American Journal of Cardiology,* 1978, *41,* 1075–1082.

Rushmer, R. F., Smith, A. O., & Lasher, E. P. Neural mechanisms of cardiac control during exertion. *Physiological Reviews,* 1960, Suppl. 4, 27–34.

Schwartz, C., & Walsh, W. J. The pathologic basis of sudden death. *Progress in Cardiovascular Diseases,* 1971, *13,* 465–481.

Skinner, J. E., Lie, J. T., & Entman, M. L. Modification of ventricular fibrillation latency following coronary artery occlusion in the conscious pig: the effects of psychological stress and beta-adrenergic blockade. *Circulation,* 1975, *51,* 656–667.

Skinner, J. E., Mohr, D. N., & Kellaway, P. Sleep-stage regulation of ventricular arrhythmias in the unanesthetized pig. *Circulation Research* 1975, *37,* 342–349.

Skinner, J. E., & Reed, J. C. Blockade of a frontocortical-brain stem pathway prevents ventricular fibrillation of ischemic heart. *American Journal of Physiology,* 1981, *240,* H156–H163.

Smith, O. A., Jabbur, S. J., Rushmer, R. F., and Lasher, E. P. Role of hypothalamic structures in cardiac control. *Physiological Reviews,* 1960, Suppl. *4,* 136–141.

Smith, R., Johnson, L., Rothfeld, D., Zir, L., and Tharp, B. Sleep and cardiac arrhythmias. *Archives of Internal Medicine,* 1972, *130,* 751–753.

Snyder, F., Hobson, J. A., & Goldfrank, F. Blood pressure changes during human sleep. *Science,* 1963, *142,* 1313–1314.

Spain, D. M., & Bradess, V. A. Sudden death from coronary heart disease. *Chest,* 1970, *58,* 107–110.

Spain, D. M. Anatomical basis for sudden cardiac death. In *Sudden Cardiac Death,* B. Surawicz, & E. D. Pellegrino (Eds.). New York: Grune & Stratton, 1964, p. 16.

Taggart, P., Carruthers, M., & Somerville, W. Electrocardiogram, plasma catecholamines and lipids, and their modification by oxprenolol when speaking before an audience. *Lancet,* 1973, *2,* 341–346.

Taggart, P., Gibbons, D., & Somerville, W. Some effects of motor-car driving on the normal and abnormal heart. *British Medical Journal,* 1969, *4,* 130–134.

Thomas, C. B. Precursors of premature disease and death: The predictive potential of habits and family attitudes. *Annals of Internal Medicine,* 1976, *85,* 653–658.

Verrier, R. L., Lombardi, F., & Lown, B. Effects of differing types of behavioral stress on coronary hemodynamics and ventricular vulnerability. *Fed. Proc.,* 1982, *41,* 1599.

Verrier, R. L., Lombardi, F., & Lown, B. Restraint of myocardial blood flow during behavioral stress. *Circulation,* 1982, *66* (Suppl. II): 258.

Verrier, R. L., Lown, B. Effects of left stellectomy on enhanced cardiac vulnerability induced by psychologic stress. *Circulation,* 1977, *55/56,* III–80.

Verrier, R. L., & Lown, B. Vagal tone and ventricular vulnerability during psychologic stress. *Circulation,* 1980, *62,* (Suppl. III): 176.

Verrier, R. L., & Lown, B. Influence of neural activity on ventricular electrical instability during acute myocardial ischemia and infarction. In: E. Sandoe, D. G. Julian, & J. W. Bell (Eds.), *Management of Ventricular Tachycardia-Role of Mexiletine.* Amsterdam: Excerpta Medica, 1978, 133–150.

Verrier, R. L., & Lown, B. Influence of psychologic stress on susceptibility to spontaneous ventricular fibrillation during acute myocardial ischemia and reperfusion. *Clinical Research,* 1979, *27,* 570A.

Verrier, J. L., & Lown, B. Sympathetic-parasympathetic interactions and ventricular electrical stability. In P. J. Schwartz, A. M. Brown, A. Malliani, & A. Zanchetti (Eds.), *Neural Mechanisms in Cardiac Arrhythmias.* New York: Raven Press, 1978, 75–85.

Voukydis, P. C., & Forwand, S. A. The effect of elicitation of the relaxation response in patients with intractable ventricular arrhythmias. *Circulation,* 1977, *55 & 56* (Suppl III): 157.

Watanabe, A. M., Besch, H. R. Interaction between cyclic adenosine monophosphate and cyclic guanosine monophosphate in guinea pig ventricular myocardium. *Circulation Research,* 1975, *37,* 309–317.

Weinblatt, E., Ruberman, W., Goldberg, J. D., Frank, C. W., Shapiro, S., and Chaudhary, B. S. Relation of education to sudden death after myocardial infarction. *New England Journal of Medicine,* 1978, *299,* 60–65.

Weinblatt, E., Shapiro, S., Frank, C. W., and Sager, R. V. Prognosis of men after first myocardial infarction. *American Journal of Public Health,* 1968, *58,* 1329–1347.

Weiss, T., & Engel, B. T. Operant conditioning of the heart in patients with premature ventricular contractions. *Psychosomatic Medicine,* 1971, *33,* 301.

Wellens, H. J. J., Vermeulen, A., & Durrer, D. Ventricular fibrillation occurring on arousal from sleep by auditory stimuli. *Circulation,* 1972, *46,* 661–665.

Wikland, B. Death from arteriosclerotic heart disease outside hospitals. *Acta Medica Scandinavica,* 1968, *184,* 129–133.

Winkle, R. A., Lopes, M. G., & Fitzgerald, J. W., et al. Arrhythmias in patients with mitral valve prolapse. *Circulation,* 1975, *52,* 73.

Yoon, M. S., Han, J., Tse, W. W., & Rogers, R. Effects of vagal stimulation, atropine, and propranolol on fibrillation threshold of normal and ischemic ventricles. *American Heart Journal,* 1977, *93,* 60–65.

6 Animal Models of Hypertension

Robert J. Campbell
James P. Henry
University of Southern California School of Medicine

GENERAL INTRODUCTION

Studies concerning the initiation, development, and maintenance of high blood pressure in animals provide much needed insight into the pathophysiology of this disease in the human population. They have been of significant benefit for understanding the various mechanisms which are of importance at different points along the course of the disorder called essential hypertension, which accounts for about 90% of the occurrence of an elevated blood pressure in humans. The etiology of human essential hypertension is, at worst, unknown, and, at best, characterized by an amalgam of current schools of thought. Thus, the contributions of each of the more well-defined animal models to determination of underlying causes should not be overlooked in terms of their applicability to studies of physiological mechanisms operating in essential hypertension.

Just as essential hypertension may be broken down by reductionist thinking into a number of coincident mechanisms of varying importance, so too can the techniques employed in producing elevated blood pressure in an animal model vary widely. Accordingly, they range, at one extreme, from the purely physical manipulation of direct interference with renal blood supply or the chemical intervention of changing the balance in ionic equilibria, to the purely psychological manipulation of introducing some type of noxious stimuli to a sensitive animal's environment. Running between these extremes are a number of other interventions in the animal's cardiovascular homeostasis. Also included along this range of models are the breeding manipulations involving spontaneous occurrence of an elevated blood pressure, or susceptibility to such, representing genetic selection for mechanisms possibly the same as, or similar to, one or more of the above. Furthermore, it appears that the physiological end results of the various techniques are interdependent, and in many cases involve the same communication pathways for information flow within the body.

The predisposition for human essential hypertension is carried polygenetically (Pickering, 1968), implying that more than one simple mechanism is involved in a sustained elevation of blood pressure. Rather, this is apparently brought on by the interaction of environmental influences with genetically linked predisposing factors. The utility of approaching the study of this disorder along homeostatically correlated but mechanistically different avenues in animal models is evidenced by the information and directions generated by a large number of independent investigations. Each of the models within the wide spectrum of experimental appraches to hypertension research provides food for thought concerning the multiple etiologic elements related to cardiovascular homeostasis that are likely to be involved in human essential hypertension.

Not all of the various models of hypertension will be detailed, but only those that are relevant to our behavioral orientation. Two have been selected for their particular interest, their respective genetic and psychosocial causation appearing to represent imcompatible opposites. Nevertheless, it will develop that the same excessive and prolonged activation of the neurohumoral controls of the cardiovascular system is important for the development of hypertension in both.

ADVANTAGES OF ANIMAL MODELS

The development of experimental techniques for inducing the hypertensive disease state in animals has demonstrated that animal studies offer certain advantages not possible in human studies. For example, the compressed life-span of infrahuman species, especially rodents, allows a survey to cover all stages of the disease in a short time, or even to follow its occurrence from generation to generation. In animals, one can investigate the etiologic aspects of the hypertension by manipulating separate variables relevant to the course of this disorder. Many times, this necessitates a manner of biological intervention, such as surgery, withholding drug therapy, behavioral constructs, etc., which would be impossible or unethical in man.

This brings up another point—the ability to control both genetic and environmental variables. When an investigator can establish conditions that will generate development of hypertensive pathophysiology in a laboratory animal, he does not have to wait for the elevated blood pressure to appear and then attempt to determine if a particular factor had been important. Instead, he can introduce that factor as a controlled variable and see if it does indeed influence the point of initiation or course of development of the disease. Experimentally controlled conditions include such factors as nutritional state and diet, social interaction, genetic composition, and pharmacological input, among others.

Finally, animal models of hypertension permit relatively more straightforward physiological and behavioral access for experimental analysis of individual components of cardiovascular homeostasis in a simpler approach toward the more complex problem that is human essential hypertension.

CATEGORIZATION OF THE VARIOUS MODELS

In the 45 years since the development of the renal ischemia model of hypertension in dogs by Goldblatt and his co-workers (Goldblatt, Lynch, Hanzal, & Summerville, 1934), the search for experimental animal models of human essential hypertension has uncovered a number and variety of models far beyond the scope of this chapter, and outside its behavioral orientation. The bulk of the chapter will concentrate on animal models of essential hypertension applicable to the study of the cognitively mediated interactions of the individual with his environment, that is, of the neuroendocrine changes that result from the interpretation by the brain of stimuli usually based on the circumstances in which they are presented. Of relevance here will be models which appear useful for experimental examination of the contribution of this interaction to idiopathic development or maintenance of a sustained elevation of blood pressure in humans. Other articles, reviews, and chapter subsections with information regarding animal models of hypertension have been published (Carretero & Romero, 1977; Folkow & Hallbäck, 1977; Weiner, 1979). For more details regarding aspects such as production, or characteristics of various types of models, or methodology of blood pressure measurement, the reader is directed to the broader reviews or to the original papers referenced in this chapter or in the publications cited above.

For the purpose of outlining a chapter on animal models of hypertension it is useful, as a tool for organization, to categorize the models according to origin. In this manner, for example, one such categorization could be hypertension of neural origin. This would include an increased blood pressure brought on by (1) direct electrophysiological or biochemical stimulation of certain areas of the central nervous system, (2) stimulation or denervation of afferent or efferent pathways involved in cardiovascular regulation by the autonomic nervous system, or (3) psychological stimulation acting by sensory or cognitive input to the central nervous system.

Another category could be hypertension of endocrine hormonal origin. This would include induction of blood pressure elevation by (1) administration of adrenocortical steroids or their pharmacological analogs, (2) large dietary intakes of NaCl, (3) combinations of (1) and (2) and sometimes including interventions described under hypertension of renal origin which follows, and (4) endogenous over-production of adrenocortical steroids due to adrenal regeneration or presence of an ACTH-producing or a catecholamine-producing tumor.

Finally, the category hypertension of renal origin would include such experimental elevations of blood pressure as are produced by (1) constriction of a renal artery, with or without removal of the contra-lateral kidney (i.e., unilateral nephrectomy), (2) occlusion of both renal arteries or of the aorta just above the renal arteries, or (3) damage of renal parenchymas by external wrap-compression, bacterial infection, or other insult.

The temptation is always there to rely on such a classification as an adequate division to simplify matters of discussion. However, there is an ever-increasing body of experimental findings in these models which suggests that animal models can not be so simply separated. Neurogenic hypertension is a case in point. Although its origin is in fact neural, the mechanisms involved could include either or both of the other two categories above, through neural influence on endocrine and renal function. The degree of interaction is at present unknown, such that a proper classification here could well be termed "mixed." Or consider, for example, a hypothetical experimental hypertension of "renal origin." Here, an event triggered in the kidney might in turn feed back to the central nervous system via a blood-borne or neural message, or both, to initiate a particular cardiovascular operation aimed at restoring homeostasis. Should this model be categorized as distinct from, and perhaps studied differently than, a hypothetical experimental hypertension of "neural origin," or one of "hormonal origin," which interacts with the cardiovascular system in much the same way?

ADEQUACY OF PRIMARY VS. SECONDARY HYPERTENSIVE ANIMAL MODELS

It seems likely that the development of essential hypertension in humans, especially when viewed against a mosaic background, as described by Page (1974), is associated with neural, renal, and hormonal factors contributing differentially along the course of this disease. In order for blood pressure to remain elevated, more than one mechanism involved in its regulation must be disturbed. Why?—In people with normal blood pressure, a perturbation of one of the components of either cardiac output or total peripheral resistance quickly sets in motion homeostatic adjustments in other components returning arterial pressure towards normal. This suggests that, in essential hypertension, some dominant control mechanism, such as the central nervous system, is able to drive any or all of the factors within the mosaic enough to maintain an increased blood pressure for some operational reason, albeit maladaptive. In recent years, two main hypotheses have stood out from this background as regards primary mechanisms involved in the pathogenesis of this disease. The first of these considers an increase in excitatory drive to the cardiovascular system, presumably of central origin, to be the initiating influence. Resulting constriction of the resistance vessels is followed by structural adaptation, which in effect narrows these vessels and reduces diastolic compliance of the heart, both through simple muscle hypertrophy in response to local pressure load (Folkow, 1978, 1982). The second hypothesis attributes to the kidney an initiating role in hypertension development, disregarding any primary stimulus occurring via the nervous system. It considers as the overriding causative event an inability of dysfunctional renal mechanisms to deal with sodium intake, with consequent elevation of fluid volume, cardiac output, and, eventually, peripheral resistance (Guyton, Coleman, Cowley, Scheel, Manning, & Norman, 1972).

On closer appraisal, these two hypotheses are not mutually exclusive, nor necessarily incompatible. This is suggested by the key role played by neurohormonal influence on kidney function. For example, increased sympathoadrenal input to the kidney, triggered centrally by repeated or chronic induction of cortical-limbic-hypothalamic alerting reactions may have a profound effect on both vascular and tubular renal mechanisms. Included here would be reduction of renal blood flow, increased renin secretion, among other effects. If these processes are influenced to a sufficient extent, renal ability to handle salt and fluid balance may be impaired. Reduction of fluid excretion would ultimately result in increased blood volume, aggravating the initial vasoconstriction. The hypertrophic and degenerative changes in heart muscle, paralleling the functional reduction in compliance, might allow resetting of the cardiac volume sensors (low pressure receptors) toward higher pressure levels. Decreased inhibition by this depressor reflex system could further reduce the fluid-excreting capacity of the kidney.

This likelihood of involvement of neurohormonal control mechanisms in generation of the essential hypertensive disorder implies that the more an animal model fits this description, the more appropriate that particular model is for study and potential understanding of the hypertensive disease processes. Many view the expression of the final cardiovascular disorder as comprising three separate but interacting parts in a complex, homeostatically controlled system: (1) a genetically predisposing capacity or constitution of an individual animal, determining its behavioral and physiological reactivity, (2) developmental determinants and ongoing environmental stimuli influencing that reactivity through cognitive processing, and (3) secondary adjustments in both (1) and (2) through mechanisms such as behavioral coping responses, physiological feedback regulation of associated processes, etc. It is appropriate, then, that any animal preparation proposed as an adequate model for essential hypertension also exhibits a somewhat similar background, insofar as another species' behavior relates to human behavior.

PREFERRED CHARACTERISTICS OF AN "IDEAL"
MODEL

Let us assume that an interaction between environment and cardiovascular controls systems is an inherent prerequisite for development of hypertension. Reactivity of cardiovascular control systems would be a measure of activation for those cognitive events mediating the interaction between environment and physiological response. Is there a difference then, in terms of end-organ response in the hypertensive cardiovascular system disorder, between: (1) a model in which the animal is genetically selected to respond with a relatively high cardiovascular control system reactivity of, say 5, to some set of environmental factors at a relatively low or normal intensity of 1, and (2) a model in which the non-predisposed animal responding at a relatively low or normal cardiovascular control system reactivity value of 1 is subjected to a set of environmental factors at a relatively high intensity of 5?

It would be helpful to have a mathematically stated theoretical relationship describing the influence of environment and central cardiovascular reactivity on development of hypertension. A strictly defined mathematical formulation similar to that quantitating the dependence of arterial pressure on the interaction of cardiac output (CO) and total peripheral resistance (TPR), i.e., $BP = CO \times TPR$, is not possible. However, an analogous treatment at the superficial level could yield a working relationship. Thus, blood pressure could be thought of in terms of a functional dependence on the interaction between environment (E) and individual reactivity (R), $BP = f (E \times R)$.

For illustrative purposes, picture, as a simplistic example, two different populations of animals (FIG. 6.1). One (IR_{ES}) is genetically selected, by systematic inbreeding, for a high degree of reactivity of central mechanisms initiating and maintaining vasoconstriction in anticipation of trouble in the environment. All individuals in this inbred population would react strongly to levels of environmental stimulation which have little or no effect, or effects in the opposite direction, on reactivity of the same systems in nonselected individuals in the outbred open population stock. Even small amounts of environmental stimulation are amplified cognitively via a constitutional hyperreactivity of central cardiovascular control systems. These inbred animals would develop high blood pressure over a wide range of environmental stimulation since, in terms of cardiovascular regulation, they are anticipating trouble and reacting maximally even at the most minute elevations or potentional elevations of environmental stimulation.

Conversely, the second population (ES_{IR}) is not genetically selected; rather, it is a free-breeding society much the same as the human population. Here, all degrees of central vasoconstrictive reactivity would be evident, "mean" reactivity would be normal, and differences would sort out according to genetically predisposed reactivity, developmentally shaped reactivity, and the interaction of

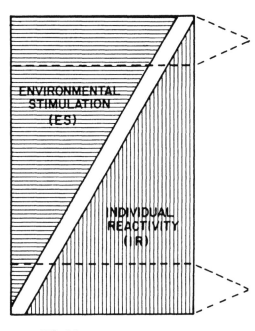

ES$_{IR}$

Almost all animals here react with elevated blood pressure because of a large magnitude, relentless environmental stimulation and continuing level of anticipation of trouble.

IR$_{ES}$

All animals here, because of genetic predisposition, react with elevated blood pressure to even small degrees of environmental stimulation as if they were large and continuing.

FIG. 6.1.

each of these with the level of environmental stimulation present over a given period of time. The degree of hypertension in these animals, as a group, would parallel the extent of environmental stimulation. If stimulation is low, there will be little or no long-term vasoconstrictor responses or associated sequelae. If, on the other hand, environmental stimulation is excessive, most, if not all, within the population become susceptible. With possible exceptions, they will react with at least some degree of vasoconstriction, leading to elevation of blood pressure over a wide range of genetic or developmental predisposition. Those most susceptible would react maximally and, therefore, exhibit the highest levels of arterial pressure.

At present, no particular model is an "ideal" model in terms of the gene-environmental interaction. While one model may stress a 100% incidence of hypertension through rigid genetic control, this does not occur in the human population. Another model may require an amount of environmental stimulation which, on the surface, appears unreasonable if trying to equate comparable environmental events in the human population without looking at the individual's response to a particular set of environmental stimuli. Nevertheless, since these two types of models represent the spectrum of gene-environmental interaction, a combination of their characteristics allows us to approach the elusive "ideal" model. It is with these types of models that this chapter concerns itself.

BEHAVIORAL FACTORS IN SPECIFIC MODELS

In many types of animal models, hypertension is experimentally induced via direct manipulation of function in a specific homeostatic system, allowing localization as to a causative event. Unlike this kind of model, the mechanism of blood pressure elevation produced indirectly through the normal cognitive interpretation of stimuli originating in the environment by the central nervous system cannot be ascribed to malfunction of a particular organ or organ system. For it is a normally developing internal stimulus resulting from the content in which the information has been presented. As such, it resembles the "primary" or idiopathic characteristics of essential hypertension in man. Indeed, some of the models found in this category may be thought of as the most appropriate for this disease.

Induction of Hypertension by Noxious Sensory Stimulation

In the early 1940s, Medoff and Farris and their co-workers reported the development of hypertension maintained under ether anesthesia in stressed, older Wistar gray Norway rats with some systolic pressures reaching more than 180 mm Hg. These blood pressure elevations were observed in rats reacting to the sound of an air blast given 5 minutes a day, 5 days a week, a procedure which had been shown previously to often result in temporary seizures typical of excessive autonomic stimulation (Medoff & Bongiovanni, 1945; Farris, Yeakel, & Medoff, 1945). Rothlin et al. (Rothlin, Cerletti, & Emmenegger, 1959) furthered these attempts to obtain hypertension in 120-day-old rats by applying chronic auditory stimulation and found that only certain types of rats were susceptible to increased blood pressure under this stress. Since they were not successful in producing hypertension in their inbred laboratory strain of albino rats, but did observe a persistent elevation in crossbred wild Norway rats, they concluded that some special disposition of the animals was important. Nevertheless, in the susceptible strain with hypertension, blood pressure values returned to control values from their high of 160 mm Hg only after removal of the stress for 4 months. These rats also exhibited a decreased renal excretory function after acute 0.9% NaCl administration, and a lethal circulatory reaction within a few days of substitution of 2% NaCl for their drinking water.

This work relating prolonged noxious sensory stimulation to the development of hypertension in rats was extented in a series of investigations beginning in the late 1950s in Buckley's laboratory (Hudak & Buckley, 1961; Rosecrans, Watzman, & Buckley, 1966; Smookler & Buckley, 1969). This group found that rats of the Wistar or Sprague-Dawley strain subjected to a randomly presented combination of loud noises of different frequencies and flashing bright lights, together with cage oscillation, developed hypertension, with systolic blood pressure reaching a maximum of 150-160 mm Hg. These elevated levels were sustained for at least a 20-week duration of chronic intermittent stress exposure, and in some tested cases, for weeks after the stress paradigm was discontinued. Among other findings, these studies showed that urinary norepinephrine and epinephrine and plasma corticosterone reach a maximum concentration in the early days of exposure to stress, but that these elevated levels return toward control values during the ensuing weeks of continued stress and increased blood pressure. No single correlation existed between the hypertensive state and adrenal catecholamine content, adrenal corticosterone content, brain norepinephrine, or brain dopamine. Of interest here also are some housing comparisions between paired and isolated control animals. Chronic isolation resulted in increased plasma corticosterone and reduced adrenal corticosterone, but no difference in blood pressure relative to housing in pairs.

In a continuation of this research, Smookler, Goebel, Siegel, and Clarke (1973) found that normal peripheral sympathetic neuronal function is absolutely essential for the increase in blood pressure induced by the noxious sensory stimulation. Adult male Sprague-Dawley rats treated repeatedly with 6-hydroxydopamine (6-OHDA) and subjected to the combination of acoustic, visual, and motion stress failed to develop the hypertension which did occur in untreated stressed animals. Based on a test of the systemic blood pressure response to stimulation of sympathetic innervation of the cardiovascular system of pithed rats, a nearly complete sympathectomy had resulted from the 6-OHDA dosage schedule in treated animals. Their responsiveness to sympathetic nerve stimulation was greatly depressed. For the nontreated rats, no significant difference between stressed and nonstressed groups was found in the frequency-response curves for sympathetic nerve stimulation, in the dose-response curves for injected norepinephrine, nor in response to isoproterenol. It was suggested, therefore, that this model of hypertension is not associated with any apparent changes in sympathetic neurotransmitter reuptake, release or receptor sensitivity, nor with adrenomedullary dysfunction. More recent work by Perhach, Ferguson, and McKinney (1976) has indicated that systolic pressures may remain elevated for 20 weeks after cessation of the combination stress paradigm. This group has also expanded the quantitative pharmacological studies of antihypertensive agents begun in this model by Buckley's laboratory (Buckley, Parham, & Smookler, 1968; Buckley, Vogin, & Kinnard, 1966).

Hall and Hall (1959a; 1959b), working with female Holtzman rats, observed that electroshock stress may produce hypertension when used alone, and will potentiate the incidence and severity of hypertension induced by unilateral nephrectomy with NaCl maintenance and treatment with desoxycorticosterone acetate (DOCA) or growth hormone. The combination of shock-stress and hormone caused more marked tissue damage in kidneys than did hormone alone in the case of DOCA, and augmented both cardiac and kidney pathology in the case of growth hormone. Stress also caused hypertrophy of adrenal and preputial glands. Lipman and Shapiro (1967) studied the effects of electric shock paired with light. In male rats infected with *E. coli* or *Proteus* and exhibiting pyelonephritis, this stress resulted in higher blood pressures, and, in the case of *Proteus,* hypertension.

Related to this model of electric-shock induced hypertension is a study by Williams and Eichelman (1971). They found that the mature male Osborne-Mendel rat, receiving footshock while alone, exhibited an increased blood pressure after his persistent but unsuccessful attempts to escape. In contrast, when paired with another rat, equivalent shock produced aggressive attack responses and decreased blood pressure. Using a similar paradigm, Conner, Vernikos-Danellis, and Levine (1971) reported that plasma ACTH levels were lower in fighting pairs of rats receiving shock than in isolated rats receiving shock of the same intensity. Thus, it should be kept in mind that different physiological responses may occur with the same physical stimulation, depending upon the cognitively mediated interaction of the animal with the psychosocial environment in which the stimulus is tested.

Besides the models described above and those to be discussed later, other methods in this category employed to induce hypertension in animals have included schedule-induced polydipsia (Falk, Tang, & Forman, 1977), immobilization (Lamprecht, Williams, & Kopin, 1973) and sound deprivation (Lockett & Marwood, 1973). In the latter case, neither salt-maintained adrenalectomized rats nor hypophysectomized rats developed the sound-withdrawal hypertension. Treatment with the glucocorticoid, methylprednisolone, restored development of hypertension in the adrenalectomized, but not the hypophysectomized rats maintained under soundproof conditions. With immobilization hypertension, the rise in blood pressure, up to 50 mm Hg above control, is accompanied by an increase in serum dopamine-β-hydroxylase activity, implying the involvement of increased sympathetic nerve activity. Falk has recently reported that limiting a rat's access to food for 5 hours a day to a schedule of intermittent delivery of small amounts generates not only excess fluid intake (polydipsia), but also other chronically exaggerated behavior, such as aggression and hyperactivity. If the rats are previously mononephrectomized and given saline to drink, they develop significantly higher blood pressure than do similarly treated animals given equivalent amounts of food at a once-per-day feeding with a matched control rate and amount of fluid intake (Falk, et al., 1977). This pressure difference was sustained even after water replaced the NaCl drinking solution for 2 weeks, such that terminal mean blood pressure for experimentals was 171 mm Hg and 142 mm Hg for controls. At autopsy, these hypertensive rats showed a slight but significantly increased heart weight and a greater kidney pathology.

Techniques used to induce hypertension in animals have also been shown to increase to even higher levels the elevated blood pressures observed in genetically hypertensive rats. Conversely, reduction of environmental stimuli has attenuated the degree of hypertension in these animals. Characteristics of such manipulation will be discussed in detail later in this chapter.

Induction of Increased Blood Pressure by Cognitive Function

Although it has been demonstrated that noxious sensory stimuli are capable of inducing hypertension in animals, these types of stimuli are not an environmental prerequisite for occurrence of essential hypertension in humans. Neither is the incidence of essential hypertension in people exposed to excessive sensory stimulation presumably any greater than in the general population not exposed to such stimuli. However, rather than being defined only in terms of environmental input, the degree to which stimuli are stressful depends on the interaction between a special set of environmental cues and a particular type of interpretation by an individual. The physiological strength of a stimulus, and therefore its potential for pathogenesis, is determined not only by its physical properties, but also by its cognitively mediated significance to the individual organism. This significance, in turn, varies from species to species and from individual to individual within a species. It is dependent not only on genetic constitution and early (postnatal) life experiences, but also, in good part, on prior learning, i.e., conditioned associations between environmental stimuli and psycho-physiological response. It is possible for stimuli which are not overtly noxious to some, to be perceived interoceptively as such by others. Not every individual animal will appraise and react to its environment in the same way. What would be a comfortable environment or even a pleasurable situation to one individual may seem threatening and evoke visceral reaction in another whose experience has "taught" him otherwise, with or without conscious memory. Even so, it is likely that the intensity and continuity of environmentally stressful stimulation can be heightened experimentally to a level sufficient to bring all individual animals into its sphere of pathogenic influence.

Throughout the literature of the past 20 years or so, there have appeared a number of reports of elevated blood pressure and development of hypertension in both classical (Pavlovian) and operant (instrumental) behavioral conditioning experiments with animals. In classical conditioning studies, the increased blood pressure occurs at first as an unconditioned reflex response to a measureable unconditioned stimulus, such as electric shock, administered independent of the subject's behavior. Subsequently, this blood pressure response appears during presentation of a conditioned stimulus, such as a buzzer, which previously had been paired repeatedly with the unconditioned stimulus. At least some of the stimulus properties of the electric shock, those responsible for induction of a rise in blood pressure, have been transferred to or acquired by the buzzer. With regard to instrumental conditioning studies, two types of relationship with blood pressure exist. In the first one, blood pressure elevations are observed incidental to or concurrent with some schedule of ongoing reinforced performance, such as bar pressing for food or avoidance of electric shock, or conflict between positive and negative reinforcement, i.e., hypertension is induced indirectly by the stress of performing a task requiring learned cognitive skills. In the second, consequent reinforcement is directly contingent upon an antecedent rise in blood pressure. The blood pressure increase itself is the instrumentally conditioned response, equivalent, to some extent, to the bar-pressing behavior of the first type, since both are maintained by the food delivery or shock-avoidance.

Once blood pressure elevations develop as an integral part of the classically or instrumentally conditioned response repertoire in an animal, stimulus generalization to environmental cues may be responsible for early maintenance of the increased pressure levels outside of the immediate milieu of the conditioning apparatus. Eventually, with gradual change in the various components of the cardiovascular system, hypertension becomes permanent. One important feature should be noted at this point concerning generalization of conditioned stimuli. Whether the hypertension is truly fixed cannot be assured in studies not reporting evidence of structural tissue change and where pressure measurements were not made outside of the environment where conditioning stress occurred. In these cases, acute arterial pressure responses to generalized environmental stimuli may be what is being measured, rather than a true permanent hypertension.

Classical (Pavlovian) Conditioning

As would be expected from its roots in the Pavlovian school of physiology, much of the early classical conditioning studies of animal models of hypertension have appeared in the Russian literature. An excellent review of this material has been presented by Simonson and Brožek (1959). They reviewed many reports of conditioned increases of arterial blood pressure after controlled presentation of sensory stimuli signaling the occurrence of an aversive event. One of the most interesting investigations described was that of Napalkov and Karas (p. 137). Not only did these workers produce hypertension by means of conditioned signals in five dogs but also abolished it by changing the conditioned activity. Conditioned signals previously paired with strong unconditioned stimuli, such as electric shock, exposure to a cat, or pistol shots, produced a greater increase in blood pressure (from 220 mm Hg to 240 mm Hg) than did the unconditioned stimuli. This exaggerated pressor response to the conditioned stimulus was continued during a period of months (900 repeat tests) without reinforcement. Hypertension was still present for a 5-month longer period of observation, following discontinuation of the experiment. However, hypertension could be abolished by, among other means, association of the conditioned stimuli producing the pressor response with feeding instead of with the noxious unconditioned stimuli.

Simon and Brožek also review reports of hypertension induced in animals subjected to a conflict situation produced by simultaneous application of positive and negative (inhibitory) conditioned signals. With this procedure blood pressure values in monkeys were raised from normal 115 to 135 mm Hg systolic and 65 to 85 mm Hg diastolic to 180 to 220 mm Hg and 110 to 120 mm Hg. Hypertension so developed was sustained in some animals up to 2 years, but was transient in others (Magakian et al., Miminoshvili et al., pp. 138–140). Other work reviewed by these authors includes production of hypertension by conditioning sensory stimuli previously associated with epinephrine or renin.

This particular experimental approach to cardiovascular physiology was strongly supported in this country by Gantt, who had previously collaborated with Bykov and others in Pavlov's laboratory. Research from Gantt's laboratory provided evidence that blood pressure increases could be classically conditioned in dogs in a quantitatively differentiated manner, according to the degree of shock previously associated with the particular tone employed. The magnitude of the conditioned blood pressure responses were directly proportional to the graded intensities of the unconditioned stimuli. Hypertensive pressure levels of 150 to 225 mm Hg were conditioned from average control values of 130 mm Hg. Elevated blood pressure in some cases persisted up to 13 months of rest without presentation of either shock or tone (Dykman & Gantt, 1960; Gantt, 1960). Other early investigations have obtained essentially similar results, including some using direct brain stimulation as unconditioned or conditioned stimuli. Another review of the initial work in this area can be found in Figar's (1965) chapter in the *Handbook of Physiology* (Figar, 1965).

More recently, Reis and his colleagues at Cornell have reported that classically conditioned increases in blood pressure are more than five times greater in cats with nucleus tractus solitarius lesions than in sham controls trained under the same conditions (Nathan, Tucker, Severini, & Reis, 1978). Bilateral electrolytic lesions of this area of the medulla oblongata abolish baroreceptor reflexes and may also interfere with function in other pathways normally serving to inhibit sympathetic vasoconstrictor activity. Lesions alone result in a mild hypertension with labile pressures, while conditioning by itself causes only slight elevation of blood pressure. The large, conditioned pressor responses in lesioned animals suggest, then, that destruction of these areas of the brain removes some central activity normally opposing or limiting the rate and level of development of a classically conditioned rise in blood pressure.

Many of the studies of classical conditioning of cardiovascular function concern autonomic regulation of heart rate. Nevertheless, although blood pressure may not be measured in these investigations, their relevance to classical conditioning of arterial pressure is indicated in a 1967 report by Yehle, Dauth, and Schneiderman. They obtained evidence suggesting that classically conditioned heart rate deceleration, at least in rabbits, reflects a compensatory reflex response to a sympathetically induced elevation of blood pressure. For additional references concerning research investigations into classical conditioning of blood pressure, the reader should consult the extensive bibliography presented by Harris and Brady (1974).

Instrumental (Operant) Conditioning

Over the past few decades, a keen interest in behavior has been generated by studies in operant or instrumental conditioning. Following up early on this emerging field for pharmacological research, Buckley's group reported in 1963 that Wistar rats subjected to the stress of an avoidance-escape operant conditioning procedure developed increased blood pressure compared to untreated controls (Aceto, Kinnard, & Buckley, 1963). In this conditioning paradigm, a rat learns to climb a pole in response to a warning tone which signals oncoming shock (i.e., avoidance), or in response to tone plus shock (i.e., escape). Presentation of tone or tone-shock combination is terminated when the rat ascends the pole. The rate of blood pressure elevation during conditioning was greater during the first 12 trials, occurring over a period of 4 weeks. Normal blood pressures within a narrow range of 112 to 120 mm Hg were increased to values between 145 and 160 mm Hg, maintained for more than 40 weeks of training. Even after rats were no longer exposed to the conditioning apparatus, blood pressure remained elevated for 5 more weeks of observation. About the same time, Meehan et al. (Meehan, Fineg, & Wheelwright, 1963; Meehan, Fineg, & Mosely, 1964) also reviewed their observations on arterial blood pressure in young chimpanzees undergoing complex operant training for orbital space flight. They found that severe hypertension developed in these animals that had been subjected to chronic bar-press avoidance conditioning, necessitating prolonged restraint. Diastolic pressure in one case ranged from 90 to 130 mm Hg. While an untrained animal exposed to similar restraint and avoidance stimuli responded with vigorous and excited objection, his acute and reversible pressure responses were far lower than those of the trained chimpanzee, whose adopted docility masked a fixed hypertension.

In Forsyth's studies of rhesus monkeys exposed to long-term, 12 to 16 hours a day Sidman shock-avoidance conditioning, almost all animals showed a steady monthly increase of systolic and diastolic blood pressure (Forsyth, 1968; 1969). This sustained increase occurred after an initial biphasic response consisting of an acute increase followed by return to normal or below normal pressure levels for months. In this type of schedule, a timer switch closes a circuit for shock delivery if allowed to complete its cycle. Pressing a lever prevents shock by resetting the timer for a new cycle (i.e., successful avoidance). The monkeys involved in these operant conditioning schedules became "increasingly and persistently emotional and excitable" compared to the controls, and had pressor responses to a number of previously neutral stimuli. Interestingly, if the schedule light was turned on in the absence of a lever to press, elevations of blood pressure ranging from 30 to 40 mm Hg could be obtained, even though no shock was delivered. No pathology specific to subjects exhibiting increased blood pressure was found. Two points could be made here concerning the biphasic nature of blood pressure conditioning in this investigation: one, that the mechanisms involved in the initiation, development, and maintenance of elevated blood pressure may differ in terms of temporal characteristics (e.g., onset, duration) as well as homeostatic direction and, two, that negative results reported in some attempts at stress-induced hypertension may be due to measures being taken during a normal phase of a biphasic response when this occurs.

These results demonstrating heightening blood pressure concurrent with operant conditioning have been verified and extended by others. Herd and his colleagues studied squirrel monkeys trained to press a key to turn off a light associated with cutaneous electric shock delivered to the tail. Over a period of 4 to 11 months, they found a distinct relationship between the rate at which each monkey pressed the key and the level of its mean arterial blood pressure (Herd, Morse, Kelleher, & Jones, 1969). Although all animals key-pressed least and were shocked most frequently during early training, their blood pressure at this time did not increase above control levels. As conditioning progressed, pressure rose gradually until it was elevated before, during, and after experimental sessions. Elevated pressure was recorded when subjects pressed the key rapidly and received relatively few shocks. This hypertension was sustained even later when the squirrel monkeys were in their home cages.

A series of studies in dogs by Anderson and Brady and their associates examined blood pressure both during avoidance performance and during a fixed-interval period preceding the avoidance session (Harris & Brady, 1974; Anderson & Brady, 1971; Anderson & Brady, 1973). During preavoidance periods of up to 15 hours, almost all dogs exhibited an increase in both systolic and diastolic blood pressures, while heart rate was either decreased or not affected. In contrast, the preparatory pattern for the period preceding a food-reinforcement schedule showed increased heart rate along with the increased pressures. Moreover, these investigators found that blood pressure elevations characteristic of the preavoidance period were associated with increased peripheral resistance, whereas increases in pressure during the avoidance session itself coincided with a decrease in peripheral resistance, but a marked increase in cardiac output. Nevertheless, interference with the elevated cardiac output response in this latter case, by pharmacological beta-adrenergic receptor blockade, does permit a rise in peripheral resistance to maintain increased blood pressure (Harris & Brady, 1974).

Operant techniques were also used by Friedman and Dahl to establish an approach-avoidance conflict situation which led to increased blood pressure in normotensive rats genetically susceptible to a NaCl-induced hypertension (Friedman & Dahl, 1975). The Dahl hypertension-sensitive strain of Sprague-Dawley rat develops severe hypertension if excess salt is ingested (see p. 178 of this chapter). Keeping their hypertensive-prone rats on a low salt diet, they trained them to press a level to obtain food pellets. However, some of these lever-presses resulted in immediate presentation of electric shock. This treatment resulted in punishment for behavioral responses necessary for food delivery and, consequently, a reduced food intake. Other hypertension-prone rats, having no lever-press contingencies, were yoked to these rats with respect to the amount of food or shock received or both, while still others served as controls exposed to none of these conditions but having free access to food. Ranking these groups from highest to lowest according to mean blood pressure indicated that those rats exposed to the punished-eating conflict generally exhibited the highest pressures (160 to 180 mm Hg), followed closely by those subjected to food deprivation and shock without conflict. Next in descending order were those rats who were food-deprived without shock, those exposed to shock, and controls (140 to 150 mm Hg). Some of the rats from different experimental groups maintained pressures elevated above control values during a posttreatment recovery period. Further-more, in a related paper, Friedman and Iwai showed that the NaCl-resistant strain of rats did not develop hypertension when subjected to this same food-shock conflict situation (Friedman & Iwai, 1976). The finding that hypertension devel-oped in the presence of reduced food intake and body weight in hypertension-susceptible animals subjected to stress suggests that any relationship between excess body weight and incidence of hypertension is not one of simple cause and effect. It is of interest here also to note that previous studies by Dahl and his colleagues failed to find chronic elevation of blood pressure in this hypertension-sensitive strain in a classical conditioning paradigm (Dahl, Knudsen, Heine, & Leitl, 1968).

A variation of these instrumental conditioning techniques has become quite important in its significance for studies of animal models of hypertension. Evi-dence from a number of laboratories has been presented that an increase in arterial blood pressure can be sustained by animals when this response per se directly produces access to food or other reinforcement, such as rewarding brain stimulation, or permits avoidance of electric shock. Following up on previous work from Miller's laboratory concerning instrumental conditioning of autonom-ic responses, DiCara and Miller reported in 1968 that curarized Sprague-Dawley rats increased their systolic blood pressure up to 22% when changes in this direction were rewarded by avoidance or escape from tail shock (DiCara & Miller, 1968). Skeletal musculature was paralyzed in these artificially respirated animals in an attempt to eliminate mediation of cardio-vascular effects by muscu-lar activity (e.g., respiratory changes). Although not directly pertinent to a consideration of hypertensive animal models, a decrease in blood pressure was also demonstrated by these investigators when changes in that direction were rewarded. Yoked controls were shocked whenever experimental animals were, regardless of the status of their arterial pressure, and as a result showed a moderate increase in systolic values.

Benson, Herd, Morse, and Kelleher (1969) modified the procedures em-ployed by Herd et al. (1969) in squirrel monkeys (described above) such that an increase in blood pressure, rather than a key press, prevented delivery of electric shock. After stable and reproducible key-pressing avoidance performance was established, the new contingency was introduced: a certain number of key presses or an increase in mean arterial pressure terminated the stimulus signaling oncoming shock delivery. Eventually, the key-press contingency itself was removed. Under this schedule, pressure increments of up to 30 mm Hg above that of controls could be obtained progressively, and maintained by appropriate presentation of stimuli according to blood pressure. Here too, as in the study by Herd et al., monkeys received the lowest number of shocks during the latter phases of the experiment, when criterion responses, in this case blood pressure increments, were most numerous. Reversals by rewarding decrements in blood pressure were also obtained.

Associates of Brady's group have employed similar instrumental conditioning techniques in their studies of learned blood pressure responses. Plumlee reported large magnitude elevations in diastolic pressure of relatively short duration in rhesus monkeys (Plumlee, 1969). For these animals, avoidance trials began with delivery of a tone followed by shock whenever their diastolic blood pressure fell below a predetermined level. An automatic adjusting schedule changed the criterion pressure requirement according to the number of shocks received. As a result, a linear relationship was observed between the minimum pressure required for avoidance and the diastolic pressure achieved, elevations of which reached up to 60 mm Hg. A yoked control monkey that simultaneously received all shocks and tones as determined by blood pressure of the experimental monkey responded with an increased blood pressure to the shock, but not to the tone. In some follow-up measurements after 7-10 weeks on this schedule for up to 22 hours a day no change in blood pressure at rest was found, nor were renal changes attributable to hypertension present. Longer-lasting large elevations in both systolic and diastolic blood pressure in baboons were obtained by Harris, Gilliam, Findley, & Brady (1973). In their investigation, increases of 30 to 40 mm Hg were sustained for more than 95% of each daily 12-hour conditioning period. Animals were required to maintain prespecified diastolic pressure levels to gain access to food and avoid shock. One interesting addition was the presence of two lights which signaled to the monkey when diastolic blood pressure was above or below the specified criterion, thus providing immediate feedback following variations in blood pressure status.

More recently, Anderson and Yingling (1979) have found in 15-16 hour sessions that increases in arterial blood pressure in the dog can be produced by making shock-avoidance a contingent consequence of prespecified levels of total peripheral resistance. When only large decreases in resistance are programmed to produce electric shock, allowing only infrequent aversive stimulation, progressive elevation of resistance is observed, along with a decrease or no change in heart rate and cardiac output and up to a 20 mm Hg rise in pressure. This cardiovascular response pattern is accompanied by inhibition of behavioral activity and a diminishing respiratory activity. As discussed by the authors, the possibility exists that renal regulation of blood volume is influenced by the chain of events initiated by respiratory suppression and reduced blood pH.

Following a different, but related, line of thought, Dworkin and his colleagues in Miller's laboratory have obtained evidence suggesting that acute elevations of blood pressure may serve to attenuate the aversiveness of noxious stimuli via a reduction of central arousal and behavioral inhibition mediated through baroreceptor pathways (Dworkin, Filewich, Miller, Craigmyle, & Pickering, 1979). Employing phenylephrine to raise arterial pressure acutely, they found that normal rats, but not rats with surgically denervated baroreceptors, ran less to avoid or escape trigeminal nucleus stimulation after infusion of this drug than after the saline vehicle. These results support their idea that baroreceptor stimulation may reinforce instrumentally conditioned blood pressure elevations, functioning as a reward by lessening the distress of reactivity to noxious stimuli.

Psychosocially Stressful Environment

The studies described above have employed electromechanical presentation of rather artificial stimuli to which inborn response patterns may never fully develop with regard to behavioral-cardiovascular interactions. Animals are genetically preprogrammed to respond to socially meaningful stimuli in a sterotyped manner as part of their inherited behavioral repertoire, which is usually strongly reinforced by early experience during development. Because of the nature of life experiences for the particular animal involved, species-specific social interaction yields an added dimension based on innate behavior. One example would be the inhibitory feedback effect on adrenocortical activity occurring as a result of the execution of sterotypic fighting behavior in rats (Conner, et al., 1971). Nevertheless, results from the preceding investigations have been supported and supplemented by experimental data concerning development of elevated blood pressure by means of manipulation of the animals' social environment. Methods here are aimed at examining the influence of temporally and spatially exaggerated environmental stimuli more closely related to the animals' natural or experiential response patterns. These studies, involving as they do the effects of social interaction on psychophysiological control mechanisms, are considered here as a proper animal model for psychosocial induction of hypertension.

In 1954, Schunk found that 50% of the cats chronically exposed to aggressive barking dogs developed hypertension with increased cardiac weight due to ventricular hypertrophy, along with renal pathology. That the psychophysiological responses involved did not appear to adapt with respect to the continuing presence of this threat without action, or extinguish due to lack of unconditioned reinforcement suggests that this response pattern is at least partially inborn.

Lapin and Cherkovich, reporting on a continuation of the work carried out in the Sukhumi monkey colony by Miminoshvili, describe techniques of experimental manipulation of social environment that serve to illustrate the degree of influence that natural stimuli have for the baboon (Lapin & Cherkovich, 1971; Miminoshvili, 1960). Having formerly lived as leader of a social grouping of male, female, and immature baboons in an open enclosure in the wild, the dominant male was transferred to a large cage together with the females with whom he had developed long-term attachment association. Later, he was separated from these females and isolated in an adjacent cage where he could view, through the wire netting, juveniles and females being fed first, a situation quite contrary to normal relationships governing this baboon group's prior social behavior in a more natural habitat. His behavior, characterized by an alert anxiety, increased to aggravated excitement when, finally, another male, a rival, was allowed into the other cage with the females again in sight of the dominant. Unable, by virtue of cage restraint, to resolve this conflict as it would be resolved in the wild, given the same circumstantial stimuli, the dominant male developed hypertension and other evidence of chronic cardiovascular disorder after 4 or 5 months of life under these conditions. Similar results were obtained in a series of related experiments.

Prompted by some of the results above and the ethological observations of others, Henry and his co-workers, starting in the mid-60s, set out along the same path to study the feasibility of induction of hypertension by manipulation of psychosocial input in mice. Concentrating on stimulation by "symbolically significant social threats," they sought to obtain evidence that the sustained psychophysiological arousal accompanying interactions such as those involved in aggregation, attachment behavior, competitive conflict, and status loss is sufficient for development and maintenance of elevated blood pressure in these social mammals (Henry, Meehan, & Stephens, 1967). Since this work embodies an ongoing systematic study of the role of such factors in the mechanisms of hypertensive etiology, and since the results may apply to many, if not all, of the foregoing models, this animal model will be discussed in somewhat more detail in the following section.

Specific Example: The CBA Mouse Psychosocial Stress Model for Study of Physiological Correlates of Behavioral State

As a starting point, Henry's group first demonstrated that males from the CBA strain of Agouti mice, raised as siblings, showed no significant change in systolic blood pressure with age. Throughout their normal life-span of 24-30 months, their arterial blood pressure, measured by tail-cuff plethysmography, remained within the range of 126 ± 12 mm Hg (Henry, Meehan, Stephens, & Santisteban, 1965). With these boxed siblings serving as controls, a number of experimental socioenvironmental manipulations were employed in an attempt to utilize their inborn and conditioned responses for initiation and development of high blood pressure. Mixing male mice previously housed in different boxes, aggregating them in smaller area boxes, exposing groups of mice to the sound, sight, and odor of a hungry cat attempting for many months to open their box, and producing territorial and mating conflict in colonies of male and female mice in interconnected boxes, result in elevations of blood pressure which are higher in males than in females. The latter group population system, stocked with 4-month-old males which had previously spent early months in isolation, produced the most intense psychosocial stimulation. Under these conditions, mean arterial blood pressure was increased more than 30 mm Hg, and sustained at this level for up to 9 months. This prolonged rise in blood pressure was maintained under ether anesthesia, but was diminished by reserpine (Henry, et al., 1967).

The objective of a continuing series of experiments emanating from these findings was to contrast certain physiological, biochemical, and behavioral parameters in one group of adult male CBA normotensive mice with the same parameters in male mice from the same genetic stock exhibiting hypertension after chronic exposure to a daily routine of brief, but repeated encounters of social confrontation. Since hypertension was observed in the males only, studies were directed toward them.

With the view that elevated blood pressure in these mice subjected to psychosocial stress in the population cages at least in part results from repeated episodes of sympatho-adrenomedullary arousal via the defense-alarm reaction, Henry's group examined the status of this system as expressed in the adrenal medulla (Henry, Stephens, Axelrod, & Mueller, 1971). The blood pressure of animals undergoing chronic conflict was significantly elevated from a mean control value of 125 ± 5 mm Hg to 168 ± 17 mm Hg (range 150 to 180 mm Hg). Both absolute and relative adrenal weights of these mice stressed by 6 months of social interaction in the population cages were more than twice those of age-matched boxed sibling control animals. Similarly, adrenal epinephrine and norepinephrine content was increased in mice experiencing the excessive psychophysiological stimulation accompanying the chronic social disorder of the multibox mixed-sex system. But long-term sustained influence on the adrenal, reflecting maintenance of its response capability, was best represented by measured increases in the biosynthetic machinery of the adrenal chromaffin cells. Tyrosine hydroxylase (TH), the rate-limiting enzyme for catecholamine synthesis, and phenylethanolamine-N-methyltransferase (PNMT), which catalyzes the N-methylation of norepinephrine to form epinephrine, were both markedly elevated in mice populating the interconnecting box environment. It is known that relatively prolonged presynaptic sympathetic nerve activity, with consequent release of acetylcholine, is a requirement for increases in the tissue levels of these two enzymes (Ciaranello, 1977; Guidotti, Hanbauer, & Costa, 1975; Thoenen, 1975; Thoenen, Mueller, & Axelrod, 1969; Thoenen, Mueller, & Axelrod, 1970). In the case of TH, this enzyme induction involves selective synthesis and accumulation of new protein and develops over a period of 1-4 days (Thoenen, et al., 1969; Thoenen, et al., 1970; Thoenen, 1975; Guidotti, et al., 1975; see Thoenen (1975) for other references). Furthermore, adrenal glu-cocorticoids have been shown to be important modulators for this transynaptic induction of TH by presynaptic cholinergic nerve activity in the sympathetic system (Mueller, Thoenen, & Axelrod, 1970; Otten & Thoenen, 1975; Thoenen & Otten, 1977). Similarly, glucocorticoids exert a significant influence on adre-nal gland PNMT activity (Ciaranello, 1977; Wurtman & Axelrod, 1966).

It was concluded from this adrenal enzyme study that these measured in-creases in TH and PNMT in mice experiencing a prolonged series of social challenges were probably attributable to mechanisms involving both the pitui-tary-ACTH and sympathetic nervous systems. In males kept in isolation for the 6 months, the adrenals were slightly enlarged. However, in this case, a different mechanism was presumably operating because despite the hypertrophy, the en-zyme levels were less in isolated animals than in boxed sibling controls (Henry, Stephens, Axelrod & Mueller, 1971).

Parallel studies with this hypertensive model detailed the incidence of result-ing pathology at the histological level (Henry, Ely, Stephens, Ratcliffe, San-tisteban, & Shapiro, 1971). Comparisons were made between distribution of le-sions in mice undergoing intense social stimulation for 6 months in the inter-communicating population cages and in similarly aged groups of control mice raised as separate sex, boxed siblings. Severity scores for interstitial nephritis, glomerular mesangial changes, myocardial fibrosis, and arteriosclerotic degener-ation of the intramural coronary vascular bed and aorta were found to be signifi-cantly higher in the psychosocially stressed animals than in controls. At the gross anatomical level, some kidneys from mice in the population cages showed changes at autopsy, such as pitting and blanching of the surface, neither of which was observed in the unstimulated control groups. It is thought that these lesions are related to some common mechanism operating in a disturbed cardiovascular regulatory state which is also expressed as the measured increase in blood pres-sure and in the increased adreno-medullary enzyme activity.

As a follow up, continuation studies along the same lines aimed at determin-ing the degree of permanence or reversibility of this pathophysiological state were reported later (Henry, Stephens, & Santisteban, 1975). If mice are returned to isolation for 1 month, after 2 months in the population cage system, systolic blood pressure and heart weight return to near normal levels. A similar but weaker reversal is seen in mice reisolated for 1 month after 5 months of psycho-social stimulation. Exposure to the stress of population conflict for 6-9 months resulted in sustained increases in heart weight and systolic blood pressure, con-firming previous results. These remained elevated despite 8 weeks of return to isolation. Neither could this reisolation reverse the development of aortic ar-teriosclerosis nor myocardial fibrosis. Indications of severe renal damage, as measured by greatly increased blood urea levels, were also observed in the socially competing males (Henry, 1976). Such degenerative structural changes, as well as the raised arterial blood pressure, parallel the progressively irreversible nature of untreated hypertension in humans (Henry, 1976). It is of interest that the adrenal PNMT levels of mice spending 6-9 months in the population cage also remained elevated in spite of prolonged return to isolation, which in some cases caused higher elevation (Henry & Stephens, 1977a). This is probably related to the finding that plasma levels of corticosterone, the primary adrenal glucocorticoid in mice, remain elevated after the first few days of population cage interaction, and are increased even more so after return of the socially stressed animals to isolation (Henry, & Stephens, 1977a).

More recently, in collaboration with Vander and his colleagues, Henry's group has addressed itself to the possibility that the renin-angiotensin system plays a participating role somewhere along the course of hypertension in these socially competing animals. Measuring plasma renin activity (PRA) in blood samples drawn by rapid retro-orbital puncture from unanesthetized mice, they sought to determine to what degree, if any, this potent pressor system might be involved in this psychosocial model (Vander, Henry, Stephens, Kay & Mouw, 1978). In a longitudinal study, within a day or two of placement in the socially competitive population cages, previously isolated males showed markedly elevated PRA levels in comparison to age-matched control males remaining in isolation. With time, and coinciding with the progressive rise and plateauing of systolic blood pressure occurring with 1 week to 2 months of social interaction, these very high initial PRA levels fell to more moderate levels of elevation. Although these values were still greater than those measured in isolates, they were not significantly different from those of normotensive males of the same age kept as boxed siblings. In later stages of excessive social stimulation, PRA increased again, to levels greater than those seen in normotensive boxed siblings. Similar results were obtained in a nonlongitudinal study using separate groups of animals. Here, psychosocially stressed males previously housed as boxed siblings also showed increased blood pressure and PRA after 3 or 10 weeks in the population cage system, as compared to controls left as boxed siblings.

In further work with this model, results confirmed that later stages of hypertension are associated with progressive impairment of renal function as well as the increased plasma renin activity (Henry & Stephens, 1979). Moreover, it was shown that administration of SQ14255, an angiotensin-converting enzyme inhibitor, produces significant reduction in blood pressure, indicating that hypertension at this point later in development is at least partially influenced by the renin-angiotensin pressor system. This agent does not lower blood pressure in nonhypertensive mice kept in isolation, nor in socially competing mice during genesis of the hypertension within the first few weeks of population cage interaction.

Although, overall, the blood pressure of males in the population cage increased relative to boxed-sibling or isolate controls, some individuals appeared to be affected more or less than others. Another series of studies was carried out to distinguish ethologically between types of animals and their responses in a slightly different social situation involving similar confrontations. Results of these studies are reported in references (Ely & Henry, 1974; Ely & Henry, 1978; Henry, Ely, Watson, & Stephens, 1975; Henry & Stephens, 1977b).

BEHAVIORAL CORRELATES OF INCREASED BLOOD PRESSURE

Several groups have developed animal models of hypertension in which apparently multifactorial genetic elements dominate the occurrence and progression of the disorder. The distinguishing characteristics of these various models, as far as experimentally determined mechanisms are concerned, illustrate well the argument that essential hypertension probably involves an interaction of different pathways influencing cardiovascular homeostasis. For example, different strains of rats develop hypertension in different ways. With sufficient cross-comparative and longitudinal study, these models would serve to broaden the information base regarding behavioral correlates of hypertension, provided certain points are kept in mind. One of these is the consideration that such a purebred animal strain is a genetically homogeneous model for a disease which occurs in the genetically heterogeneous human population. Another is the frequency with which certain characteristics may appear as inbred traits accompanying the hypertension, but having nothing to do with the elevation of blood pressure per se; these may also occur in the normotensive parent strain from which the hypertensive animals are derived.

By means of these genetic animal models, we can potentially answer such questions as: What are the behavioral or "personality" characteristics that are associated with a particular animal's constitutional predisposition to high blood pressure? Unfortunately, too few of the many investigations dealing with these models address such questions. For the three out of four genetic models about which there has been published little or no behavioral data, only a very brief description follows, since these models have been adequately reviewed for their other characteristics in a recent chapter by Folkow and Hallbäck (1977). The fourth model seems a more fertile area for a behaviorally oriented review.

New Zealand Genetically Hypertensive Rats

This earliest of the successful genetic models of animal hypertension was developed by Smirk and his group in New Zealand. It began as the result of a mating, in 1955, between a pair of random bred Wistar-derived albino rats showing above average blood pressures within the University of Otago foundation colony (Smirk & Hall, 1958). Designated GHR, this hypertensive strain has now been inbred by brother-sister mating for over 40 generations. Mean systolic blood pressures run close to 180 mm Hg for males, and over 165 mm Hg for females, while normotensive controls average 120 mm Hg, and rarely exceed 140 mm Hg. In summarizing current thinking about the GHR, it is safe to say that mechanisms operating in the early stages appear to involve sympathetic control of the cardiovascular system, with later increasing involvement of structural properties of the blood vessels. No readily apparent renal or adrenocortical primary dysfunction has been measured, but prostaglandin metabolism may play a role (Clark & Phelan, 1976; Folkow, & Hallbäck, 1977; Phelan, Simpson, & Smirk, 1976).

Dahl Hypertensive-Sensitive Rats

Having noticed in studies of salt-induced hypertension that some Sprague-Dawley rats are more resistant to NaCl loading than others, which often succumbed to a severe hypertension relatively rapidly, Dahl and his associates selectively bred the rats in each of these directions. This approach yielded two separate strains in which blood pressure response to different levels of salt ingestion is thus an inherited characteristic (Dahl, Heine, & Tassinari, 1962). One, which developed systolic pressures of up to 200 mm Hg after 8% NaCl dietary intake, is called the hypertension sensitive (or susceptible) rat (HSR). The other, which did not develop hypertension in response to high salt loading, is termed the hypertension resistant rat (HRR). Both strains are normotensive at "normal" dietary salt levels. As compared to HRR, the sensitive animals exhibit an exaggerated vascular reactivity to vasopressor agents, such as norepinephrine and angiotensin, even before the onset of measureable hypertension, and renal mechanisms play an important role. Moreover, for this particular model, over-production of the mineralocorticoid 18-hydroxy-11-deoxycorticosterone, appears to be one other predisposing component within a polygenic mode of inheritance (Dahl, Heine, & Tassinari, 1964; Folkow, & Hallbäck, 1977; Rapp & Iwai, 1976).

Milan Hypertensive Rats

When rats with elevated blood pressure were sporadically observed in their stock colony of Wistars, Bianchi and his co-workers bred them to establish another strain of hypertensive rats, abbreviated MHS (Bianchi, Fox, & Imbasciati, 1974). High blood pressure develops in these rats about 2-4 weeks after weaning, and plateaus at 160 to 170 mm Hg between 45-60 days of age. Compared to normotensive controls bred from the same stock, MHS rats showing this 30% to 40% pressure elevation also exhibit a significantly higher heart/body weight ratio. Research with this model indicates that MHS rats may be primarily characterized by inherent renal disturbances of blood volume control, presumably due to a reduction of effectively filtering glomeruli (Bianchi & Baer, 1976). Nevertheless, it is of interest to note some additional behaviorally oriented observations made by Bianchi et al. (1974). They have reported that by leaving the mother and offspring together for longer than 25 days, the onset of the blood pressure difference between MHS and normotensive control rats is delayed. In addition, blood pressure of both males and females is reduced during mating, climbs later, but does not reach premating levels. They further observed that MHS rats left alone in individual cages tend to have higher blood pressure than those living in group cages.

Spontaneously Hypertensive Rats (SHR)

Also approaching the development of a spontaneously hypertensive animal model from the standpoint of genetic selection, Okamoto and Aoki in the early 1960s employed controlled successive brother-sister inbreeding of those rats of the Kyoto-Wistar strain exhibiting elevated blood pressures (Okamoto & Aoki, 1963). Within a few generations, offspring showed significantly higher arterial pressures than members of the parent strain. The Kyoto spontaneously hypertensive rats differ from the New Zealand genetically hypertensive rats in that they exhibited this more rapid generation-to-generation pressure rise, the blood pressure levels reached are higher, and hypertension is present in 100% of the animal population, frequently developing a malignant phase. At present, offspring of this inbred strain, commonly designated SHR for spontaneously hypertensive rat(s), are beyond the F_{45} generation at Kyoto University, and have been further differentiated genealogically into several substrains with distinguishing characteristics (Okamoto, 1969; Okamoto, 1972; US, DHEW, NIH, 1977).

Among the various animal models of human essential hypertension, the SHR represents the most extensively studied model. The SHR model exhibits many close similarities to essential hypertension in man. As such, it is of great value as an experimental research probe into essential hypertension mechanisms and appears to be one of the most sensitive animal models for detecting the therapeutic hypotensive activity of current and potential antihypertensive agents (ILAR, 1976; Onesti, Fernandes, & Kim, 1976; Yamori, 1977). Since the introduction of this model to the hypertension research community, there have been a very large number of studies concerning the biochemical and physiological correlates of predisposition to or occurrence of high blood pressure in SHRs. In comparison, there have been relatively few investigations dealing with ongoing behavioral correlates. But, when compared to behaviorally oriented research done with the other genetic models described above, the information obtained for SHRs is substantially more complete and sufficient for correlative studies. For that reason, the Okamoto-Aoki spontaneously hypertensive rat model will be discussed in more detail in the following section.

Specific Example: The SHR Model for the Study of Behavioral Correlates of Physiological State

According to most evidence, development or maintenance, or both, of elevated blood pressure in the SHR is associated genetically with a relative functional hyperreactivity of neural and hormonal cardiovascular control systems. These, in turn, appear to trigger subsequent autoregulatory structural adaptation characteristic of cardiac and vascular responses to pressure load in the hypertensive state. These conclusions are drawn in comparison to the lower activity of these systems in rats of the Wistar-Kyoto foundation stock from which SHRs were derived and which exhibit lower blood pressures, although supportive evidence comes also from studies using other normotensive rats as controls. For hemodynamic and related considerations, the reader is referred to the excellent treatment given this subject by Folkow and his group (1978, 1982).

Early work, done soon after introduction of this model, suggested existence of an increased activity in central regulation of not only the sympathetic-adrenomedullary and pituitary-adrenocortical systems, but also the pituitary-thyroid axis (Okamoto, 1969; Okamoto, 1972). For example, sympathetic firing frequency, measured directly in splanchnic nerves, was 2-3 times greater in SHRs than in WKY rats (Okamoto, Nosaka, Yamori, & Matsumoto, 1967). In addition to evidence from these many earlier studies, later work provides more experimental support for this contention. Iriuchijima reported that sympathetic splanchnic vasoconstrictor discharge was elevated in SHRs (Iriuchijima, 1973). The neurophysiological findings of Judy et al (1976) indicate that the sympathetic nervous system (SNS) plays a major role in the development and maintenance of hypertension in the SHR. Along with other evidence, they cite the striking correlation between blood pressure and sympathetic nerve activity (renal) in SHRs of varying ages. No correlation was seen in normotensive rats whose pressures, but not nerve activity, increased slightly with age. Of great importance also, they report that in back-bred SHRs genetically selected for normal blood pressures, sympathetic nerve activity is identical to that of Wistar control rats. Continuing research from this laboratory, using the Kyoto-Wistar as a control comparison, demonstrated that mean sympathetic nerve activity in the cervical sympathetic, greater and lesser splanchnic, and splenic, as well as the renal nerves, was greater in SHRs than in WKYs or back-crossed SHRs (Judy, Watanabe, Murphy, Aprison, & Yu, 1979; Judy & Farrell, 1979). Moreover, they found that the amount of renal sympathetic nerve activity left uninhibited by high pressure baroreceptors increases with age in SHRs. Similar evidence was obtained by Schramm and his associates (Schramm & Barton, 1979). Elevated sympathetic nerve activity, as measured reciprocally by the strength of the splanchnic nerve silent period after central excitation, is present both during the development before measurable high blood pressure and during maintenance of hypertension is SHRs. No such elevation is seen in age-matched weanling and adult control WKY rats. Additional findings in physiological and pharmacological studies reported by Tucker and Johnson (1980a, b) also suggest that significant elevations of SNS activity seen during the second week of development in SHRs but not WKYs are responsible for the hypertensive course taken by SHRs.

Experimental data from sympathectomized animal preparations also indicated that an intact SNS appears to be essential in the development of SHR hypertension. Reporting on work done in 1971, Folkow's group presented evidence of a 40% reduction in blood pressure of adult SHRs following treatment with antiserum to nerve growth factor (NGF-AS) injected for the first 5 days of life (Folkow, Hallbäck, Lundgren, & Weiss, 1972). This "immunosympathectomy" in newborn animals is known to effectively diminish SNS function as measured later, both biochemically and physiologically in adults (Steiner & Schonbaum, 1972; Zaimis & Knight, 1972). Similar results are obtained after chemical sympathectomy in neonatal SHRs. Treating these rat pups with the sympathetic neurotoxin, 6-hydroxydopamine (6OHDA), for 14 days after birth almost completely prevented the development of hypertension as measured at 6, 8, 10, and 12 weeks of age (Finch, Cohen, & Horst, 1973). Neonatal administration of this agent has been shown to produce a permanent destruction of a large fraction of sympathetic neurons, resulting in widespread reduction of noradrenergic innervation to many tissues and organs (Malmfors & Thoenen, 1971). Additional research confirming the dependence of SHR hypertension on the integrity of sympathetic innervation comes from the laboratories of Vapaatalo et al. (Vapaatolo, Hackman, Antilla, Vainionpää, & Neuvonen, 1974), Provoost and De Jong (Provoost, Bohus, & De Jong, 1977), Ikeda et al. (Ikeda, Shibota, Shino, Nagaoka, & Fujita, 1976), and Johnson (Johnson & Macia, 1979). The first three of these groups reported a reduction of blood pressure in adult SHRs which had been chemically sympathectomized with 6OHDA shortly after birth. The latter group reported that SHRs did not become hypertensive if almost completely sympathectomized by a combined treatment of newborn with guanethidine and NGF-AS both at concentrations which were ineffective or only moderately effective alone.

Biochemical assessment of sympathoadrenomedullary activity has yielded additional strong supportive evidence for an increase in this cardiovascular control system in SHRs. Soon after Ozaki et al. reported that adrenomedullary norepinephrine content of adult SHRs was twice that of normotensive control rats (Ozaki, Suzuki, Yamori, & Okamoto, 1968), Nagatsu's group also found increased levels of tyrosine hydroxylase and dopamine-β-hydroxylase in the adrenals of adult SHRs (Nagatsu, Nagatsu, Mizutani, Umezawa, Matsuzaki, & Takeuchi, 1971). Strengthening the interpretation of results from previous biochemical investigations (Okamoto, 1969; Okamoto, 1972), Yamori and his coworkers found an increased turnover of norepinephrine in the hearts of young SHRs, as compared to age-matched WKY control rats (Yamori, 1974). This measured difference, which suggests an enhanced sympathetic drive to the heart in SHRs, was evidence at the prehypertensive and early hypertensive stages (30 and 60 days old), but was no longer present at 100 days of age, when hypertension was stabilized. Possibly related to this, cardiac monoamine oxidase activity in SHRs is consistently above that in WKY rats at various ages (Kumagai, Sejima, Yamada, Yamori, & Okamoto, 1976).

Further research at the biochemical level provided more evidence for sympathetic nervous system involvement, but indicated that observed increases in activity may be subdivided into different pathways according to the stage of development of the blood pressure elevation, in turn dependent on the age of the animals. Overall, results have demonstrated that measures indicative of increased sympathetic neuronal discharge appear particularly before onset and during incipient stages of hypertension. These measures include elevated dopamine-β-hydroxylase (DBH) activity in serum and mesenteric vessels and increased norepinephrine in plasma from SHRs sacrified by decapitation (Grobecker, Roizen, Weise, Saavedra, & Kopin, 1975; Nagatsu, Ikuta, Numata, Kato, Sano, Nagatsu, Umezawa, Matsuzaki, & Takeucki, 1976; Nagatsu, Kato, Numata, Ikuta, Umezawa, Matsuzaki, & Takeuchi, 1974; Nagaoka & Lovenberg, 1976). Young SHRs, as compared to age-matched normotensive WKY rats, also exhibit elevated activity of choline acetyltransferase and tyrosine hydroxylase in sympathetic celiac ganglia, which contain greater amounts of norepinephrine (Lütold, Karoum, & Neff, 1979; Nakamura & Nakamura, 1977). During these early stages, there appears to be less of an increase in adrenomedullary contribution. In later stages, the adrenal medulla is especially involved, as suggested by data from a number of laboratories (Nagatsu, et al., 1971; Nagatsu, Kato, Numata, Ikuta, Sano, Nagatsu, Umezawa, Matsuzaki, & Takeuchi, 1977; Nakamura, Nakamura, & Suzuki, 1977; Roizen, Weise, Grobecker, & Kopin, 1975). At this time, sympathetic innervation to the vas deferens also appears to be differentially activated (Nagatsu, et al., 1977), although in contrast to the earlier stages, plasma levels of norepinephrine in SHRs with fixed hypertension do not differ significantly from those of adult WKY rats (Nagaoka, et al., 1976; Roizen, et al., 1975). Plasma epinephrine during this phase is apparently elevated (Roizen, et al., 1975). However, as will be discussed below, many of the results regarding plasma levels of catecholamines are dependent on the state of the animal immediately prior to blood sampling.

Likewise, recent evidence supports previous findings (Okamoto, 1969; Okamoto, 1972) of pituitary involvement in the course of SHR hypertension. For example, early workers obtained morphological evidence of increased ACTH release. Later, both Yamori et al. (Yamori, Ohta, Horie, & Sato, 1976) and Freeman et al. (Freeman, Davis, Varsano-Abaron, Vlick, & Weinberger, 1975) obtained results suggesting that dexamethasone does not effectively suppress pituitary ACTH secretion in SHRs as it does in WKY rats. Pituitary, adrenal, and thyroid weights are significantly higher in SHRs than in age-matched WKYs (Yamada, Kojima, Kubota, Aizawa, Tawata, Koizumi, Yamori, & Okamoto,

1977). Plasma arginine-vasopressin concentrations in SHRs are almost twice those in WKY rats at 24 weeks of age (Möhring, Kintz, & Schoun, 1978). Elevated levels of mineralocorticoids such as corticosterone, deoxycorticosterone, 18-hydroxydexycorticosterone, and aldosterone have been reported for young SHRs (Tan & Mulrow, 1977), but not in all studies (Nakamura, et al., 1977) possibly because of age or control differences. In fact, results of basal plasma corticosterone level comparisons between SHRs and WKY rats have not been consistent even when measured in the same laboratory (McCarty, Kvetňanský, Lake, Thoa, & Kopin, 1978). Both higher and lower levels of this steroid in SHRs have been found as compared to WKYs. Elevated levels of other adrenocortical steroids in response to increased ACTH stimulation have not been ruled out. Since corticosterone is able to diminish ACTH release by negative feedback inhibition, it is of interest here that administration of corticosterone to young SHRs can slow the development of hypertension (Baer, Knowlton, & Laragh, 1972). This suggests that ACTH may be playing at least a partial role. Indirect evidence suggesting the involvement of ACTH-related opioid peptides, or their receptors has also been presented by Wendel and Bennett (1981).

Greater activation of these neural and hormonal pathways in SHRs than in WKY rats lends support to the likelihood of involvement of cortico-limbic and hypothalamic control systems in blood pressure elevation in SHRs. That these central cardiovascular regulatory influences are involved was first suggested by early results reported by Yamori and Okamoto (1969). They found that the decrease in blood pressure after surgical section of the descending posterior hypothalamic-mesencephalic pressor pathway was significantly larger in SHRs than in WKYs. More recent investigations have broadened the basis of support for this interpretation. Data from Buñag's laboratory has shown that posterior hypothalamic lesions produce a significantly greater reduction in blood pressure in SHRs than in normotensive or DOCA-hypertensive rats (Buñag & Eferakeya, 1976). In response to posterior hypothalamic stimulation at a number of different frequencies, SHRs show greater increases in efferent sympathetic nerve activity and arterial pressure than do WKYs or other controls (Buñag, Eferakeya, & Langdon, 1975; Buñag & Takeda, 1979; Campbell, Robinson, & Whitehorn, 1976; Juskevich, Robinson, & Whitehorn, 1978). This enhanced sympathetic and blood pressure response is an inherent characteristic of the SHRs and is not secondary to sustained hypertension for two reasons. First, SHRs maintained normotensive by drug therapy showed similar responses, i.e., greater than those in untreated or drug-treated WKYs (Juskevich, et al., 1978). Second, this heightened response of the sympathetic nervous system and cardiovascular pressor activity occurs not only in adult (18-20 weeks) SHRs with established hypertension, but even in 9-week old SHRs, whose pressure elevation is still developing (Buñag & Takeda, 1979).

The existence of differences between the SHR and its control, the WKY rat, in terms of central nervous system mechanisms operating in each is also supported by biochemical evidence from a number of laboratories. Although reports are too numerous to allow adequate review or discussion of discrepancies, a few can be noted as examples. Compared to age-matched WKY controls, SHRs have: lower levels of DBH in locus ceruleus at 3 weeks of age (Nagatsu, et al., 1976); delayed disappearance rate for brainstem ^{3}H norepinephrine after intra-ventricular injection at 6 weeks (Yamori, Oshima, & Okamoto, 1973); higher norepinephrine content in medulla-pons at 7 and 10 weeks, and in spinal cord at 4, 7, and 10 weeks (De Jong, Nijkamp, & Bohus, 1975); and in telencephalon at 10 weeks (Yamori, et al., 1973); elevated PNMT in brainstem at 4 weeks (Saavedra, Grobecker, & Axelrod, 1976); higher TH in hypothalamus and cor-pus striatum, higher DBH in hypothalamus and medulla-pons, and higher tryp-tophan hydroxylase in hypothalamus at 5 weeks (Nagaoka & Lovenberg, 1977); decreased norepinephrine and dopamine-β-hyrroxylase in specific hypothalamic nuclei at 4 and 14 weeks (Saavedra, Grobecker, & Axelrod, 1978); higher serotonin levels in telencephalon and brainstem at 26-30 weeks (Takaori, Tan-aka, & Okamoto, 1972). Other differences in individual brain regions have been reported (McCrorey, Bulman, & Hendley, 1977; Myers, Whittemore, & Hendley, 1979; Versteeg, Palkovits, van der Gugten, Wijnen, Smeets, & De Jong, 1976; Zukowska-Grójec, 1979). It should be kept in mind that some variations or lack of variations, in comparison to non-WKY controls, are thought to arise from genetic factors unrelated to pathogenesis of hypertension and are shared by both the SHR and its parent strain the WKY.

Highly integrated central nervous system cardiovascular mechanisms for pat-terned circulatory responses are located in brain regions known to subserve specific behavioral functions (Cohen & Obrist, 1975; Gunn, Wolf, Block, & Person, 1972; Hilton & Spyer, 1980; Reis & Doba, 1974; Smith, 1974; Zanchet-ti, Baccelli, & Mancia, 1976). Given the above evidence for existence of differ-entiated activity levels of SHR and WKY cardiovascular control centers for peripheral neural and hormonal output, it would not be surprising to find dis-tinguishing behavioral characteristics associated with the development of hyper-tension in SHRs. That this seems to be the case is indicated by a number of investigations. In one of the first studies comparing SHR and WKY rat behavior, Takaori et al. found that 60% of the total normotensive WKY rats trained in a standard Sidman nondiscriminated avoidance paradigm were poor performers or nonperformers. In contrast, almost all SHRs were good avoiders (Takaori, et al., 1972). Furthermore, they observed that decreasing brain serotonin concentra-tions (using p-chlorophenylalanine) increased both blood pressure and avoidance performance in WKY rats, while intraperitoneal administration of the serotonin precursor, L-5-hydroxytryptophan, decreased both blood pressure and avoidance performance in SHR and WKY rats.

Other studies, in attempts to examine any possible relationship between hy-pertension and repressed hostility or aggression, tested for differences in shock-induced fighting or in mouse-killing behavior. After 1 week of isolation, SHRs killed mice more frequently than did normotensive Wistar (not WKY) control rats, but hypertensive killers had a somewhat lower blood pressure than did hypertensive nonkillers (Rifkin, Silverman, Chavez, & Frankl, 1974). If compared to WKY controls, however, this difference in muricide was not evident (Eichelman, De Jong, & Williams, 1973). Eichelman et al. described a study in which female SHRs and WKY rats were subjected to four daily sessions of paired, foot shock-induced fighting (Eichelman, et al., 1973). Counting the number of attack responses made toward an opponent, they reported that SHRs fought about four times more than normotensive WKYs, but significantly less than NIH Wistar rats. Furthermore, the SHR jump threshold, i.e., the lowest current intensity at which the rat jumps 50% of the time, was significantly lower than that of the WKY, but higher than that of the NIH Wistar. As in previous biochemical investigations, these results demonstrate the need for appropriate controls. In this case, no clearly defined association between hypertension and aggression emerges, since strain differences appear to be genetically separate and unrelated to the hypertension.

More information concerning behavior in this animal model is contained in studies which include measurements of locomotor activity. In general, SHRs exhibit a higher level of locomotor activity in both open-field and running-wheel test situations. But, here again, normotensive rats other than WKY have been used as controls in some of the studies, and slight variations in results may be attributed to strain differences, as well as differences in testing procedures. For example, Pappas et al. described a greater motor activity of SHRs in both open field and activity wheel, including greater rearing, as compared to non-WKY Wistar controls (Pappas, Peters, Saari, Sobrian, & Minch, 1974). Later, Rosecrans and Adams, measuring spontaneous activity including rearing, reported that SHRs were less active than normotensive Wistar (not WKY) controls (Rosecrans & Adams, 1976). However, on repeated testing, activity in the normotensive rats declined more (54%-73%) between initial and final exposure than did activity in SHRs (17%-36%). Thus, during final testing, the SHRs displayed greater activity. Similar results were obtained in open-field testing. Although normotensive Wistars exhibited more open-field activity initially, their activity was markedly reduced in subsequent exposure to levels much below those of SHRs. In more recent work with WKY controls, Tucker and Johnson (1980b) found that SHR and WKY rats did not differ in open-field activity when measured at 16 days of age. Rosecrans and Adams (1976) found also that spontaneous motor activity of SHRs was suppressed less than that of normotensive Wistars by a conditioned stimulus, while they showed an enhanced performance in an unsignaled shuttle avoidance paradigm. This diminished conditioned (shock) suppression found here is consistent with the results of Saari and Pappas (1973), who found that foot shock-induced suppression of drinking behavior was less in SHRs than in normotensive Wistars.

This lesser conditioned suppression of ongoing behavior does not appear to extend to pharmacological reduction of motor activity. As shown by Tilson et al., although both WKYs and SHRs exhibited lower 2-hour motor activity scores than either Sprague-Dawley albino or Long-Evans hooded rats, the scores for SHRs were significantly higher than those for WKY rats (Tilson, Chamberlain, Gylys, & Buyniski, 1977). In the same work, it was found that the ED_{50} (mg/kg) for depression of that motor activity, by the centrally acting antihypertensive agent clonidine, was considerably less for SHRs than for WKYs. Numerous other investigations have demonstrated a greater motor activity in SHRs as compared to the appropriate genetic control, the WKY rat (Campbell & DiCara, 1977; McCarty & Kopin, 1979; Myers, et al., 1977; Sasagawa & Yamori, 1975; Shimamoto & Nagaoka, 1977). Perhaps related to these findings are the interesting data of Hall et al. (Hall, Ayachi, & Hall, 1976). These workers found that SHRs are more resistant to the induction of pentobarbital and barbital anesthesia than normotensive WKY or COBS Wistar rats. Furthermore, SHRs awaken more quickly than either Wistar strains after pentobarbital or α-chloralose anesthesia. However, although these differences may be due to a variation in sensitivity of central neuronal systems, differences in hepatic inactiviation or renal excretion cannot be excluded.

The results of a study by Campbell and DiCara and their co-workers demonstrated that lower blood pressure is associated with lower conditioned active avoidance responding in a combined group of SHRs and WKYs (Campbell & Di Cara, 1977). This associative relationship between avoidance performance and blood pressure was observed over a wide pressure range which was due to genetic differences between the animals. It was of interest, therefore, to ascertain if a similar relationship might hold in a genetically homogeneous, but pharmacologically heterogeneous, group of SHRs exhibiting a similar wide range of blood pressure. That is, an attempt was made to lower the pressures of SHRs by pharmacological manipulation to the level of WKY rats and to determine if avoidance responding would be lowered accordingly. This was of special interest in the case of those agents believed to lower arterial pressure by a central mechanism and which were known to cause behavioral effects as well. The results of this additional study demonstrated that lower avoidance performance was associated with lower pressure obtained by therapeutic intervention (R. J. Campbell, L. V. DiCara, and H. A. Ferguson, unpublished observations).

Based in part on these results and in part on the findings of earlier studies, a working hypothesis regarding the SHR model was developed on the assumption that SHR "personality" factors and the elevated blood pressure are the expression of a third variable—a genetic one. More specifically, this hypothesis attributes an interdependent, somatic-psychoemotional profile of high blood pressure-high conditioned avoidance responding to a common genetic characterization for the SHR (Campbell & Di Cara, 1977). Increased availability of certain central and pituitary polypeptides, coinciding with increased sympathoadrenomedullary activity, is genetically determined as a psychogenic anticipatory hyperreactivity (to environmental stimuli) in hypertensive rats of the Wistar-Kyoto foundation stock (cf. Weiner's "vigilance" in man (Weiner,

1970)). This is responsible, at least in part, for the superior active avoidance conditioning, and is a major contributing factor in the development of hypertension, given the vascular autoregulatory reactivity under increased pressure loads (Folkow, 1978, 1982).

Much recent evidence from Kopin's laboratory supports this hypothesis. First, workers in his laboratory determined that if chronic indwelling catheters are employed, rather than acute sampling of blood necessitating animal handling, no strain differences in plasma norepinephrine or epinephrine are found in undisturbed SHRs and age-matched WKY rats while in their home cages (Chiueh & Kopin, 1978; McCarty & Kopin, 1978; McCarty & Kopin, 1977). These results strongly suggest that true basal sympathetic-adrenomedullary activity is similar for both the SHR model and its parent strain. Nevertheless, their additional findings show that stress, such as foot shock or immobilization, or the anticipation of such stress, or even such a mild environmental change as being placed in another cage, produces a greater increase in both catecholamines in SHRs at various ages. This greater catecholamine response continues during recovery from stress for a longer duration in SHRs than in WKYs, taking longer to return to basal prestress levels (McCarty, Chiueh, & Kopin 1978; Chiueh & Kopin 1978; McCarty & Kopin, 1977; McCarty & Kopin, 1978; Kvetnansky, McCarty, Thoa, Lake, & Kopin, 1979). Plasma corticosterone also appears to be increased by immobilization stress more in SHRs than in WKY rats (Kvetnansky, et al., 1979), but this was not a consistent finding (McCarty, Kvetnansky, Lake, Thoa & Kopin, 1978).

Additional evidence corroborates this hyperreactivity of SHRs to stress. Berkowitz and Hahn recently reported that agitation in a cold environment caused a greater release of norepinephrine from the mesenteric vein, mesenteric artery, and inferior vena cava in SHRs (Berkowitz & Hahn, 1979). Similarly, after immobilization stress, DBH activity in serum, adrenals, and other sympathetically innervated tissues was more elevated in SHRs than in WKY rats (Nagatsu, Kato, Fujita, & Takahashi, 1979). Futher data from McCarty and Chiueh (1980) suggest that SHRs are hyperactive in their sympathetic-adrenal responses to some but not all types of stressful stimulation. Significantly greater and longer lasting increments in plasma levels of norepinephrine and epinephrine in SHRs than in WKYs results after exposure to intermittent inescapable shock but not to cold. Presumably it is this greater catecholaminergic reactivity to environmental stimulation that is responsible for the elevated levels of related biosynthetic enzymes mentioned previously.

This heightened reactivity to environmental stimuli perceived as stressful might explain why others had earlier found that reduction of environmental stimulation significantly slowed development of high blood pressure in SHRs, while a stressful environment produced even higher levels of pressure than those found in nonstressed SHRs. It has been shown that blood pressures of SHRs reared in near-total darkness or in social isolation are lower than those of control

SHRs (Lais, Bhatnagar, & Brody, 1974; Hallbäck, 1975). In contrast, SHRs subjected to acute or chronic stress, such as immobilization, or a combination of aversive sensory stimuli, or cold exposure, exhibit further increases in their already high arterial pressure (Folkow, Hallbäck & Weiss, 1973; Yamori, Matsumoto, Yamabe, & Okamoto, 1969). These changes are greater in SHRs than in normotensive control rats in these earlier studies, although later work has demonstrated that this difference between them may only be observed under certain conditions. These conditions apply to duration or recurrence of the stress and are related to difference in vasomotor reaction to norepinephrine as compared to epinephrine (Kvetnansky, et al., 1979).

CONCLUSION

Although generalizations leave something lacking in terms of mechanistic definition, when made from a large body of evidence, they at least provide a potential for understanding some of the characteristics of a problem under study. For the most part, evidence from the animal models reviewed in this chapter supports the premise that behavioral processes are intimately related to genesis of the multiple pathological mechanisms operating in production of an elevated arterial pressure. Included are those models most extensively studied within the framework of psychology as applied to occurrence of disease. We have only touched upon what can be learned from animal studies as they apply to models of essential hypertension in man, yet the questions generated and directions aimed seem to be significant for carry-over to the clinical setting. Two animal models of hypertension have been examined in detail in this chapter. They represent seemingly opposite ends of a wide spectrum of causation of high blood pressure, one genetic and one psychosocial. Still, workers familiar with these models have concluded, for both, that excessive and prolonged activation of neurohormonal cardiovascular control systems, environmentally triggered and behaviorally modulated, is an important factor in the etiology of their hypertension. Experiments with the psychosocial stress model of hypertension have demonstrated the power of socioenvironmental variables to produce severe hypertension and its sequelae in an otherwise healthy mouse population. Experiments with the spontaneously hypertensive rat model of hypertension have demonstrated the contibution of psychophysiological constitution to this cardiovascular disorder. It is difficult to believe that such behavioral processes are important for this disease in rodents but not for essential hypertension in humans, whose cognitive interaction with the environment would surely involve complex psychological factors as influential as those of mice and rats. The recent appearance of similar clinical formulations for prevention and therapy support this reasoning.

Results obtained from research with these animal models of hypertension suggest that profitable future research will be directed toward monitoring various parameters prior to onset of measurable hypertension. It is in these types of studies that noncausal associative relationships might be separated from possible cause-and-effect relationships which can be investigated further for verification of a causal status. A parallel course of study would seem profitable in the human population, where physiological and behavioral data shown relevant to animal models is collected from a large human population before the onset of hypertension in whatever proportion of that population later develops this disorder.

REFERENCES

Aceto, M. D. G., Kinnard, W. J., & Buckley, J. P. Effect of compounds on blood pressure and behavioral responses of rats chronically subjected to an avoidance-escape situation. *Archives Internationales de Pharmacodynamie et de Therapie, 1963, 144,* 214–225.

Anderson, D. E., & Brady, J. V. Pre-avoidance blood pressure elevations accompanied by heart rate decreases in the dog. *Science,* 1971, *172,* 595–597.

Anderson, D. E., & Brady, J. V. Prolonged pre-avoidance upon blood pressure and heart rate in the dog. *Psychosomatic Medicine* (1973, *35,* 4–12.

Anderson, D. E., & Yingling, J. E. Aversive conditioning of elevations in total peripheral resistance in dogs. *American Journal of Physiology* 1979, *236,* H880–H887.

Baer, L., Knowlton, A., & Laragh, J. H. The role of sodium balance and the pituitary-adrenal axis in the hypertension of spontaneously hypertensive rats. In *Spontaneous Hypertension: Its Pathogenesis and Complications (Proc. 1st Int. Sympos. SHR),* 1972, Okamoto, K. (Ed.), Springer-Verlag, New York, pp. 203–209.

Benson, H., Herd, J. A., Morse, W. H., & Kelleher, R. T. Behavioral induction of arterial hypertension and its reversal. *American Journal of Physiology,* 1969, *217,* 30–34.

Berkowitz, B., & Hahn, R. Blood vessel catecholamines, stress and vascular disease (abstr.). *Second International Symposium on Catecholamines and Stress, September 12–16, 1979, Smolenice Castle, Czechoslovakia, Abstracts,* 1979, p. 105.

Bianchi, G., Fox, U. and Imbasciati, E. The development of a new strain of spontaneously hypertensive rats. *Life Sciences,* 1974, 14:339–347.

Bianchi, G. and Baer, P. G. Characteristics of the Milan hypertensive strain (MHS) of rat. *Clinical and Experimental Pharmacology and Physiology,* 1976, Suppl. 3:15–20.

Buckley, J. P., Parham, C., & Smookler, H. H. Effects of reserpine on rats subjected to prolonged experimental stress. *Archives Internationales de Pharmacodynamie et de Therapie* 1968, *172,* 292–300.

Buckley, J. P., Vogin, F. E., & Kinnard, W. J. Effects of pentobarbital, acetylsalicylic acid, and reserpine on blood pressure and survival of rats subjected to experimental stress. *Journal of Pharmaceutical Sciences* 1966, *55,* 572–575.

Buñag, R. D., & Eferakeya, A. E. Immediate hypotensive atter-effects of posterior hypothalamic lesions in awake rats with spontaneous, renal or DOCA hypertension. *Cardiovascular Research,* 1976, *10,* 663–671.

Buñag, R. D., Eferakeya, A. E., & Langdon, D. S. Enhancement of hypothalamic pressor responses in spontaneously hypertensive rats. *American Journal Physiology* 1975, *228,* 217–222.

Buñag, R. D. & Takeda, K. Sympathetic hyperresponsiveness to hypothalamic stimulation in young hypertensive rats. *American Journal of Physiology,* 1979, *237,* 39–44.

Campbell, R. J. & DiCara, L. V. Running wheel avoidance behavior in the Wistar-Kyoto spontaneously hypertensive rat. *Physiology and Behavior,* 1977, *19,* 473–480.

Campbell, J. C., Robinson, D. S., & Whitehorn, D. Differences in central nervous system regulation of blood pressure in spontaneously hypertensive and matched control rats (abstr.). *Physiologist*, 1976, *19*, 147.

Carretero, O. A., & Romero, J. C. Production and characteristics of experimental hypertension in animals. In *Hypertension: Physiopathology and Treatment*, 1977, Genest, J., Koiw, E., & Kuchel, O. (Eds). McGraw-Hill, New York, pp. 485–507.

Chiueh, C. C., & Kopin, I. J. Hyperresponsivity of spontaneously hypertensive rat to indirect measurement of blood pressure. *American Journal of Physiology*, 1978, *234*, 690–695.

Ciaranello, R. D. Regulation of phenylethanolamine-N-methyltransferase synthesis and degradation. In *Structure and Function of Monamine Enzymes*, (1977), Usdin, E., Weiner, N., & Youdim, M. B. H. (Eds.). Marcel Dekker, New York, pp. 497–525.

Clark, D. W. J., & Phelan, E. L. The role of the sympathetic nervous system in the pathogenesis of genetic hypertension (GH) in rats: A brief review. *Clinical and Experimental Pharmacology and Physiology*, 1976, Suppl. 3, 65–68.

Cohen, D. H., & Obrist, P. A. Interaction between behavior and the cardiovascular system. *Circulation Research*, (1975) *37*: 693–706.

Conner, R. L., Vernikos-Danellis, J., & Levine, S. Stress, fighting and neuroendocrine function. *Nature*, 1971, *234*, 564–566.

Dahl, L. K., Heine, M. and Tassinari, L. Effects of chronic excess salt ingestion. Evidence that genetic factors play an important role in susceptibility to experimental hypertension. *Journal of Experimental Medicine* 1962, 115:1173–1190.

Dahl, L. K., Heine, M. and Tassinari, L. J. Effects of chronic excess salt ingestion. Vascular reactivity in two strains of rats with opposite genetic susceptibility to experimental hypertension. *Circulation* (Suppl. 2) 1964, 29/30:11–22.

Dahl, L. K., Knudsen, K. D., Heine, M., & Leitl, G. Hypertension and stress. *Nature* (1968) *219*: 735–736.

De Jong, W., Nijkamp, F. P., & Bohus, B. Role of noradrenaline and serotonin in the central control of blood pressure in normotensive and spontaneously hypertensive rats. *Arch. Int. Pharmacodyn. Ther.*, 1975, *213*, 272–284.

DiCara, L. V., & Miller, N. E. Instrumental learning of systolic blood pressure responses by curarized rats: Dissociation of cardiac and vascular changes. *Psychosomatic Medicine* 1968, *30*, 489–494.

Dworkin, B. R., Filewich, R. J., Miller, N. E., Craigmyle, N., & Pickering, T. G. Baroreceptor activation reduces reactivity to noxious stimulation: Implications for hypertension. *Science*, 1979, *205*, 1299–1301.

Dykman, R. A., & Gantt, W. H. Experimental psychogenic hypertension: Blood pressure changes conditioned to painful stimuli (schizokinesis). *Bulletin of the Johns Hopkins Hospital*, 1960, *107*, 72–89.

Eichelman, B., De Jong, W., & Williams, R. B. Aggressive behavior in hypertensive and normotensive rat strains. *Physiology and Behavior*, 1973, *10*, 301–304.

Ely, D. L., & Henry, J. P. Effects of prolonged social deprivation on murine behavior patterns, blood pressure, and adrenal weight. *Journal of Comparative Physiological Psychology*, 1974, *87*, 733–740.

Ely, D. L., & Henry, J. P. Neuroendocrine response patterns in dominant and subordinate mice. *Hormones and Behavior*, 1978, *10*, 156–169.

Falk, J. L., Tang, M., & Forman, S. Schedule-induced chronic hypertension. *Psychosomatic Medicine*, 1977, *39*, 252–263.

Farris, E. J., Yeakel, E. H., & Medoff, H. S. Development of hypertension in emotional gray Norway rats after air blasting. *American Journal of Physiology*, 1945, *144*, 331–333.

Figar, S. Conditional circulatory responses in men and animals. *Handbook of Physiology: Circulation (Section 2)*, 1965, *3*, 1991–2035.

Finch, L., Cohen, M., & Horst, W. D. Effects of 6-hydroxydopamine at birth on the development of hypertension in the rat. *Life Sciences*, 1973, *13*, 1403–1410.

Folkow, B. Cardiovascular structural adaptation; its role in the initiation and maintenance of primary hypertension (The Fourth Volhard Lecture). *Clinical Sciences and Molecular Medicine*, 1978, *55*, 3s–22s.

Folkow, B. Physiological aspects of primary hypertension. *Physiological Reviews*, 1982, 62:347–504.

Folkow, B., & Hallbäck, M. Physiopathology of spontaneous hypertension in rats. In *Hypertension: Physiopathology and Treatment*, 1977, Genest, J., Koiw, E., & Kuchel, O. (Eds.). McGraw-Hill, New York, pp. 507–529.

Folkow, B., Hallbäck, M., Lundgren, Y, & Weiss, L. The effects of "immunosympathectomy" on blood pressure and vascular "reactivity" in normal and spontaneously hypertensive rats. *Acta Physiologica Scandanavica*, 1972 *84*, 512–523.

Folkow, B., Hallbäck, M., & Weiss, L. Cardiovascular responses to acute mental 'stress' in spontaneously hypertensive rats. *Clincal Sciences and Molecular Medicine* 1973, *45*, 131–133.

Forsyth, R. P. Blood pressure and avoidance conditioning: A study of 15-day trials in the rhesus monkey. *Psychosomatic Medicine*, 1968, *30*, 125–135.

Forsyth, R. P. Blood pressure responses to long-term avoidance schedules in the restrained rhesus monkey. *Psychosomatic Medicine*, 1969, *31*, 300–309.

Freeman, R. H., Davis, J. O., Varsano-Abaron, N., Vlick, S., & Weinberger, M. H. Control of aldosterone secretion in spontaneously hypertensive rat. *Circulation Research* (1975) *37*, 66–71.

Friedman, R. & Dahl, L. K. The effect of chronic conflict on the blood pressure of rats with a genetic susceptibility to experimental hypertension. *Psychosomatic Medicine*, 1975, *37*, 402–416.

Friedman, R. & Iwai, J. Genetic predisposition and stress-induced hypertension. *Science*, 1976, *193*, 161–162.

Gantt, W. H. Cardiovascular component of the conditional reflex to pain, food and other stimuli. *Physiological Reviews*, 1960, *40*, (Suppl. 4): 266–291.

Goldblatt, H., Lynch, J., Hanzal, R. F., & Summerville, W. W. Studies on experimental hypertension: I. The production of persistent elevation of systolic blood pressure by means of renal ischemia. *Journal of Experimental Medicine*, 1934, *59*, 347–379.

Grobecker, H., Roizen, M., Weise, V., Saavedra, J. M., & Kopin, I. J. Sympathoadrenal medullary activity in young spontaneously hypertensive rats. *Nature*, 1975, *258*, 267–268.

Guidotti, A., Hanbaurer, I., & Costa, E. Role of cyclic nucleotides in the induction of tyrosine hydroxylase. In *Advances in Cyclic Nucleotide Research, Vol 5*, 1975, Dummond, G. I., Greengard, P., and Robison, G. A. (Eds.). Raven Press, New York, pp. 619–639.

Gunn, C. G., Wolf, S., Block, R. T., & Person, R. J. Psychophysiology of the cardiovascular system. In *Handbook of Psychophysiology*, 1972, Greenfield, N. S. & Sternbach, R. A. (Eds.). Holt, Rinehart, and Winston, New York, pp. 457–489.

Guyton, A. C., Coleman, T. G., Cowley, A. W., Scheel, K. W., Manning, D., & Norman, R. A. Arterial pressure regulation. Overriding dominance of the kidneys in long-term regulation and in hypertension. *American Journal of Medicine*, 1972 *52* 584–594.

Hall, C. E., Ayachi, S., & Hall, O. Differential sensitivity of spontaneously hypertensive (SHR) and control rats to various anesthetic agents. *Clincal and Experimental Pharmacology and Physiology*, 1976, Suppl. 3, 83–86.

Hall, C. E., & Hall, O. Augmentation of hormone-induced hypertensive cardiovascular disease by simultaneous exposure to stress. *Acta Endocrinologica*, 1959, *30*, 557–566.(a)

Hall, C. E., & Hall, O. Enhancement of somatotrophic hormone-induced hypertensive cardiovascular disease by stress. *American Journal of Physiology*, 1959, *197*, 702–704.(b)

Hallbäck, M. Consequence of social isolation on blood pressure, cardiovascular reactivity and design in spontaneously hypertensive rats. *Acta Physiologica Scandanavica* 1975, *93*, 455–465.

Harris, A. H., & Brady, J. V. Animal learning—visceral and autonomic conditioning. *Annual Review of Psychology*, 1974, *25*, 107–132.

Harris, A. H., Gilliam, W. J., Findley, J. D., & Brady, J. V. Instrumental conditioning of large-magnitude, daily, 12-hour blood pressure elevations in the baboon. *Science*, 1973, *182;* 175–177.

Henry, J. P. Understanding the early pathophysiology of essential hypertension. *Geriatrics*, 1976, *31*, 59–72.

Henry, J. P., Ely, D. L., Stephens, P. M., Ratcliffe, H. L., Santisteban, G. A., & Shapiro, A. P. The role of psychosocial factors in the development of arteriosclerosis in CBA mice. *Atherosclerosis*, 1971, *14*, 203–218.

Henry, J. P., Ely, D. L., Watson, F. M. C., & Stephens, P. M. Ethological methods as applied to the measurement of emotion. In *Emotions—Their Parameters and Measurement*, 1975, Levi, L. (Ed.). Raven Press, New York, pp. 469–497.

Henry J. P., Meehan, J. P., & Stephens, P. M. The use of psychosocial stimuli to induce prolonged systolic hypertension in mice. *Psychosomatic Medicine* 1967, *29*, 408–432.

Henry, J. P., Meehan, J. P., Stephens, P., & Santisteban, G. A. Arterial pressure in CBA mice as related to age. *Journal of Gerontology*, 1965, *20*, 239–243.

Henry, J. P., & Stephens, P. M. The social environment and essential hypertension in mice: Possible role of the innervation of the adrenal cortex. *Progress in Brain Research*, 1977, *47*, 263–276.(a)

Henry, J. P., & Stephens, P. M. *Stress, Health, and the Social Environment. A Sociobiologic Approach to Medicine*, 1977. Springer-Verlag, New York. (b)

Henry, J. P., & Stephens, P. M. An animal model of neuropsychological factors in hypertension. In *Prophylactic Approach to Hypertensive Diseases (Perspectives in Cardiovascular Research Series, Vol. 4)*, 1979, Yamori, Y., Lovenberg, W., & Freis, W. (Eds.). Raven Press, New York, pp. 299–307.

Henry, J. P., Stephens, P. M., Axelrod, J., & Mueller, R. A. Effects of psychosocial stimulation on the enzymes involved in the biosynthesis and metabolism of noradrenaline and adrenaline. *Psychosomatic Medicine*, 1971, *33*, 227–237.

Henry, J. P., Stephens, P. M., & Santisteban, G. A. A model of psychosocial hypertension showing reversibility and progression of cardiovascular complications. *Circulation Research*, 1975, *36*, 156–164.

Herd, J. A., Morse, W. H., Kelleher, R. T., & Jones L. G. Arterial hypertension in the squirrel monkey during behavioral experiments. *American Journal of Physiology*, 1969, *217*, 24–29.

Hilton, S. M., & Spyer, K. M. Central nervous system regulation of vascular resistance. *Annual Review of Physiology*, 1980, *42*, 399–411.

Hudak, W. J., & Buckley, J. P. Production of hypertensive rats of experimental stress. *Journal of Pharmaceutical Sciences* 1961, *50*, 263–264.

Ikeda, H., Shibota, M., Shino, A., Nagaoka, A., & Fujita, T. Effect of chemical sympathectomy on development of hypertension in stroke-prone and stroke-resistant SHR. *Japanese Heart Journal*, 1976 *17*, 420–421.

Iriuchijima, J. Sympathetic discharge rate in spontaneously hypertensive rats. *Japanese Heart Journal*, 1973 *14*, 350–356.

Johnson, E. M. & Macia, R. A. Unique resistance to guanethidine-induced chemical sympathectomy of spontaneously hypertensive rats. A resistance overcome by treatment with antibody to nerve growth factor. *Circulation Research*, 1979, *45*, 243–249.

Judy, W. V., & Farrell, S. K. Arterial baroreceptor reflex control of sympathetic nerve activity in the spontaneously hypertensive rat. *Hypertension*, 1979, *1*, 605–614.

Judy, W. V., Watanabe, A. M., Henry, D. P., Besch, H. R., Jr., Murphy, W. R., & Hockel, G. M. Sympathetic nerve activity: Role in regulation of blood pressure in the spontaneously hypertensive rat. *Circulation Research*, 1976, *38*, (Suppl. 2): 21–29.

Judy, W. V., Watanabe, A. M., Murphy, W. R., Aprison, B. S., & Yu, P. Sympathetic nerve activity and blood pressure in normotensive backcross rats genetically related to the spontaneously hypertensive rat. *Hypertension,* 1979, *1,* 598–604.

Juskevich, J. C., Robinson, D. S., & Whitehorn, D. Effect of hypothalamic stimulation in spontaneously hypertensive and Wistar-Kyoto rats. *European Journal of Pharmacology,* 1978, *51,* 429–439.

Kumagai, H., Sejima, S., Yamada, H., Yamori, Y., & Okamoto, K. Studies on the monoamine oxidase in spontaneously hypertensive rats. *Japanese Heart Journal,* 1976 *17:* 414–415.

Kvetñanský, R., McCarty, R., Thoa, N. B., Lake, C. R., & Kopin, I. J. Sympatho-adrenal responses of spontaneously hypertensive rats to immobilization stress. *American Journal of Physiology,* 1979, *236,* 457–462.

Lais, L. T., Bhatnagar, R. A., & Brody, M. J. Inhibition by dark adaptation of the progress of hypertension in the spontaneously hypertensive rat (SHR). *Circulation Research,* 1974, *34–35* (Suppl. 1): 155–160.

Lamprecht, F., Williams, R. B., & Kopin, I. J. Serum dopamine-B-hydroxylase during development of immobilization-induced hypertension. *Endocrinology* (1973) *92:* 953–956.

Lapin, B. A., & Cherkovich, G. M. Environmental changes causing the development of neuroses and corticovisceral pathology in monkeys. In *Society, Stress and Disease: The Psychosocial Environment and Psychosomatic Disease,* 1971, Levi, L. (Ed.). Oxford University Press, London, pp. 266–280.

Lipman, R. L., & Shapiro, A. P. Effects of a behavioral stimulus on blood pressure of rats with experimental pyelonephritis. *Psychosomatic Medicine,* 1967, *29,* 612–620.

Lockett, M. F., & Marwood, J. F. Sound deprivation causes hypertension in rats. *Federation Proceedings,* 1973 *32,* 2111–2114.

Lütold, B. E., Karoum, F., & Neff, N. H. Deficient dopamine metabolism in the celiac ganglion of spontaneously hypertensive rats. *Circulation Research,* 1979, *44,* 467–471.

Malmfors, T., & Thoenen, H. (Eds.) *6-Hydroxydopamine and Catecholamine Neurons* (1971). Elsevier, New York.

McCarty, R. and Chiueh, C. C. SHR rats: Adrenergic hyperresponsivity to footshock stress but not to cold exposure. *Society for Neuroscience Abstracts,* 1980, 12: 862.

McCarty, R., Chiueh, C. C., & Kopin, I. J. Spontaneously hypertensive rats: Adrenergic hyperresponsivity to anticipation of electric shock. *Behavioral Biology* 1978, *23,* 180–188.

McCarty, R., & Kopin, I. J. Excessive elevation of plasma catecholamines during stress in spontaneously hypertensive rats (abstr.). *Society for Neuroscience Abstracts,* 1977, *3,* 255.

McCarty, R., & Kopin, I. J. Alterations in plasma catecholamines and behavior during acute stress in spontaneously hypertensive and Wistar-Kyoto normotensive rats. *Life Sciences* 1978 *22,* 997–1006.

McCarty, R., & Kopin, I. J. Patterns of behavioral development in spontaneously hypertensive rats and Wistar-Kyoto normotensive controls. *Developmental Psychobiology,* (1979) *12:* 239–243.

McCarty, R., Kventñanský, R., Lake, C. R., Thoa, N. B., & Kopin, I. J. Sympatho-adrenal activity of SHR and WKY rats recovery from forced immobilization. *Physiology and Behavior* 1978, *21,* 951–955.

Medoff, H. S. & Bongiovanni, A. M. Blood pressure in rats subjected to audiogenic stimulation. *American Journal of Physiology,* 1945, *143,* 300–305.

Meehan, J. P., Fineg, J., & Mosely, J. D. The effect of restraint and training on the arterial pressure of the immature chimpanzee (abstr.). *Federation Proceedings,* 1964, *23,* 515.

Meehan, J. P., Fineg, J., & Wheelwright, D. D. Blood pressure instrumentation for the MA-5 flight. In *Results of the Project Mercury Ballistic and Orbital Chimpanzee Flights, NASA Report No. SP-39,* 1963, Henry, J. P., & Mosely, J. D. (Eds.). National Aeronautics and Space Administration, Manned Spacecraft Center, Houston, Texas, pp. 59–68.

Miminoshvili, D. I. Experimental neuroses in monkeys. In *Theoretical and Practical Problems of Medicine and Biology in Experiments on Monkeys,* 1960, Utkin, I. A. (Ed.). Pergamon Press, New York, pp. 53–67.

Möhring, J., Kintz, J., and Schoun, J. Role of vasopressin in blood pressure control of spontaneously hypertensive rats. *Clinical Science and Molecular Medicine* (1978) *55:* 247s–250s.

Mueller, R. A., Thoenen, H., & Axelrod, J. Effect of pituitary and ACTH on the maintenance of basal tyrosine hydroxylase activity in the rat adrenal gland. *Endocrinology* 1970, *86,* 751–755.

Myers, M. M., McCrorey, D., Bulman, C. A., & Hendley, E. D. Open field behavior and brain norepinephrine uptake in spontaneously hypertensive rats and Wistar-Kyoto normotensive controls (abstr.). *Federation Proceedings,* 1977, *36,* 4079.

Myers, M. M., Whittemore, S. R., & Hendley, E. D. Forebrain catecholamine mechanisms in the spontaneously hypertensive rat (abstr.). *Second International Symposium on Catecholamines and Stress, September 12–16, 1979, Smolenice Castle, Czechoslovakia, Abstracts,* (1979) p. 52.

Nagaoka, A., & Lovenberg, W. Plasma norepinephrine and dopamine-β-hydroxylase in genetic hypertensive rats. *Life Sciences,* 1976, *19,* 29–34.

Nagaoka, A., & Lovenberg, W. Regional changes in the activities of aminergic biosynthetic enzymes in the brains of hypertensive rats. *European Journal of Pharmacology,* 1977, *43,* 297–306.

Nagatsu, T., Ikuta, K., Numata (Sudo), Y., Kato, T., Sano, M., Nagatsu, I., Umezawa, H., Matsuzaki, M., & Takeuchi, T. Vascular and brain dopamine-β-hydroxylase activity in young spontaneously hypertensive rats. *Science,* 1976, *191,* 290–291.

Nagatsu, T., Kato, T., Fujita, K., and Takahashi, I. Catecholamine enzymes of spontaneously hypertensive rats under stress (abstr.). *Second International Symposium on Catecholamines and Stress, September 12–16, 1979, Smolenice Castle, Czechoslovakia, Abstracts,* (1979) p. 53.

Nagatsu, T., Kato, T., Numata (Sudo), Y., Ikuta, K., Sano, M., Nagatsu, I., Umezawa, H., Matsuzaki, M., & Takeuchi, T. Norepinephrine synthesizing enzymes in brain, adrenals, and peripheral sympathetic nerves of spontaneously hypertensive rats. *Japanese Journal of Pharmacology,* 1977, *27,* 531–535.

Nagatsu, T., Kato, T., Numata (Sudo), Y., Ikuta, K., Umezawa, H., Matsuzaki, M., & Takeuchi, T. Serum dopamine-β-hydroxylase activity in developing hypertensive rats. *Nature,* 1974, *251,* 630–631.

Nagatsu, J., Nagatsu, T., Mizutani, K., Umezawa, H., Matsuzaki, M., & Takeuchi, T. Adrenal tyrosine hydroxylase and dopamine-β-hydroxylase in spontaneously hypertensive rats. *Nature,* 1971, *230,* 381–382.

Nakamura, K., & Nakamura, K. Selective activation of sympathetic ganglia in young spontaneously hypertensive rats. *Nature,* 1977, *266,* 265–266.

Nakamura, K., Nakamura, K., & Suzuki, T. Reciprocal changes in adreno-medullary and cortical functions in spontaneously hypertensive rats. In *Proceedings of the 2nd International Symposium on the Spontaneously Hypertensive Rat,* 1977. U.S. Department of Health, Education, and Welfare Publication NIH 77–1179, pp. 149–158.

Nathan, M. A., Tucker, L. W., Severini, W. H., & Reis, D. J. Enhancement of conditioned arterial pressure responses in cats after brainstem lesions. *Science,* 1978, *201,* 71–73.

Okamoto, K. Spontaneous hypertension in rats. *International Review of Experimental Pathology,* 1969, *7,* 22–270.

Okamoto, K. (Ed.) *Spontaneous Hypertension: Its Pathogenesis and Complications (Proceedings of the 1st International Symposium on SHR)* (1972). Springer-Verlag, New York.

Okamoto, K. and Aoki, K. Development of a strain of spontaneously hypertensive *Japanese Circulation Journal,* 1963, 27:282–293.

Okamoto, K., Nosaka, S., Yamori, Y., & Matsumoto, M. Participation of neural factors in the pathogenesis of hypertension in the spontaneously hypertensive rat. *Japanese Heart Journal,* 1967, *8,* 168–180.

Onesti, G., Fernandes, M., & Kim, K. E. (Eds.). *Regulation of Blood Pressure by the Central Nervous System, 1976.* Grune and Stratton, New York.

Otten, V., & Thoenen, H. Circadian rhythm of tyrosine hydroxylase induction by short-term cold stress: Modulatory action of glucocorticoids in newborn and adult rats. *Proceedings of the National Academy of Sciences USA,* 1975 72, 1415–1419.

Ozaki, M., Suzuki, Y., Yamori, Y., & Okamoto, K. Adrenal catecholamine content in the spontaneously hypertensive rat. *Japanese Circulation Journal* 1968, *32,* 1367–1372.

Page, I. H. Arterial hypertension in retrospect. *Circulation Research,* 1974, *34,* 133–142.

Pappas, B. A., Peters, D. A. V., Saari, M., Sobrian, S. K., & Minch, E. Neonatal 6-hydroxydopamine sympathectomy in normotensive and spontaneously hypertensive rat. *Pharmacology Biochemistry and Behavior,* 1974 2, 381–386.

Perhach, J. L., Jr., Ferguson, H. C., & McKinney, G. R. Evaluation of antihypertensive agents in the stress-induced hypertensive rat. *Life Sciences,* 1976, *16,* 1731–1736.

Phelan, E. L., Simpson, F. O., & Smirk, F. H. Characteristics of the New Zealand strain of genetically hypertensive (GH) rats. *Clinical and Experimental Pharmacology and Physiology,* 1976, Suppl. 3: 5–10.

Pickering, G. *High Blood Pressure.* Churchill, London, 1968.

Plumlee, L. A. Operant conditioning of increases in blood pressure. *Psychophysiology,* 1969, *6,* 283–290.

Proceedings of the 2nd International Symposium on the Spontaneously Hypertensive Rat, 1977. U.S. Department of Health, Education, and Welfare Publication NIH 77-1179.

Provoost, A. P., Bohus, B., & De Jong, W. Differential influence of neonatal sympathectomy on the development of DOCA-salt and spontaneous hypertension in the rat. *Progress in Brain Research,* 1977, *47,* 417–424.

Rapp, J. P. and Iwai, J. Characteristics of rats selectively bred for susceptibility or resistance to the hypertensive effect on high salt diet. *Clinical and Experimental Pharmacology and Physiology,* 1976, Suppl 3:11–14.

Reis, D. J., & Doba, N. The central nervous system and neurogenic hypertension. *Progress in Cardiovascular Disease,* 1974 *17,* 51–71.

Rifkin, R. J., Silverman, J. M., Chavez, F. T., & Frankl, G. Intensified mouse killing in the spontaneously hypertensive rat. *Life Sciences* 1974, *14,* 985–992.

Roizen, M. F., Weise, V., Grobecker, H., & Kopin, I. J. Plasma catecholamines and dopamine-β-hydroxylase activity in spontaneously hypertensive rats. *Life Sciences,* 1975, *17,* 283–288.

Rosecrans, J. A., & Adams, M. D. Brain 5-hydroxytryptamine correlates of behavior: Studies involving spontaneously hypertensive (SHR) and normotensive Wistar rats. *Pharmacology Biochemistry and Behavior,* 1976, *5,* 559–564.

Rosecrans, J. A., Watzman, N., & Buckley, J. P. The production of hypertension in male albino rats subjected to experimental stress. *Biochemical Pharmacology,* 1966 *15,* 1701–1718.

Rothlin, E., Cerletti, A., & Emmenegger, H. Experimental psycho-neurogenic hypertension and its treatment with hydrogenated ergot alkaloids (Hydergine). *Acta Medica Scandanavica* 1959, (Suppl) *312,* 27–35.

Saari, M., & Pappas, B. A. Neonatal 6-hydroxydopamine sympathectomy reduces foot shock-induced suppression in normotensive and hypertensive rats. *Nature (New Biol.),* 1973, *244,* 181–183.

Saavedra, J. M., Grobecker, H., & Axelrod, J. Adrenaline-forming enzyme in brainstem: Elevation in genetic and experimental hypertension. *Science,* 1976, *191,* 483–484.

Saavedra, J. M., Grobecker, H., & Axelrod, J. Changes in central catechol-aminergic neurons in the spontaneously (genetic) hypertensive rat. *Circulaton Research,* 1978, *42,* 529–534.

Sasagawa, S., & Yamori, Y. Quantitative analysis on the behavior of spontaneously hypertensive rats (SHR) and stroke-prone SHR. *Japanese Heart Journal,* 1975, *16,* 313–315.

Schramm, L. P. & Barton, G. N. Diminished sympathetic silent period in spontaneously hypertensive rats. *American Journal of Physiology,* 1979, 147–152.

Schunk, J. Emotionale Faktoren in der Pathogenese der essentiellen Hypertonie. *Zeitschrift fur Klinische Medizin,* 1954 152–251.

Shimamoto, K., & Nagaoka, A. Behavioral and pharmacological characteristics of the spontaneously hypertensive rat. In *Spontaneous Hypertension: Its Pathogenesis and Complications (Proc. 1st Int. Sympos. SHR),* 1977, Okamoto, K. (Ed.). Springer-Verlag, New York, pp. 86–88.

Simonson, E., & Brožek, J. Russian research on arterial hypertension. *Annals of Internal Medicine,* 1959 *50,* 129–178.

Smirk, F. H., & Hall, W. H. Inherited hypertension in rats. *Nature,* 1958), *182,* 727–728.

Smith, O. A. Reflex and central mechanisms involved in the control of the heart and circulation. *Annual Review of Physiology,* 1974, *36,* 93–123.

Smookler, H. H., & Buckley, J. P. Relationships between brain catecholamines synthesis, pituitary adrenal formation and the production of hypertension during prolonged exposure to environmental stress. *International Journal of Neuropharmacology* 1969, *8,* 33–41.

Smookler, H. H., Goebel, K. H., Siegel, M. I., & Clarke, D. E. Hypertensive effects of prolonged auditory, visual, and motion stimulation. *Federation Proceedings,* 1973, *32,* 2105–2110.

Spontaneously Hypertensive (SHR) Rats: Guidelines For Breeding, Care and Use, 1976. Committee on Care and Use of Spontaneously Hypertensive Rats (SHR), Institute of Laboratory Animal Resources (ILAR).

Steiner, G., & Schonbaum, E. (Eds.). *Immunosympathectomy.* Elsevier, Amsterdam. 1972.

Takaori, S., Tanaka, C., & Okamoto, K. Relationship between behavior and brain monoamines in spontaneously hypertensive rats. In *Spontaneous Hypertension: Its Pathogenesis and Complications (Proc. 1st. Int. Sympos. SHR),* 1972, Okamoto, K. (Ed.). Springer-Verlag, New York, pp. 89–92.

Tan, S. Y., & Mulrow, P. J. Renin, prostaglandins, and mineralocorticoids in the spontaneously hypertensive rate at various stages of development. In: *Proceedings of the 2nd International Symposium on the Spontaneously Hypertensive Rat,* 1977. U.S. Department of Health, Education, and Welfare Publication NIH 77–1179, pp. 452–459.

Thoenen, H. Trans-synaptic regulation of neuronal enzyme synthesis. In *Handbook of Psychopharmacology, Vol. 3, Biochemistry of Biogenic Amines,* 1975, Iverson, L. L., Iverson, S. D., and Synder, S. H. (eds.), Plenum Press, New York, pp. 443–475.

Thoenen, H., Mueller, R. A., & Axelrod, J. Trans-synaptic induction of adrenal tyrosine hydroxylase. *Journal of Pharmacology and Experimental Therapeutics,* 1969 *169,* 249–254.

Thoenen, H., Mueller, R. A., & Axelrod, J. Neuronally dependent induction of adrenal phenylethanolamine-N-methyltransferase by 6-hydroxydopamine. *Biochemical Pharmacology,* 1970, *19,* 669–673.

Thoenen, H., & Otten V. Trans-synaptic enzyme induction: Ionic requirements and modulatory role of glucocorticoids. In *Structure and Function of Monoamine Enzymes,* 1977, Usdin, E., Weiner, N., & Youdim, M. B. H. (Eds.). Marcel Dekker, New York, pp. 439–464.

Tilson, H. A., Chamberlain, J. H., Gylys, J. A., & Buyniski, J. P. Behavioral suppressant effects of clonidine in strains of normotensive and hypertensive rats. *European Journal of Pharmacology,* 1977, *43,* 99–105.

Tucker, D. C. and Johnson, A. K. Elevated sympathetic tone in neonatal SHR. *Society for Neuroscience Abstracts,* 1980a, 12:633.

Tucker, D. C. and Johnson, A. K. The ontogenesis of cardiac and behavioral hyperreactivity in spontaneously hypertensive rats. *Society for Neuroscience Abstracts,* 1980b, 12:856.

Vander, A. J. Henry, J. P., Stephens, P. M., Kay, L. L., & Mouw, D. R. Plasma renin activity in psychosocial hypertension of CBA mice. *Circulation Research,* 1978 *42,* 496–502.

Vapaatalo, H., Hackman, R., Antilla, P., Vainionpää, V., & Neuvonen, P. J. Effects of 6-hydroxydopamine on spontaneously hypertensive rats. *Nauyn-Schmiedegergs Archives of Pharmacology,* 1974 *284,* 1–13.

Versteeg, D. H. G., Palkovits, M., van der Gugten, J., Wijnen, H. L. J. M., Smeets, G. W. M., & De Jong, W. Catecholamine content of individual brain regions of spontaneously hypertensive rats (SH-rats). *Brain Research,* 1976, *112,* 429–434.

Weiner, H. Psychosomatic research in essential hypertension: Retrospect and prospect. In *Psychosomatics in Essential Hypertension,* 1970, Koster, M., Musaph, H., & Visser, P. (Eds.) (Bibliotheca Psychiatrica, No. 144). S. Karger, New York, pp. 58–116.

Weiner, H. *Psychobiology of Essential Hypertension.* Elsevier, New York, 1979 pp. 41–52.

Wendel, O. T. and Bennett, B. The occurrence of analgesia in an animal model of hypertension. *Life Sciences,* 1981, 29: 515–521.

Williams, R. B., & Eichelman, B. Social setting: Influence on the physiological response to electric shock in the rat. *Science,* 1971, *174,* 613–614.

Wurtman, R. J., & Axelrod, J. Control of enzymatic synthesis of adrenaline in the adrenal medulla by adrenal cortical steroids. *Journal of Biological Chemistry,* 1966, *241,* 2301–2305.

Yamada, T., Kojima, A., Kubota, T., Aizawa, T., Tawata, M., Koizumi, Y., Yamori, Y., & Okamoto, K. Evaluation of thyroid function in rats with spontaneous hypertension and in patients with essential hypertension. In *Proceedings of the 2nd International Syposium on the Spontaneously Hypertensive Rat (1977).* U.S. Department of Health, Education, and Welfare Publication NIH 77-1179, pp. 140–148.

Yamori, Y. Contribution of cardiovascular factors to the development of hypertension in spontaneously hypertensive rats. *Japanese Heart Journal,* 1974, *15,* 194–196.

Yamori, Y. Pathogenesis of spontaneous hypertension. *Japanese Circulation Journal,* 1977, 4:259–266.

Yamori, Y., Matsumoto, M., Yamabe, H., & Okamoto, K. Augmentation of spontaneous hypertension by chronic stress in rats. *Japanese Circulation Journal,* 1969, *33,* 399–409.

Yamori, Y., Ohta, K., Korie, R., & Sato, M. Hypophyseal function in SHR: Lysine incorporation and ACTH content. *Japanese Heart Journal,* 1976, *17,* 407–409.

Yamori, Y., & Okamoto, K. Hypothalamic tonic regulation of blood pressure in spontaneously hypertensive rats. *Japanese Circulation Journal,* 1969, *33,* 509–519.

Yamori, Y., Ooshima, A., & Okamoto, K. Deviation of central norepinephrine metabolism in hypertensive rats. *Japanese Circulation Journal,* 1973, *37,* 1235–1245.

Yehle, A., Dauth, G., & Schneiderman, N. Correlates of heart-rate classical conditioning in curarized rabbits. *Journal of Comparative and Physiological Psychology,* 1967, *64,* 98–104.

Zaimis, E., & Knight, J. (Eds.) *Nerve Growth Factor and Its Antiserum* Athlone, London, 1972.

Zanchetti, A., Baccelli, G., & Mancia, G. Fighting emotions and exercise: Cardiovascular effects in the cat. In *Regulation of Blood Pressure by the Central Nervous System,* 1976, Onesti, G., Fernandes, M., & Kim, K. E. (Eds.). Grune and Stratton, New York, pp. 87–103.

Zukowska-Grójec, Z. Metabolism of 3H-tyrosine to catecholamines in brain tissue of spontaneously hypertensive and normotensive rats at rest and during running stress. *Second International Symposium on Catecholamines and Stress, September 12–16, 1979, Smolenice Castle, Czechoslovakia, Abstracts,* 1979, p. 92.

7 Behavioral-Cardiac Interactions in Hypertension

Paul A. Obrist   Alan W. Langer

Alberto Grignolo   Kathleen C. Light

Janice L. Hastrup   James A. McCubbin

John P. Koepke   Michael H. Pollak
Medical School University of North Carolina Chapel Hill

INTRODUCTION[1]

There is abundant evidence that the arterial blood pressure (BP) is influenced by the individual's interaction with the environment. A most dramatic example of this is represented by those studies where continuous intraarterial recordings of BP were made over periods of up to 24 hours in normotensive individuals where the range of the systolic blood pressure (SBP) was found to vary up to 100 mm Hg from sleep to emotional excitement (Bevan, Honour, & Stott, 1969). Of more direct relevance to the role of behavioral factors in the etiology of essential hypertension are reports of the development of elevated BP's in animals exposed to environmental events such as shock avoidance (Forsyth, 1969; Morse, Herd, Kelleher, & Grose, 1971), social isolation followed by crowding (Henry, Stephens, & Santisteban, 1975) and experimental conflict (Lawler, Barker, Hubbard, & Allen, 1980). In humans, cultural factors such as social structure (Henry & Cassel, 1969) or socioeconomic status (Tyroler, 1977) are reported to relate to an elevated BP. While these various lines of evidence implicate behavioral

---

[1]This chapter is not intended to provide a comprehensive overview of research concerning behavior and hypertension. These can be found in the following sources: Weiner, 1977; Frumkin, Nathan, Prout, & Cohen, 1978; Shapiro, Schwartz, Ferguson, Redmond, & Weiss, 1977; Henry & Cassell, 1969.

events in the etiological process in the sense that they are necessary first steps, they are not all that informative in certain other respects. For example, they do not indicate in any definitive manner why only a certain percentage of the population ever becomes hypertensive, thus preventing us from identifying such individuals with any confidence until the BP is elevated and sustained. In addition, they fail to delineate the hemodynamic basis (mechanisms) responsible for the development of hypertension and the manner they interact with behavioral events. It must be emphasized that an elevation of the BP is only a symptom indicating a derangement of one or more of the mechanisms which control it. It does not tell us which mechanisms are involved, how the derangement came about, or how it should be treated and prevented. An analogous situation is seen with another common sympton: the presence of a fever does not reveal what the infecting organism is, the site of the infection, the events and circumstances that led up to it, nor the appropriate treatment and preventative measures. The analogy can be extended to those treatments of an elevated BP which focus just on the BP, as is common with any behavioral intervention technique. This is no different in principle from treating a fever with aspirin. The necessity to delineate the mechanisms and the behavioral input is also indicated by the possibility that an elevated BP may reflect different etiological processes among individuals and that behavioral influences may be of greater significance with some etiologies than with others. Insight into the etiological process thus is fundamental for any effort in prevention or treatment.

When dealing with an already established hypertension, we are faced with still another problem, namely that the mechanisms now maintaining the elevated pressure may be different from those which initially triggered the chain of events leading up to the present condition (Brown, Fraser, Lever, Morton, Robertson, Schalekamp, 1977). This should become clearer later in this chapter. For now, it suffices to be aware that hypertension is a progressive condition and that if we are to shed light on the etiological process, particularly behavioral influences, then we must focus our energies at the beginning not the culmination of the disease. In turn, this creates the problem of where to start and with whom. The purpose of this chapter is to propose a model which will guide such efforts. This model may ultimately prove relevant to the etiological process in only a certain percentage of hypertensives. Also, it is no doubt incomplete consisting of partial truths. Nonetheless, in evaluating the model, we should obtain insight into the means by which the BP is controlled in the behaving organism and in turn shed greater insight into the etiological process.

THE MODEL

There is evidence indicating that in the development of a hypertension, the BP progresses over a period of years from moderately elevated, or boderline levels, to more appreciably elevated values, a state commonly referred to as established hypertension.[2] While the presence of of a borderline hypertension in early adulthood is far from a perfect predictor of an eventual established hypertension (Julius, 1977b), it offers a starting point for developing some working hypothesis concerning the etiological process.

The first of these hypotheses concerns the hemodynamic control in hypertension. Individuals evidencing borderline hypertension are commonly observed to have an elevated cardiac output (CO) but as yet no elevation of the vascular resistance (Lund-Johansen, 1967; Safar, Weiss, Levenson, London, & Milliez, 1973; Sannerstedt, 1966). The elevated CO is mediated by sympathetic (beta-adrenergic) influences on the myocardium (Julius & Esler, 1975; Julius, Pascual, & London, 1971). On the other hand, in older individuals with a more established hypertension, the CO is either normal or depressed while the vascular resistance is elevated. These are age related effects and are clearly demonstrated in the Lund-Johansen (1967) study. Here hypertensives were divided into four age groups, < 30, $30-39$, $40-49$ and > 50. Resting state BP and hemodynamics were ascertained in both the four subgroups of hypertensives and age matched normotensives (except that no normotensives were older than 50). With the hypertensives, the BP was lower in the youngest group (averaging $150/92$) than the oldest group (averaging $184/104$) while no BP differences were seen among the normotensive groups. Cardiac output was above the age matched normotensive average in 14 of the 19 youngest hypertensives but in only 2 of 16 of the oldest hypertensives. Such observations thus suggest that in its progression, hypertension initially involves a beta-adrenergically mediated increase in the CO. Over time, this hemodynamic picture changes with an increase in vascular resistance gradually becoming a more dominant influence.[3]

There are in fact some longitudinal data supporting the existence of such a transition. For example, Lund-Johansen (1967, 1979) did a 10 year follow-up on 29 of his youngest subjects and found that over this time span that their mean CO had significantly decreased while their vascular resistance had significantly in-

---

[2]Deciding what BP values constitute borderline versus established hypertension can be somewhat arbitrary. We shall use the criterion suggested by Julius (1977a) who considered BP values of 160/100 or greater as indicative of established hypertension and values between 140/90 and 160/100 mm Hg in individuals between ages 17-40 as indicative of borderline hypertension. Also, borderline hypertension is sometimes referred to as labile hypertension. This indicates that the BP values are found to exceed the given cutoff value (like 140/90) on some occasions but not on others. In this chapter, we shall only use the designation "borderline hypertension."

[3]A note a caution is necessary. We do not wish to imply that a beta-adrenergically mediated elevated CO is invariably the precursor of a more established hypertension. This caution is clearly suggested by the Safar et al. (1973) study which dealt with 85 borderline hypertensives, all less than 30 years of age. Approximately two-thirds (58 of 85) of the subjects evidenced an elevated output. Where a normal CO was found, it was not clear whether the transition from a high to a normal CO had already occurred (these subjects were significantly older, i.e., 27.0 vs. 23.5 years of age) or whether their marginally elevated BP never involved an elevated output in the first place. Rather, it could have reflected another etiological process involving only the vasculature.

creased (also see Eich, Cuddy, Smulyan, & Lyons, 1966; Pfeffer & Frohlich, 1973.

A second aspect of our conceptual scheme invokes the concept of metabolic inefficiency. We propose that in order for the behavioral cardiac interaction to prove relevant to the etiological process, it must result in a breakdown of the efficiency with which the cardiovascular system adjusts to the demands of metabolic activity. Otherwise, it is hard to make a case that we are dealing with anything out of the ordinary. For example, the extensive cardiovascular adjustments associated with the metabolic demands of exercise are not normally viewed in the healthy individual as having pathophysiological consequences. Increases in HR, CO, and BP which occur are in direct proportion to increased tissue requirements. However, under conditions other than exercise, cardiovascular adjustments sometimes occur which appear to exceed the concurrent metabolic demands associated with energy production. This would be seen, for example, when an increase in the CO in a given situation is excessive relative to any increase in O_2 consumption. In turn, this excessive increase in the CO has been proposed to result eventually in an elevation of vascular resistance, and hence its pathophysiological consequence. This has been thought to come about in two manners which could act either as alternative or complimentary mechanisms. One, the tissues become overperfused with blood; this triggers autoregulation of blood flow which returns flow to metabolically warranted levels. This is an intrinsic mechanism (not neurogenic) which causes the arterioles to constrict increasing their resistance. In turn, the CO is decreased because the venous return is now lessened but the arterial pressure stays elevated because of the increased vascular resistance (Coleman, Granger, & Guyton, 1971; Coleman, Samer, & Murphy, 1979). A second mechanism which is also intrinsic, involves structural changes of the vasculature in the form of a hypertrophy of the smooth muscles resulting from the elevated BP in conjunction with either an elevated CO or vascular resistance. This too acts to elevate further the vascular resistance and perpetuate the elevation of the BP (Folkow, Hallback, Lundgren, Sivertsson, & Weiss, 1973; Folkow & Neil, 1971; Friedman, 1977). Both mechanisms could be considered to be responsible for the changing hemodynamic picture previously discussed as hypertension progresses from a high CO state to an elevated vascular resistance.

A second manner by which metabolic efficiency could be compromised involves the kidney and the control of water and electrolyte balance. The situation is schematized as follows. It has been hypothesized (e.g., Brown, et al., 1977; Guyton, 1977) that established fixed hypertension is dependent on a kidney abnormality because sustained high levels of BP would normally be expected to deplete the body of both water (pressure diuresis) and sodium (Na)(pressure natriuresis). But since water and electrolyte balance is maintained in hypertension, it is proposed that kidney functioning at normal pressure is impaired and that the higher pressure is necessary to maintain balance. Or as Brown, et al.

(1977, p. 539) state with respect to Na ". . . the rise in pressure is the price paid to maintain sodium balance." It should be emphasized that fluid and Na homeostasis is being achieved but only thanks to a pathologically high BP. Guyton (1977) depicts the sequence of events as first involving Na retention which results in an increase in the blood volume and hence an increase in the CO. The elevated CO acts as previously described to trigger autoregulation and an elevation of BP which then acts to facilitate Na excretion. Thus, similar mechanisms may be involved in both of these hypothesized schemes by which we suggest that hypertension may evolve. Only the triggering mechanisms differ, i.e., the elevated CO resulting from increased beta-adrenergic drive in one instance and an expanded blood volume in the other. It is also believed that vascular reactivity is enhanced by Na retention hence further influencing the BP (Brown, et al. 1977).

While an elevated CO due to increased beta-adrenergic drive clearly implicates a neural mechanism, neurogenic influences are as yet uncertain with regard to the proposed kidney abnormality. However, neural influences are suggested by the evidence that Na balance can involve both alpha- and beta-adrenergic mechanisms (Zanchetti, Stella, Leonetti, Morganti, & Terzoli, 1976; Bello-Reuss, Trevino, & Gottschalk, 1976; Grignolo, 1980). For example, beta-adrenergic excitation can influence the release of renin—a kidney hormone involved in the control of Na balance. If so, then the behavioral-cardiac interaction may extend to the kidney and its control of Na balance and hence the blood pressure. Thus, it is conceivable that beta-adrenergic processes influence the myocardium directly as well as indirectly via the kidney; that is, these are not mutually exclusive but rather complimentary influences.

Finally, the concept of metabolic inefficiency can be viewed in still another manner. We know the BP can be quite labile reaching hypertensive values on occasion in individuals who never develop established hypertension, while some others will. How can we understand this? The concept of metabolic inefficiency can help on this account. We propose that an acute elevation of the BP is a potentially ominous symptom only when it is the result of mechanisms indicative of metabolic inefficiency such as Na retention or excessive beta-adrenergic drive on the myocardium. When it is not, such as many be the case when an elevation of the BP results directly from alpha-adrenergic influences on the vasculature, it has no particular significance with respect to established hypertension. Of course, direct neurogenic influences on the vasculature could eventually result in structural changes but structural changes may also be dependent on Na retention (Brown, et al. 1977) and in the absence of the latter, structural changes would be minimal.

In summary, it is proposed that in some individuals the etiology of hypertension may initially involve excessive beta-adrenergic drive on the myocardium resulting in an elevated CO and hence an elevated BP. At this stage, the BP is only marginally elevated and commonly labile. With time, the vascular resistance becomes elevated, the CO normalizes and the BP becomes more elevated and sustained (established hypertension). The transition may involve at least two mechanisms. One, the initial elevated CO, because it is metabolically unwarranted, initiates such events as autoregulation of the vasculature and smooth muscle hypertrophy, all of which elevate vascular resistance. Possibly complimenting this are renal mechanisms involving Na retention which have a similar influence on the myocardium and vasculature. In this case, the elevated BP acts to facilitate Na excretion and bring Na intake and output into balance. With this in mind, we would next like to review studies which provide evidence as to the merit of this scheme and which specifically implicate the behavioral-cardiac interaction in the etiological process.

TESTING THE MODEL

Historical Antecedents

Before reviewing our more recent efforts where the focus is on myocardial events as well as the BP, it is helpful to overview some of our earlier efforts since they place the more current work in perspective. Our initial studies focused on phasic HR changes during classical aversive conditioning. In humans, the anticipatory HR response was not supportive of the notion that the behavioral-cardiac interaction was relevant to pathophysiology in two respects. First, the anticipatory HR changes were demonstrated to be under parasympathetic control which masked sympathetic effects (Obrist, Wood, & Perez-Reyes, 1965). This is illustrated in Figure 7.1, which depicts HR changes on non-reinforced test trials (the UCS is omitted) with an intact and pharmacologically blocked (atropine) vagal innervation. Note that with the vagal innervation intact, there is a biphasic anticipatory response; first, an acceleration then a deceleration peaking about where the UCS would have occurred. This biphasic response is vagally mediated, reflecting an initial loss then an increase in vagal tone, since with the innervation blocked, there is only a uniphasic acceleration which is coincident in time with the anticipatory deceleration. This vagal dominance cannot be attributed to using insufficiently threatening procedures, since the intensity of the UCS was set considerably above a level the subjects first judged to be very painful. Such vagal dominance is not very conforting to our hypothesis involving beta-adrenergic influences nor for that matter with any view that relegates vagal influences to states of rest and vegetation. It is instead in line with data demonstrating appreciable decreases in HR in desert rodents in a threatening open field situation (Hofer, 1970) and in rats trained to avoid shock by decreasing HR (Brener, Phillips, & Connally, 1977).

A second line of evidence embarrassing to our metabolic inefficiency hypothesis also emanates from the classical conditioning paradigm. This is the observation that concomitant with these vagally mediated HR changes are directionally consistent phasic changes in non-extensive somatic or striate muscle activity. These include such acts as mouth and ocular movements, subtle postural changes

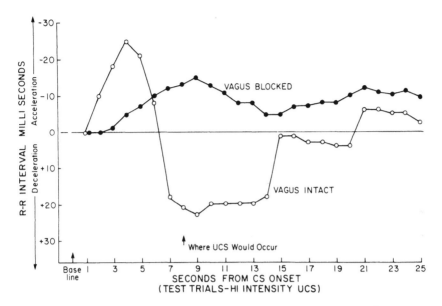

FIG. 7.1.   Second-by-second changes in HR on test trials (UCS omitted) during classical aversive conditioning in humans with an intact (open circles) and blocked (closed circles) vagal innervations (Obrist, et al., 1965). Copyright, 1965, by the American Psychological Association. Reprinted by permission.

and respiratory activities (Obrist, 1968; Obrist, Webb, & Sutterer, 1969). Their relationship with HR is depicted in Figure 7.2 which again uses only non-reinforced test trials and shows two aspects of somatomotor activity, chin EMG (mouth movements) and eye blinks and movements. In effect, what we see in association with the phasic anticipatory deceleration of HR is a momentary state of somatic immobilization. This covariation has been observed under a variety of circumstances and experimental procedures. For example, experimental manipulations such as of the CS-UCS interval during aversive conditioning and of the preparatory interval during a signaled reaction time (RT) task, which modified phasic HR changes, influenced somatic activity in a like manner (Obrist, 1968; Webb & Obrist, 1970). Phasic anticipatory decreases in HR are also observed in cats in conjunction with a decrease in electrical activity of the pyramidal tract (Howard, Obrist, Gaebelein, & Galosy, 1974).

These various lines of data along with some neurophysiological considerations led to the hypothesis that these vagally mediated HR changes and concomitant somatic effects reflect a common central nervous system integrating mechanism, similar to that involved in more extensive somatomotor activity such as exercise (Obrist, Webb, Sutterer, & Howard, 1970; Obrist, Howard, Lawler, Galosy, Meyers, & Gaebelein, 1974a). To the extent that this is a valid position, it argues for the metabolic appropriateness of these HR changes. In all, our efforts up to this point do not support the model, nor for that matter the more

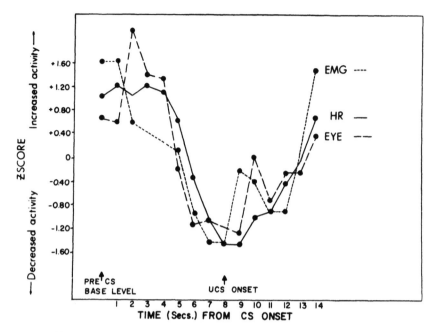

FIG. 7.2.   Second-by-second changes in HR, chin EMG and occular activity on test trials (UCS omitted) during classical aversive conditioning in humans—values converted to Z scores (Obrist, et al., 1969). Copyright 1969 by the Society for Psychophysiological Research. Reprinted with permission.

generalized belief that behavioral-cardiac interactions can have eventual pathophysiological consequences with regard to cardiovascular function.

Coping and the Heart: A Beta-Adrenergic Link

This picture began to change first when the experimental paradigm was modified and even more when the focus shifted from phasic to tonic changes in myocardial activity. At this point, attention began to be given the BP in a systematic manner because for the first time a case could be made that these data were relevant to hypertension and the etiological process.

The first important step was the demonstration that by changing the experimental paradigm from one where the individual had no control to one where some control was possible over the experimental stimuli and events[4] (in these

---

[4]This stimulus parameter has been referred to as an active-passive coping dimension. Passive coping is exemplified by classical aversive conditioning where escape or avoidance from the aversive stimuli is not possible. Active coping is characterized by shock avoidance where the individual can exert some control over the receipt of aversive stimuli contingent on some aspect of its behavior, such as performance on a reaction time task.

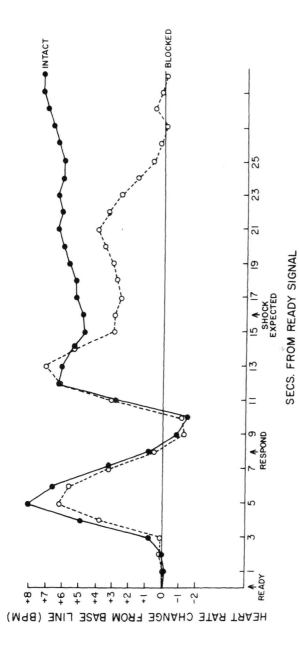

FIG. 7.3. Second-by-second changes in HR with an intact and blocked sympathetic innervation during a signaled shock avoidance reaction time task. Based on trials when shock was not delivered (Obrist, et al., 1974b). Copyright 1974 by the Society for Psychophysiological Research. Reprinted with permission.

207

first studies, electric shock) sympathetic effects on the myocardium were evoked and were independent of concomitant somatic activities. The first study (Obrist, Lawler, Howard, Smithson, Martin, & Manning, 1974b) evaluated only phasic myocardial events (not the BP) using a signaled RT task, with the sympathetic innervation intact in some individuals and blocked in others. The HR changes are shown in Figure 7.3 which indicates that HR is under predominately vagal control during the 8-second preparatory interval of the task. Sympathetic influences became evidenced toward the end of the next 8-second period between response execution and when shock might occur (shock was not administered on the trials shown) and continued to be seen during the remainder of the measurement period. With the innervation blocked, HR returned to baseline following response execution. Three different aspects of somatic activity were evaluated. Each was found to directionally covary with HR when vagal influences were evident, such as during the preparatory interval and at response execution, and throughout the remainder of the measurement period when the sympathetic innervation was blocked. With an intact innervation, increased sympathetic excitation was associated with a decrease in somatic activity in the form of a return to baseline.

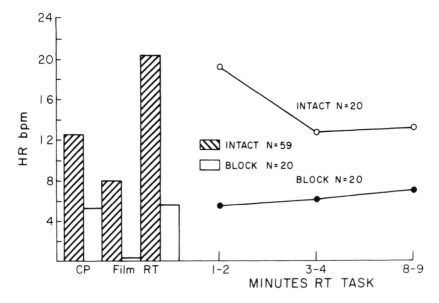

FIG. 7.4.   Change from baseline in tonic levels of HR with an intact and blocked sympathetic innervation. Left: changes averaged over 90 seconds of cold pressor, and first 2 minutes of film and shock avoidance task. Right: changes in first 9 minutes of shock avoidance task (Obrist, et al., 1978). Copyright 1978 by the Society for Psychophysiological Research. Reprinted with permission.

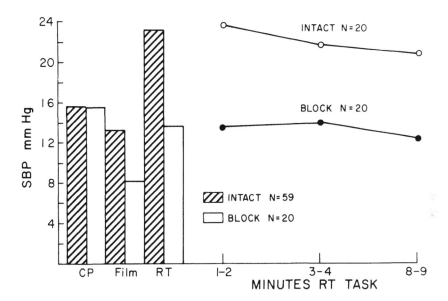

FIG. 7.5.   Change from baseline in tonic levels of systolic blood pressure with an
intact and blocked sympathetic innervation as in Figure 7.4 (Obrist, et al., 1978).
Copyright (1978) by the Society for Psychophysiological Research. Reprinted
with permission.

The next studies evaluated tonic levels of myocardial performance as well as
BP, such as average HR in blocks of one or two minutes. The shift to tonic levels
was suggested by the observation in some individuals that tonic activity during
the task was appreciably elevated above baseline (e.g., 30–40 bpm). Phasic
effects are typically smaller and superimposed on these. Also, when the concern
is hypertension, tonic events are more relevant than phasic changes. These
studies (Obrist, Gaebelein, Teller, Langer, Grignolo, Light, & McCubbin, 1978;
Obrist, Light, McCubbin, Hutcheson & Hoffer 1979a) used an unsignaled shock
avoidance RT task and two conditions in which the subjects were more passively
engaged: the cold pressor (submerging the foot in iced water) and viewing an
erotic film. The important observations relevant to the present discussion are that
sympathetic influences on the myocardium were most evident for the shock
avoidance task. Figure 7.4 depicts the HR data which shows that HR is most
accelerated with an intact innervation and most attenuated by sympathetic blockade during the first minutes of the avoidance task than during comparable time
periods of the cold pressor and erotic movie. Blood pressure was influenced in a
more complex manner (Figures 7.5 and 7.6). Systolic blood pressure (SBP, Fig.
7.5) like HR, was most elevated with an intact innervation and more attenuated
by pharmacological blockade during shock avoidance than the other two tasks.
With the latter, pharmacological blockade had either no effect (cold pressor) or a

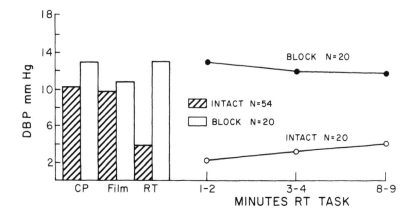

FIG. 7.6.   Change from baseline in tonic levels of diastolic blood pressure with an intact and blocked sympathetic innervation as in Figure 7.4 (Obrist, et al., 1978). Copyright (1978) by the Society for Psychophysiological Research. Reprinted with permission.

slight attenuating effect (film). Diastolic blood pressure (DBP, Fig. 7.6) during shock avoidance, on the other hand, evidenced just the opposite effect from SBP. As compared to the other two tasks, it increased least with an intact innervation. Pharmacological blockade had little effect on DBP during the cold pressor and film but resulted in a significantly greater increase during shock avoidance than with an intact innervation[5] (see Fig. 7.6).

In summary, these studies not only serve the purpose of demonstrating a sympathetic influence on the myocardium which appears independent of concurrent somatomotor activity (suggestive of a metabolically inefficient response), but represent the first step of implicating the behavioral-cardiac interaction in the etiological process. That is to say, our working hypothesis (conceptual model) proposes that in the early stages, exececssive sympathetic drive on the heart

---

[5]The DBP effect during shock avoidance can be understood as follows. There is evidence (Ahlquist, 1976) that in certain vascular beds (e.g., striate muscle) beta-adrenergic receptors result in vasodilation upon stimulation. Thus, simultaneous with increased beta-adrenergic drive on the myocardium would be a vasodilation in these beds. Because this vasodilation largely offsets any alpha-adrenergic vasoconstriction in still other vascular beds, there is little change in vascular resistance. Pharmacological blockade, however, minimizes this vasodilation while leaving unchecked the alpha-adrenergic vasoconstriction. Thus, the vascular resistance is now more increased, resulting in a greater increase in DBP. Forsyth (1976) directly assessed the vascular resistance and regional blood flows in rhesus monkeys during shock avoidance with and without beta-adrenergic blockade, and observed effects consistent with this interpretation. It should also be noted that in young borderline hypertensives who commonly demonstrate increased beta-adrenergic drive even when resting, it is the SBP, not DBP, that is elevated (e.g., Safar, et al., 1973, where the resting BP averaged 143/73), which is also suggestive of beta-adrenergic vasodilation.

among other things triggers the hypertensive process. This suggestion was derived from clinical research (e.g., Lund-Johansen, 1967) where one cannot definitively ascertain the relevance of any behavioral influence. The present research demonstrates a behaviorally-evoked beta-adrenergic influence on the myocardium. This influenced the SBP likely through an increase in CO and contractility. There is, to our knowledge, little other available evidence of this nature involving human study subjects. Brod (1963) did observe an increase in the CO during a demanding mental arithmetic task but did not assess neurogenic mechanisms. A beta-adrenergic influence on both HR and CO was reported during simulated flying of an air craft (Eliasch, Rosen, & Scott, 1967) as well as during shock avoidance on CO in monkeys (Forsyth, 1976) and HR in dogs (Anderson & Brady, 1976). We also recently observed beta-adrenergic influence on both HR and intraventricular dP/dt during shock avoidance in dogs[6] (Grignolo, Light, & Obrist, 1981. In all, it now seems reasonably established that the behavioral cardiac interaction can under certain circumstances evoke beta-adrenergic mechanisms.

Cardiac and Renal Inefficiency

The next necessary steps in evaluating the significance of the behavioral-cardiac interaction in humans involve a series of observations which lend further credence to our conceptual scheme. But before describing these, it is appropriate to present additional data on the metabolic inefficiency scheme with regard to myocardial performance and renal functioning in association with a shock avoidance task using dogs.

A problem faced is how to determine whether a given myocardial or renal adjustment associated with a given behavioral task, is metabolically inefficient. One needs a reference point. For this purpose, we used the adjustments made to exercise on a treadmill. It was reasoned that both the myocardial and renal adjustment to exercise should reflect a reasonably efficient adjustment to a metabolic load providing the animal is not unduly upset by the procedure. Thus, one could then compare the adjustments made to a signaled shock avoidance task to see if the resulting CO change was excessive relative to any change in O_2 consumption and whether renal function deviated in a manner indicative of inappropriate functioning.

The first study (Langer, 1978; Langer, Obrist, & McCubbin, 1979) evaluated during both exercise and shock avoidance, the CO and the arterial-venous blood oxygen content difference (A-V O_2d). The latter was used, rather than the O_2

---

[6]Intraventricular dP/dt refers to the rate of pressure development in the ventricle during the isovolumic contraction phase (prior to the ejection of blood). It is considered a reasonably valid measure of sympathetic influences on myocardial contractility (Randall & Smith, 1974).

consumption, since a behavioral disruption of the metabolic adjustment would be more apparent. As expected, the A-V O_2d was found to be directly related to the CO and HR during exercise, with each increasing as the metabolic load increased. The shock avoidance task disrupted this relationship between A-V O_2d and CO in four of five dogs and with HR in five of six dogs and in a manner indicative of a metabolic inefficient act and suggestive of tissue overperfusion. This is illustrated for one dog in Figure 7.7 and table 7.1. The figure shows that at any given level of CO during both conditions, the A-V O_2d is significantly less during avoidance than exercise. An efficient adjustment would demonstrate comparable A-V O_2d at similar levels of output. Rather, the output is excessive during avoidance. The table demonstrates that at a level of exercise which evokes an increase in the CO comparable to that generated during avoidance, the A-V

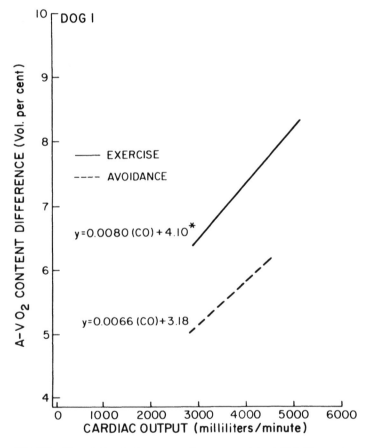

FIG. 7.7.   The relationship between cardiac output and the A-V O_2d in one dog during exercise and a shock avoidance task. Derived from Langer, 1978.

TABLE 7.1
Relationship Between Cardiac Output and HR to the A-V O_2d
During Exercise and Avoidance in One Dog.

		Rest	Exercise 3 mph	Avoidance
CO L/min	x̄	2.0	3.8	3.5
	S.E.Est.	0.24	0.16	0.09
HR bpm	x̄	127	177	195
	S.E.Est.	35	26	22
A-V O_2d Vol %	x̄	5.2	7.1	5.4
	S.E.Est.	0.24	0.30	0.22

O_2d during avoidance is 24% less than exercise and comparable to the resting state, where the output is noticeably less. We have not as yet evaluated whether this excessive output during avoidance is mediated by beta-adrenergic mechanisms, since we are awaiting an improvement in our methodology in measuring the A-V O_2d. However, it would not be unexpected since, as previously indicated, we have observed beta-adrenergic influences on intraventricular dP/dt, HR and CO in dogs during shock avoidance (Grignolo, Light & Obrist 1981).

The second study (Grignolo, 1980; Grignolo, Koepke, & Obrist, 1982) evaluated renal function by measuring water and Na excretion at rest and during both exercise and avoidance. Under all conditions, the six dogs used were volume expanded with physiological saline so as to amplify excretion rates by placing a load on the kidney. Not surprisingly, excretion rates at rest increased up to 9 times after volume expansion. Exercise acted to increase excretion rates further but rather modestly.[7] Shock avoidance, on the other hand, most commonly acted to decrease excretion rates although to varying degrees in different animals. In the dog showing the largest HR increases, excretion rates decreased by up to 50%. This is illustrated in Figure 7.8 which depicts the change from a baseline in HR, and water and Na excretion while the dog rested for 30 minutes and then during both 30 minutes of exercise and shock avoidance. During rest, there is no change but note that while exercise and avoidance had very comparable effects on HR (increasing it in excess of 60 bpm on most of 6 occasions of measurement under each condition) they had diametrically opposite effects on water and Na excretion. The glomerular filtration rate was also evaluated and found to increase some during exercise but not change during shock avoidance, suggesting that the

_____

[7]There are reports (Poortmans, 1977) that exercise commonly results in both water and Na retention which is in contrast to our observations. The reason for this discrepancy is not clear, although we suspect that the fact that the dogs were volume loaded is likely responsible. In any case, it is not critical to our observations since we also have the resting state as a reference point.

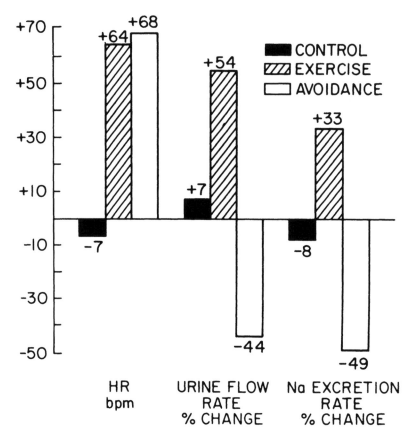

FIG. 7.8.   Average change in HR (bpm) and urine fluid volume and Na (%), from baseline in one dog for three control (C) six exercise (E) and six avoidance (A) sessions. Derived from Grignolo, 1980.

increased excretion rate during exercise is due to increased filtration while the decrease during avoidance is due to increased tubular reabsorption. The latter is influenced by neurohumoral mechanisms including the renin-angiotensin system (Zanchetti, et al., 1976) which acts to facilitate Na reabsorption. This mechanism has drawn considerable attention in hypertension research (Page & McCubbin, 1966, Page, 1977). We are only beginning to evaluate the mechanisms involved in the decrease in water and Na excretion during shock avoidance. In the dog whose data are depicted in Figure 7.8, we have observed no change in Na excretion rates during avoidance on three occasions following beta-adrenergic blockade. The involvement of a beta-adrenergic mechanism is also suggested by the observation that in the other dogs, appreciable decreases in water and Na excretion were only consistently observed on those avoidance days where HR was most accelerated (i.e., > 30 bpm increase over base-line). Also, suggestive of a beta-adrenergic involvement is the report that plasma renin is elevated in those borderline hypertensives who demonstrate increased sympathetic drive on the myocardium (Esler, Julius, Zweifler, Randall, Harburg, Gardiner, & De-Quattro, 1977).

In summary, we now have evidence in the chronic dog preparation that behavioral influences, one acting through the heart, the other through the kidney, can disrupt two basic metabolic processes. In one, the heart pumps excessive amounts of blood, in the other, the kidney reabsorbs excessive amounts of Na.[8] A case can be made that common to each event are beta-adrenergic mechanisms, although this awaits further study in the dog preparation. Although still speculative since the mechanisms are not known with any degree of certainty, the consequence of both is proposed to be an elevated BP. In the case of tissue overperfusion, the elevated pressure is a consequence of returning perfusion to more normal levels through autoregulation. In the case of Na, the elevated pressure acts directly to restore balance between intake and output. Finally, these data suggest that beta-adrenergic influences act directly on the myocardium as well as indirectly through renal processes. If this is the case, then we have two metabolically inappropriate adjustments literally working hand in hand to alter the control of the BP, which would be a very powerful demonstration of the potential role of the behavioral-cardiac interaction in the etiological process.

In closing this section, it should be noted that a disruption in these two metabolic processes was suggested by a number of previous reports. For example, individuals with both a high resting CO and HR were observed to have appreciably lower A-V O_2d than individuals with lower resting outputs and heart rates (Stead, Warren, Merrill, & Brannon 1945). In field studies with humans, both water and Na excretion have been reported as depressed on days when individuals claimed to be involved in threatening situations requiring increased alertness in contrast to more tranquil situations (Schottstaedt, Grace, & Wolff, 1956; see Langer, 1978 and Grignolo, 1980 for a review of this literature). Such studies, while providing very suggestive observations, did not propel us far since they did not evaluate mechanisms, they were isolated from any conceptual framework, and were not performed in the context of the etiology of hypertension.

---

[8]For those not familiar with renal physiology, it should be noted that the tubules of the kidney are continually reabsorbing Na to one degree or another from the glomerular filtrate since the Na excreted is but a fraction (1-3%) of the Na filtered. It is tubular reabsorption that largely maintains balance. Thus, our observation of a decrease in the excretion of Na via an increase in tubular reabsorption during shock avoidance reflects an exaggeration of a process that is occurring all the time, much like the elevated CO reflects an exaggeration of an event that occurs continuously.

ASPECTS OF BEHAVIORAL INFLUENCES ON BP IN
HUMANS

This chapter will close by detailing some additional observations in our young adult human subject population which further demonstrates behavioral influences on the BP and in turn lends further credence to the hypothesis that excessive sympathetic drive on the heart is one of the early events in the etiological process (see Obrist, 1981 for more details).

Individual Differences

There are appreciable individual differences in beta-adrenergic myocardial reactivity, as indexed by HR[9], and SBP reactivity. The presence of individual differences is a necessary condition if behaviorally evoked beta-adrenergic reactivity is relevant to the etiological process. This is because if most subjects were to react in a similar quantitative manner, the relevance of these effects to the etiology would be questioned. Also, it gives us a handle to work with since it raises the question of whether the more reactive in contrast to less reactive subjects are at risk with regard to hypertension later in life.

Initially, reactivity was evaluated by obtaining the difference between a baseline (pre-task rest) while the subject rested just prior to being exposed to the experimental procedures, and the first 2 minutes of the shock avoidance task. The onset of the later procedure was selected because beta-adrenergic reactivity was greatest at this point. Of the 154 subjects for whom we have HR data, the range of change scores extends from -5 to $+74$ bpm, with 32 (21%) exceeding a 30 bpm change. With SBP, data were available on 138 of these subjects. The range extended from -3 to 60 mm Hg with 10 (7%) exceeding a 40 mm Hg change. Furthermore, subjects who demonstrated the largest HR changes not surprisingly also demonstrated the largest SBP changes. For example, when the 154 subjects were divided into quintiles on the basis of HR reactivity, those in the upper quintile whose HR increase averaged 42 bpm, demonstrated a SBP increase of 34 mm Hg. On the other hand, subjects in the lowest quintile of HR

---

[9]We are reasonably confident that HR changes during the shock avoidance task reliably reflect beta-adrenergic influences, and for two reasons. One, the average change in tonic HR between the baseline obtained just before the onset of the first task and the first 2 minutes of the shock avoidance task averaged 21 bpm when the sympathetic innervation was intact but only 5 bpm with the innervation blocked. Second, the subjects are usually somatically quiet during this task other than when releasing the respond key. This assures us that there is likely a minimal contribution of a loss of vagal restraint due to somatic activity. A loss of vagal restraint might be expected under these conditions but as a synergistic effect due to increased sympathetic excitation (see Julius, et al., 1971a). Also, another reason to use HR is that HR data are available on more subjects than are other indices of sympathetic influences on the myocardium such as R wave to pulse wave interval (see Obrist, Light, McCubbin, Hutcheson, & Hoffer, 1979a).

reactivity who averaged a HR change of but 4 bpm, averaged a SBP increase of 11 mm Hg. The intermediate quintiles on HR reactivity were distributed with regard to SBP in a similarly consistent manner.

These individual differences and the apparent relationship between beta-adrenergic influences on the heart and SBP reactivity compelled us to focus on the question of whether beta-adrenergic hyperresponsiveness was one of the early events in the etiological process. A definitive answer to this question awaits a longitudinal study. Such an effort is costly with respect to time, energy and monies. In order to justify such an effort, we have raised several questions with this subject population which if answered affirmatively would encourage such an effort. Up until now, questions have been focused on two issues. One is whether beta-adrenergic reactivity is a reasonably stable characteristic of an individual under a variety of circumstances; the other is whether beta-adrenergic reactivity relates to hypertension in the family, particularly the parents.

Stability of Reactivity

We assume that if beta-adrenergic hyperreactivity is a precursor of established hypertension, then it should be characteristic of the individual under a variety of personally important circumstances other than shock avoidance. Thus, it seemed important to verify that high cardiovascular reactivity is a stable characteristic of some individuals. The first data indicating that reactivity does generalize to other circumstances were obtained with the use of a second baseline. Resting HR and SBP were obtained in 56 of the subjects previously exposed to the cold pressor, film, and shock avoidance task who returned to the laboratory on two separate occasions just to relax, and informed that they would not be exposed to any other experimental procedure. This baseline is henceforth referred to as the relaxation baseline in contrast to the pretask baseline previously described. Not surprisingly, the two base-lines differed, with the relaxation baseline evidencing lower HR and SBP values. Somewhat surprisingly though, the magnitude of the difference was a function of reactivity to the shock avoidance task and this difference generalized across the other two experimental procedures, i.e., the cold pressor and film as well as the pretask baseline. This is illustrated in Table 7.2a for HR and 7.2b for SBP. The 56 subjects were first divided into quartiles on the basis of the difference in HR reactivity between the relaxation baseline and the first two minutes of the shock avoidance task. Table 7.2a presents the average HR values under all five conditions for each quartile while Table 7.2b presents the mean SBP values under all five conditions based on HR reactivity. That is, the same 14 subjects are in the same quartile in both parts of the table. With regard to HR, the individual differences in reactivity to the onset of the shock avoidance are even more pronounced using the relaxation baseline. They now range from −11 to 104 bpm. Subjects in the upper quartile demonstrate on the average a 90% increase in HR between the relaxation baseline and shock avoidance. But note

TABLE 7.2-a
Mean HR During Two Types of Baselines and Experimental Tasks
with the Innervations Intact. Data Quartiled on the Basis of HR
Reactivity During Shock Avoidance. N = 56 (see text for details).
Percent Change in ( ).

Heart Rate Reactivity	Relaxation Baseline	Pre-task Baseline		Cold Pressor		Film		Shock Avoidance	
Most	63	80	(26)	96	(51)	86	(35)	120	(90)
↓	65	78	(20)	92	(40)	80	(23)	103	(57)
↓	68	75	(11)	88	(29)	80	(18)	93	(37)
Least	67	66	(−2)	80	(19)	72	(7)	76	(13)
x̄ =	66	75		89		79		98	

how these most reactive subjects also demonstrate an appreciably more accelerated HR during the pre-task baseline, cold pressor and film. Yet their average
HR during the relaxation baseline is not different from the other three groups. At
the other extreme, the 14 least reactive subjects demonstrated no difference
between baselines and minimal reactivity to the cold pressor and film. Another
indication that HR reactivity is a fairly stable phenomenon is the observation that
reactivity to one condition like the cold pressor correlates appreciably with
reactivity to any other condition like shock avoidance providng the reference
point is the relaxation baseline (range of r values +.53 to +.58). Thus, in regard
to HR, through the use of the relaxation baseline, we see the most reactive
subjects on the shock avoidance task, show greater HR changes in three other
conditions indicating that it is not unique to the one task and is in contrast to a
previous conclusion (Obrist, Langer, Grignolo, Sutterer, Light, & McCubbin,
1979b) where we had remarked that beta-adrenergic hyperractivity was unique to
shock avoidance. This was because the pre-task baseline was used as the refer-

TABLE 7.2-b
Mean SBP During Two Types of Baselines and Experimental
Tasks with the Myocardial Innervations Intact. Data Quartiled on
the Basis of HR Reactivity During Shock Avoidance. N = 56.
Percent Change in ( ).

Heart Rate Reactivity	Relaxation Baseline	Pre-task Baseline		Cold Pressor		Film		Shock Avoidance	
Most	124	137	(10)	157	(26)	149	(20)	170	(37)
↓	121	130	(7)	142	(17)	137	(13)	154	(27)
↓	124	126	(2)	137	(11)	137	(11)	150	(22)
Least	121	124	(2)	141	(17)	133	(9)	137	(13)
x̄ =	123	129		144		139		153	

ence point to obtain difference scores. Since it is already elevated in the more reactive individuals, it obscures the fact that such individuals also are more reactive to the cold pressor and film. Obviously, in such individuals, the choice of baseline is important. These baseline differences and their relationship to reactivity have been replicated in 72 subjects in a follow-up study (Light & Obrist, 1980b) as well as in another 18 subjects from a pilot study. In all, it appears that the reactive subjects had a propensity to respond to any novel or challenging event, a condition further implicating beta-adrenergic hyperresponsivity in the etiological process. What is still needed are relatively controlled field studies evaluating beta-adrenergic responsivity under more naturalistic conditions. We do have data indicating that reactivity is a stable characteristic of the individual over periods of up to 1 year and that more naturalistic laboratory tasks, such as difficult mental arithmetic problems, games, challenging reaction time tasks using financial incentives and the preparation and then making a speech to a TV camera, evoke appreciable individual differences in HR reactivity.

There were appreciable parallels between the HR and SBP effects which too were replicated in follow-up studies. As indicated in Table 7.2b, the more HR reactive subjects demonstrate greater levels of SBP under all conditions except the relaxation baseline, the most pronounced effect, as with HR, being to the shock avoidance task. The SBP effect is most clearly seen when one compares the two extreme groups on HR reactivity. This is depicted in Figure 7.9, which shows the difference in SBP levels between the highest and lowest quartiles of HR reactivity. The difference during the relaxation baseline is but 3 mm Hg, increasing to 13 mm Hg during the pre-task baseline, 16 mm Hg during the cold pressor and film and then peaking at 33 mm Hg during shock avoidance. Such data clearly implicate the behavioral cardiac interaction in the control of SBP responsiveness. This is seen in still another manner.

When we include another 82 subjects on whom we also collected a follow-up or relaxation baseline, we find that 33 of the 138 subjects demonstrate a SBP level during the pre-task baseline of 140 mm Hg or more, averaging 146 mm Hg. By some standards, such resting values are considered borderline hypertensive. The behavioral-myocardial influences on these elevated SBP values is indicated in the following manner. First, in these same 33 subjects, the SBP during the relaxation baseline decreases in 27, the mean now being 131 mm Hg. Second, the magnitude of the decrease in SBP was directly correlated with the HR decrease between these two baselines ($r = +.52$). Finally, the level of the SBP during the pre-task baseline was directly related to both HR as well as SBP reactivity to shock avoidance in the first study and a variation on the shock avoidance task in the second study. Such observations bear similarities to the clinical studies evaluating hemodynamics during 'rest' with borderline hypertensives. With both types of studies, the elevated resting SBP blood pressure is in association with circumstances that are novel and can have threatening qualities, e.g., insertion of catheters. But in our case, we are in a better position to

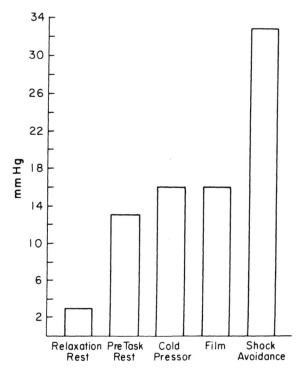

FIG. 7.9.   Differences in SBP between HR reactors and nonreactors (upper and lowest quartile) during two baselines and three experimental procedures. (Unpublished data.)

conclude that the borderline hypertensive values are related to the behavioral-cardiac interaction because of the use of the follow-up baseline.

Parental History and Reactivity

Another manner in which we have evaluated the significance of beta-adrenergic reactivity is to ascertain the relationship of HR and SBP in our subject population to the presence or absence of hypertension in their parents. Since there is evidence that hypertension tends to be familial (Pickering, 1977; Paul, 1977), it would be expected that beta-adrenergic reactivity, if of significance in the etiological process as well as SBP, would relate to the incidence of hypertension in our subjects' parents. We sent out a reasonably detailed family health questionnaire to the parents of 137 of the subjects on whom we had data from both the relaxation and pre-task baseline as well as the shock avoidance task or some variation of it (see Hastrup, Light, & Obrist, 1982. One hundred seventeen (85%) were returned of which 104 provided usable data on both parents (75% of our original sample). On the basis of the information provided, we considered 34 of the 208 parents involved as hypertensive, primarily because they indicated they were involved in anti-hypertensive regimes such as diet and medication. The incidence of hypertension in the parents was found to relate to HR reactivity to the shock avoidance task using either baseline as the reference point as well as to the tonic level of HR at the onset of the task. For example, when the subjects are broken down by quartiles with regard to tonic levels of HR during task onset, 18 of the hypertensive parents had sons in the upper quartile and 12 in the next quartile, or 30 of the 34 parents had sons in the upper half of the HR distribution. Similar effects were seen with SBP, with mean levels of SBP during the pre-task baseline and onset of the avoidance task relating most appreciably to parental history.

This relationship can be seen in still another manner which illustrates the interactive nature of family history and a behavioral influence. Average HR and SBP was determined during both baselines and RT task onset as a function of whether no parent was hypertensive (N = 74), one parent was hypertensive (N = 16) or both parents were hypertensive (N = 9). With both HR (Figure 7.10) and SBP (Figure 7.11) when neither parent had hypertension, the average values at all three data points were always less but nore appreciably so at RT task onset.

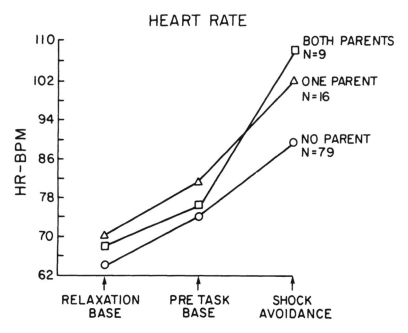

FIG 7.10.   Mean HR during relaxation and pre-task baseline, and the onset of the shock avoidance task. Displayed as a function of whether no parent, one parent, or both parents are hypertensive. Hastrup, et al., 1982.

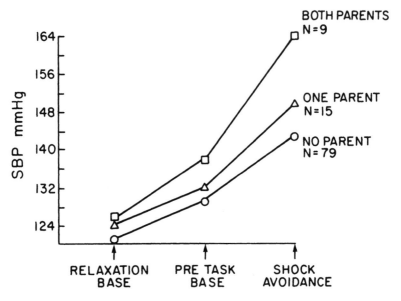

FIG. 7.11.   Mean SBP during relaxation and pre-task baselines, and the onset of the shock avoidance task. Displayed as in Figure 7.10. Hastrup, et al., 1982. Note: SBP was not available on one subject who had one hypertensive parent.

The interaction between conditions and family history was significant for both measures. Subjects with one hypertensive parent were not consistently differentiated from those with two hypertensive parents with HR while with SBP, the two parent subjects always had higher values, the difference being least during the relaxation baseline and most during the RT task.

There are two other facets of the family history data to note. Blood pressure reactivity to the cold pressor has been evaluated as a possible prognostic tool in normotensives and in early hypertension. The results have been inconsistent, leading Weiner (1970) to conclude that it was not a reliable predictor; Julius and Schork (1971) came to a similar conclusion with regard to vascular reactivity to this event in borderline hypertension. There are two problems with the use of the cold pressor. One, if increased beta-adrenergic reactivity is of significance in the etiological process, then it is not too surprising that the cold pressor does not have much in the line of predictive powers since it does not evoke as appreciable a beta-adrenergic effect as do other tasks such as shock avoidance. To evaluate this possibility, we had available HR data during the cold pressor on 45 of our subjects on whom we also had parental histories. Of the 90 parents, 21 were considered hypertensive. We could find no relationship to parental history of HR (tonic levels or reactivity) during the cold pressor. This is likely not due just to the reduced sample size since we still found the same relationship between family history and HR during the RT task with these 45 subjects as with the entire sample.

A second problem faced with the cold pressor when evaluating SBP reactivity is that with individuals with an already elevated pre-task base level, reactivity may be minimized (an initial value effect). Since we also had the follow-up or relaxation baseline (a natural way to correct for base level effects) SBP to the cold pressor was evaluated with respect to parental history using both baselines. There was a trend for SBP reactivity to relate to hypertension when the relaxation baseline was used as the baseline (14 of the 20 hypertensive parents had sons whose SBP reactivity was above the median) while no such trend was observed with the pre-task baseline (a 10-10 median split). Should this trend be strengthened with additional data, it underscores the significance of which baseline is used but in turn creates another problem. It suggests that a vascular component may be of importance in the etiological process. That is to say, since the SBP response during the cold pressor is primarily due to vascular responsiveness (remember how uneffected SBP responsivity was to beta-adrenergic blockade) a vascular contribution independent of a myocardial influence may be of importance.

Another facet of the parental history data to note was a spin off from our first attempt to evaluate SBP in the field (Light & Obrist, 1980a). When we first observed appreciable individual differences in beta-adrenergic reactivity, the question was raised whether the more reactive subjects evidenced greater SBP values under a variety of other conditions such as the relaxation baseline, in their student health records, and at a campus blood pressure screening booth. Overall, the SBP values obtained under these conditions were unrelated to HR reactivity to the shock avoidance task. However, a relationship was observed between field values and HR reactivity, and both SBP reactivity in the laboratory and parental history of hypertension. In the 60 subjects involved in this effort, 29 showed an occasional SBP value in the the clinic or relaxation baseline of 135 mm Hg, a value arbitrarily designated as marginally elevated, while the remaining 31 subjects never evidenced a value this high. Although HR reactors to shock avoidance were equally distributed among those two sub-groups, those subjects who were both HR reactors and demonstrated an occasional marginally elevated SBP value in the clinic or during the relaxation baseline demonstrated appreciably greater SBP reactivity during the pre-task baseline, the cold pressor, film and shock avoidance, and a greater incidence of hypertension among their parents. Although we are dealing with small numbers of hypertensive parents (17 of 74 parents), the trend suggests that the occurrence of a marginally elevated SBP pressure on some occasions does not impart much information about its potential consequences. What are also necessary conditions are a propensity to overreact myocardially and possibly an elevated plasma renin as an index of possible kidney function (Esler et al., 1977).

There are two other matters to discuss in regard to these parental history data. It is not too surprising that a relationship is observed between parental history and levels of SBP in our subjects. There is evidence that BP in parents and children are directly though modestly correlated (Feinleib, 1979). Thus, a parent with an elevated pressure might be expected to have offspring evidencing higher BP values at any age than offspring whose parents have lower BP values. Of greater importance is the observation that HR and parental history are related because this bears on the etiological process and, as just discussed, might improve our predictive ability. Secondly, a relationship between parental hypertension and behavioral influences has been demonstrated in two recently published studies. In one (Falkner, Onesti, Angelakos, Fernandes, & Langman, 1979), 14 and 15-year-old adolescents were exposed to challenging mental arithmetic problems. Individuals who had at least one hypertensive parent demonstrated greater increases in HR, SBP, and DBP than those with no hypertensive parent, with the effect being more pronounced (particularly sustained) in those adolescents demonstrating marginally elevated resting DBP. There is one aspect of the data which is at variance with some of our own observations and conceptual schemes. This is the DBP effects. We observe minimal changes in DBP when beta-adrenergic influences are maximal (see Figure 7.6) and only a non-significant association between DBP and parental history. There is no obvious explanation for this discrepancy. Their borderline subjects were selected on the basis of elevated resting DBP values, which could account for an overall elevated values but not for greater reactivity. At best, one can conclude that there may be differing etiological processes. A second study (Lawler, Barker, Hubbard & Allen, 1980) bred rats to be predisposed to hypertension by crossing spontnaeous hypertensive with normotensive rats. When the resulting offspring are subjected to a shock-avoidance, conflict paradigm, they demonstrate a gradually escalating level of SBP over the 15-week course of the experiment. However, offspring who were not exposed to this procedure show no change in SBP over the same time period. This demonstrates, as we have seen in our young adult human subjects, that the predisposition as indicated by the family history becomes manifest as a result of the behavioral-cardiac interaction.

SOME FINAL COMMENTS

There are two matters that should be addressed before summarizing. One concerns our DBP data where in contrast to SBP, we rarely find it elevated, and on occasion inversely related to the SBP. This, it could be argued, weakens our model since an elevation of the DBP in some circles is considered to herald the arrival of established hypertension (Kannel, 1977). There are, however, two considerations which counter this argument. First, the model suggests that an elevated SBP would preceed an elevated DBP because: (1) the elevated CO and increased myocardial contractility would more apt to influence SBP than DBP; (2) the vascular resistance has not as yet noticeably increased since autoregulation or vascular changes take place over time. The DBP would most clearly indicate vascular involvement. Secondly, and as might be recalled, clinical studies evaluating hemodynamics in borderline hypertension commonly report an elevated SBP but not an elevated DBP (e.g., Safar, et al., 1973).

A final matter is that we don't understand the basis for the individual differences in myocardial reactivity. An effort has been made to see if they relate to some contemporary behavioral metrics like the type A-B dimension without success (Dembroski, Weiss, Shields, Feinleib, & Haynes, 1978). Some evidence suggests that the more reactive subjects become more engaged in the performance tasks but this is hardly the whole story (Light & Obrist, 1980b). For example, it does not account for the generalization of reactivity to conditions requiring no particular task involvement, such as the painful cold pressor. Also, the subject population is quite homogenous with respect to age, educational background and career aspirations, variables that could influence attitude involvement, etc. Perhaps the necessary strategy to use in evaluating a behavioral influence on these individual differences is suggested by Lazarus (1978) who indicated that in any given situation one must consider both how the individual appraises the situation, for example, is it important or threatening, and then how the individual copes with it.

SUMMARY

Behavioral influences on the BP have been demonstrated ranging from acute effects associated with moment to moment interaction of the organism with its environment to more long term effects as indicated by epidemiological studies as well as with chronic animal preparations. While such observations suggest the probable significance of the behavioral-cardiac interaction in the etiology of essential hypertension, they do not delineate the means by which this influence comes about and why hypertension strikes only a certain percentage of the population, necessary information for both treatment and prevention. On the basis of several lines of evidence, we have begun to assess some working hypotheses which link both myocardial and renal events to the etiological process. In chronically prepared dogs, evidence has accrued indicating that a behavioral task (shock avoidance) can evoke an increase in the CO which is excessive relative to any increase in oxygen consumption and an aberrant renal response characterized by Na retention. Such results suggest two interacting beta-adrenergic mechanisms by which a more sustained elevated BP may result. In humans, we believe it is necessary to focus our efforts on a young adult population who is not as yet hypertensive but who may demonstrate a pre-hypertensive condition involving the same mechanisms. While renal function and the CO have not yet been assessed other evidence suggests the relevance of these mechanisms. For one thing, beta-adrenergic influences on the myocardium are observed under certain conditions which also influence the SBP. Appreciable individual differences in myocardial reactivity are also seen which raises the question of whether such hyperresponsive individuals are pre-hypertensive. This possibility is suggested by the observations thay hyperresponsiveness appears to generalize to a variety of challenging circumstances and to the incidence of hypertension in their parents. More definitive efforts will necessitate a longitudinal study and further assessment of myocardial (the CO) and renal function. In conclusion, the theme of this chapter is to emphasize the need to refocus our efforts from a symptom oriented approach in hypertension research, to one delineating mechanisms. This is because the etiological process is complex, it likely varies among individuals as likely does the relative influence of the behavioral-cardiac interaction. The proposed working hypotheses are intended as one means to accomplish this end.

ACKNOWLDEGMENTS

Research cited and performed by the authors was supported by the following research grants: MH 07995 National Institute of Mental Health (PAO); HL 18976 (PAO); HL 23718 (KCL), HL 24643 (AWL) National Heart, Lung, and Blood Institute; National Service Awards F-32-HL 05531 (KCL), F-32 HL 05671 (JLH) and F-32 HL 05713 (MHP) National Heart, Lung and Blood Institute.

REFERENCES

Ahlquist, R. P. Adrenergic receptors in the cardiovascular systems. In P. R. Saxen & R. P. Forsyth (Eds.), *Beta-adrenoceptor blocking agents*. New York: American Elsevier, 1976, pp. 29–34.

Anderson, D. E., & Brady, J. V. Cardiovascular responses to avoidance conditioning in the dog. *Psychosomatic Medicine*, 1976, *38*, 181–189.

Bello-Reuss, E., Trevino, D. L., & Gottschalk, C. W. Effect of renal sympathetic nerve stimulation on proximal water and sodium transport. *Journal of Clinical Investigation*, 1976, *57*, 1104–1107.

Bevan, A. T., Honour, A. J., & Stott, F. H. Direct arterial pressure recording in unrestricted man. *Clinical Science*, 1969, *36*, 329–344.

Brener, J., Phillips, K., & Connally, S. Oxygen consumption and ambulation during operant conditioning of heart rate increases and decreases in rats. *Psychophysiology*, 1977, *14*, 483–491.

Brod, J. Hemodynamic basis of acute pressor reactions and hypertension. *British Heart Journal*, 1963, *25*, 227–245.

Brown, J. J., Fraser, R., Lever, A. F., Morton, J. J., Robertson, J. I. S., & Schalekamp, M. A. D. H. Mechanisms in hypertension: A personal view. In J. Genest, E. Koiw, & O. Kuchel (Eds.), *Hypertension: Physiopathology and treatment*. New York: McGraw-Hill, 1977, pp. 529–548.

Coleman, T. G., Granger, H. J., & Guyton, A. C. Whole body circulatory, autoregulation and hypertension. *Circulation Research*, 1971, *29*, (Suppl 2, II-76-II-86).

Coleman, T. G., Samar, R. E., & Murphy, W. R. Autoregulation versus other vaso-constrictors in hypertension—A critical review. *Hypertension*, 1979, 1, 324–330.

Dembroski, T. M., Weiss, S. M., Shields, J. L., Feinleib, M., & Haynes, S. G. *Coronary-prone behavior*. New York: Springer-Verlag, 1978.

Eich, R. H., Cuddy, R. P., Smulyan, H., & Lyons, R. H. Hemodynamics in labile hypertension: A follow up study. *Circulation*, 1966, *34*, 299–307.

Eliasch, H., Rosen, A., & Scott, H. M. Systemic circulatory response to stress of simulated flight and to physical exercise before and after propranolol block. *British Heart Journal*, 1967, 29, 617–683.

Esler, M., Julius, J., Zweifler, A., Randall, O., Harburg, E., Gardiner, H., & DeQuattro, V. Mild high-renin essential hypertension-Neurogenic hypertension? *New England Journal of Medicine*, 1977, *296*, 405–411.

Falkner, B., Onesti, G., Angelakos, E. T., Fernandes, M., & Langman, C. Cardiovascular response to mental stress in normal adolescents with hypertensive parents. Hemodynamics and mental stress in adolescents. *Hypertension*, 1979, *1*, 23–30.

Feinleib, M. Genetics and familial aggregation of blood pressure. In Onesti, G. & Klimt, C. R.(Eds), *Hypertension - Determinants, Complications and Intervention*, New York: Grune & Stratton, 1979, 35–48.

Folkow, B. U. G., Hallback, M. I. L., Lundgren, Y., Sivertsson, R., & Weiss, L. Importance of adaptive changes in vascular design for establishment of primary hypertension, studied in man and in spontaneously hypertensive rat. *Circulation Research*, 1973, *32–33*, (Suppl 1, I-2-I-16).

Folkow, B., & Neil, E. *Circulation*. New York: Oxford University Press, 1971.

Forsyth, R. P. Blood pressure response to long-term avoidance schedules in the restrained rhesus monkey. *Psychosomatic Medicine*, 1969, *31*, 300–309.

Forsyth, R. P. Effect of propranolol on stress-induced hemodynamic changes in monkeys. In P. R. Saxena & R. P. Forsyth (Eds.), *Beta-adrenoceptor blocking agents*. New York: American Elsevier, 1976, pp. 317–322.

Freidman, S. M. Arterial contractility and reactivity. In J. Genest, E. Koiw & O. Kuchel (Eds.), *Hypertension: Physiopathology and treatment*. New York: McGraw-Hill, 1977, pp. 470–485.

Frumkin, K., Nathan, R. J., Prout, M. F., & Cohen, M. L. Nonpharmocological control of essential hypertension in man: A critical review of the experimental literature. *Psychosomatic Medicine*, 1978, *40*, 294–320.

Grignolo, A. *Renal function and cardiovascular dynamics during tread-mill exercise and shock-avoidance in dogs*. Unpublished doctoral dissertation, University of North Carolina at Chapel Hill, 1980.

Grignolo A., Koepke, J. P. & Obrist, P. A. *Renal function, heart rate and blood pressure during exercise and avoidance in dogs*. American Journal of Physiology, 1982, *242*, R482–R490.

Grignolo, A., Light, K. C., & Obrist, P. A. *Beta adrenergic influences on the canine myocardium: A behavioral and pharmacological study*. Pharmacology, Biochemistry and Behavior, 1981, 5, 313–319.

Guyton, A. C. Personal views on mechanisms of hypertension. In J. Genest, E. Koiw & O. Kuchel (Eds.), *Hypertension: Physiopathology and treatment*. New York: McGraw-Hill, 1977, pp. 566–575.

Hastrup, J. L., Light, K. C., & Obrist, P. A. *Parental hypertension and cardiovascular response to stress in healthy young adults* Psychophysiology 1982, 19, In Press

Henry, J. P., & Cassel, J. C. Psychosocial factors in essential hypertension: Recent epidemiologic and animal literature evidence. *American Journal of Epidemiology*, 1969, *90*, 171–200.

Henry, J. P., Stephens, P. M., & Santisteban, G. A. A model of psycho-social hypertension showing reversibility and progression of cardiovascular complications. *Circulation Research*, 1975, *36*, 156–164.

Hofer, M. A. Cardiac and respiratory function during sudden prolonged immobility in wild rodents. *Psychosomatic Medicine*, 1970, *32*, 633–647.

Howard, J. L., Obrist, P. A., Gaebelein, C. J., & Galosy R. A. Multiple somatic measures and heart rate during classical aversive conditioning in the cat. *Journal of Comparative & Physiological Psychology*, 1974, *87*. 228–236.

Julius, S. Classification of hypertension. In Genest J., Koiw, E. & Kuchel, O. (Eds.). *Hypertension- Physiopathology and treatment*. New York: McGraw-Hill, 1977, pp. 9–12. (a)

Julius, S. Borderline hypertension: Epidemiologic and clinical implications. In J. Genest, E. Koiw & O, Kuchel (Eds.), *Hypertension: Physiopathology and treatment*. New York: McGraw-Hill, 1977, pp. 630–640. (b)

Julius, S., & Esler, M. D. Autonomic nervous cardiovascular regulation in borderline hypertension. *American Journal of Cardiology*, 1975, *36*, 685–696.

Julius, S., Pascual, A. V., & London, R. Role of parasympathetic inhibition in the hyperkenetic type of hypertension. *Circulation*, 1971, *64*, 413–418.

Julius, S., & Schork, M. A. Borderline hypertension: A critical review. *Journal of Chronic Disease*, 1971, *23*, 723–754.

Kannel, W. B. Importance of hypertension as a major risk factor in cardiovascular disease. In J. Genest, E. Koiw & O. Kuchel (Eds.), *Hypertension: Physiopathology and treatment*. New York: McGraw-Hill, 1977, pp. 888–910.

Langer, A. W. *A comparison of the effects of treadmill exercise and signaled shock avoidance training on hemodynamic processes and the arterial-mixed venous oxygen content difference in conscious dogs*. Unpublished doctoral dissertation, University of North Carolina, Chapel Hill, 1978.

Langer, A. W., Obrist, P. A., & McCubbin, J. A. Hemodynamic and metabolic adjustments during exercise and shock avoidance in dogs. *American Journal of Physiology*, 1979, *236*, H225–H230.

Lawler, J. E., Barker, G. F., Hubbard, J. W., & Allen, M. T. The effects of conflict on tonic levels of blood pressure in the genetically borderline hypertensive rat. *Psychophysiology*, 1980, *17*, 363–370.

Lazarus, R. S. A strategy for research on psychological and social factors in hypertension. *Journal of Human Stress*, 1978, *4*, 35–40.

Light, K. C., & Obrist, P. A. Cardiovascular response to stress: Effects of opportunity to avoid, shock experience and performance feedback. *Psychophysiology*, 1980, *17*, 243–252. (b)

Light, K. C., & Obrist, P. A. Cardiovascular reactivity to behavioral stress in young males with and without marginally elevated systolic pressures: Comparison of clinic, home and laboratory measures. *Hypertension*, 1980, *2*, 802–808 (a) (a).

Lund-Johansen, P. Hemodynamics in early essential hypertension. *Acta Medica Scandinavica*, 1967, (Suppl 482, 1–101).

Lund-Johansen, P. Spontaneous changes in central hemodynamics in essential hypertension—a 10-year follow-up study. In G. Onesti & C. R. Klimt (Eds.), *Hypertension—determinants, complications and intervention*. New York: Grune & Stratton, 1979, pp. 201–209.

Morse, W. H., Herd, J. A., Kelleher, R. T., & Grose, S. A. Schedule-controlled modulation of arterial blood pressure in the squirrel monkey. In H. D. Kimmal (Ed.), *Experimental psychopathology - recent research and theory*. New York: Academic Press, 1971, pp. 147–163.

Obrist, P. A. Heart rate and somatic-motor coupling during classical aversive conditioning in humans. *Journal of Experimental Psychology*, 1968, *77*, 180–193.

Obrist, P. A. *Cardiovascular Psycho-physiology—A perspective*. New York: Plenum, 1981, pp. 236.

Obrist, P. A., Howard, J. L., Lawler, J. E., Galosy, R. A., Meyers, K. A., & Gaebelein, C. J. The cardiac somatic interaction. In P. A. Obrist, A. H. Black, J. Brener & L. V. DiCara (Eds.), *Cardiovascular psychophysiology: Current issues in response mechanisms, biofeedback and methodology*. Chicago: Aldine, 1974, 136–162. (a)

Obrist, P. A., Lawler, J. E., Howard, J. L., Smithson, K. W., Martin, P. L., & Manning, J. Smypathetic influences on cardiac rate and contractility during acute stress in humans. *Psychophysiology,* 1974, *11*. 405–427. (b)

Obrist, P. A., Gaebelein, C. J., Teller, E. S., Langer, A. W., Gringnolo, A., Light, K. C., & McCubbin, J. A. The relationship among heart rate, carotid dp/dt and blood pressure in humans as a function of the type of stress. *Psychophysiology,* 1978, *15*, 102–115.

Obrist, P. A., Langer, A. W., Grignolo, A., Sutterer, J. R., Light, K. C., & McCubbin, J. A. Blood pressure control mechanisms and stress: Implications for the etiology of hypertension. In G. Onesti & L. R. Klimt (Eds.), *Hypertension: Determinants, complications and intervention.* New York: Grune & Stratton, 1979, 69–94. (b)

Obrist, P. A., Light, K. C., McCubbin, J. A., Hutcheson, J. S., & Hoffer, J. L. Pulse transit time: Relationship to blood pressure and myocardial performance. *Psychophysiology,* 1979, *16*, 292–301. (a)

Obrist, P. A., Webb, R. A., & Sutterer, J. R. Heart rate and somatic changes during aversive conditioning and a simple reaction time task. *Psychophysiology,* 1969, *5*, 696–723.

Obrist, P. A., Webb, R. A., Sutterer, J. R., & Howard, J. L. The cardiac-somatic relationship: Some reformulations. *Psychophysiology,* 1970, *6*, 569–587.

Obrist, P. A., Wood, D. M., & Perez-Reyes, M. Heart rate during conditioning in humans: Effects of UCS intensity, vagal blockade and adrenergic block of vasomotor activity. Journal of *Experimental Psychology,* 1965, *70*, 32–42.

Page, I. H. Some regulatory mechanisms of renovascular and essential arterial hypertension. In J. Genest, E. Koiw & O. Kuchel (Eds.), *Hypertension: Physiopathology and treatment.* New York: McGraw-Hill, 1977, 576–587.

Page, I. H., & McCubbin, J. W. The physiology of arterial hypertension. In W. F. Hamilton & P. Dow (Eds.), *Handbook of physiology: Circulation.* Section 2, Volume 1. Washington, D.C.: American Physiological Society, 1966, 2163–2208.

Paul, O. Epidemiology of hypertension. In J. Genest, E. Koiw & O. Kuchel (Eds.), *Hypertension: Physiopathology and treatment.* New York: McGraw-Hill, 1977, 613–629.

Pfeffer, M. A., & Frohlich, E. D. Hemodynamic and myocardial function in young and old normotensive and spontaneously hypertensive rats. *Circulation Research,* 1973, *32*, (Supp 1, I-28-I-38).

Pickering, T. G. Personal views on mechanisms of hypertension. In J. Genest, E. Koiw & O, Kuchel (Eds.), *Hypertension: Physiopathology and treatment.* New York: McGraw-Hill, 1977, 598–605.

Poortmans, J. R. Exercise and renal function. *Exercise and Sport Science Reviews,* 1977, *5*, 255–294.

Randall, D. C., & Smith, O. A. Ventricular contractility during controlled exercise and emotion in the primate. *American Journal of Physiology,* 1974, *226*, 1051–1059.

Safar, M. E., Weiss, Y. A., Levenson, J. A., London, G. M., & Milliez, P. L. Hemodynamic study of 85 patients with borderline hypertension. *The American Journal of Cardiology,* 1973, *31*, 315–319.

Sannerstedt, R. Hemodynamic response to exercise in patients with arterial hypertension. *Acta Medica Scandinavica,* 1966, (Suppl *458*, 1–83).

Schottstaedt, W. W., Grace, W. J., & Wolff, H. G. Life situations, behavior, attitudes, emotions and renal excretion of fluid and electrolytes. *Journal of Psychosomatic Research,* 1956, *1*, 75–83; 147–159; 203–211; 287–291; 292–298.

Shaprio, A. P., Schwartz, G. E., Ferguson, D. C. E., Redmond, D. P., & Weiss, S. M. Behavioral methods in the treatment of hypertension I. Review of their clinical status. *Annals of Internal Medicine,* 1977, *86*, 626–636.

Stead, E. A., Warren, J. V., Merrill, A. J., & Brannon, E. S. The cardiac output in male subjects as measured by the technique of atrial catherization. Normal values with observations on the effects of anxiety and tilting. *Journal of Clinical Investigation,* 1945, *24,* 326–331.

Tyroler, H. A. The Detroit project studies of blood pressure: A prologue and review of related studies and epidemiological issues. *Journal of Chronic Diseases,* 1977, *30,* 613–624.

Webb, R. A., & Obrist, P. A. The physiological consomitants of reaction time performance as a function of preparatory interval series. *Psychophysiology,* 1970, *6,* 389–403.

Weiner, H. Psychosomatic research in essential hypertension. In M. Koster, H. Musaph & P. Viser (Eds.), *Psychosomatics in essential hypertension,* Bibliotheca Psychiatica No. 144, 1970, 58–115.

Weiner, H. *Psychobiology and human disease.* New York: Elsevier, 1977.

Zanchetti, A., Stella, A., Leonetti, G., Morganti, A., & Terzoli, L. Control of renin release: A review of experimental evidence and clinical implications. *The American Journal of Cardiology,* 1976, *37,* 675–691.

8 Modification of Coronary-Risk Behavior

Ethel Roskies
University of Montreal

INTRODUCTION

Although a few of the risk factors for coronary heart disease (CHD) are clearly beyond the control of the individual, a goodly number are directly linked to personal habits and lifestyle. Sex, advanced age, and family propensity are risk factors outside individual control, but contrasting with these is the risk attributed to serum cholesterol (dietary lipid quantity and quality), high blood pressure, smoking, sedentary lifestyle and type A behavior. In prospective epidemiological studies, fully half of the observed incidence of coronary heart disease is accounted for by the presence of only three of the controllable factors: arterial blood pressure, serum cholesterol, and smoking (Report of the Inter-Society Commission for Heart Disease Resources, 1970).

The growing recognition of the health dangers posed by the "American way of life" (Farquhar, 1978a) has led many individuals to change their lifestyle, either on their own initiative, or by seeking professional help. In the U.S. over the last 20 years there has been a sharp decline in cigarette smoking (particularly among middle-aged men), a shift in diet from animal to vegetable fats, and an increased interest in recreational exercise. There has also been a corresponding decline in cardiovascular mortality, though the relationship between the lifestyle changes and the improved health status is still being debated (Cooper, Dyer, Moss, Stamler, Soltero, Liu, & Stamler, 1978; Dwyer & Hetzel, 1980; Levy, 1978; Stamler, 1978; Stern, 1979; Vaisrub, 1980; Walker, 1977).

Ironically, professional activity in fostering and evaluating coronary risk reduction has lagged behind individual initiative. Although there has been a tremendous spurt in new knowledge of the epidemiology of coronary arteriosclerosis since the early 1950s, the medical establishment has been cautious in applying this knowledge to coronary risk reduction. In part, the slow growth of preventive cardiology can be explained by the fact that dramatic improvements in coronary diagnosis and treatment were attracting much of the attention and funding during this time period. But much of the delay has also come from the belief held by many that further knowledge of risk factors was required before any intervention could be responsibly undertaken (Ahrens, 1976; Borhani, 1977; Corday & Corday, 1975; Corday, 1978).

The debate between further knowledge verus immediate intervention has not been fully resolved to this date, but since the early 70s the balance has begun to weigh in favor of intervention efforts. In 1970 the Inter-Society Commission for Heart Disease Resources (Report of the Inter-Society Commission for Heart Disease Resources, 1970) strongly recommended that ''a strategy of primary prevention of premature atherosclerotic diseases be adopted as a long term national policy for the United States.'' More to the point, one year later a task force of this commission recommended that the National Heart and Lung Institute develop and support preventive trials in high-risk subjects with multiple risk factors. (National Heart and Lung Institute Task Force on Arteriosclerosis, 1971). In 1973 the American Heart Association entered the area of prevention with a slightly different emphasis, that of fostering bio-behavioral collaboration. It formed a committee on Motivation for Risk Factor Reduction and charged it with the responsibility ''for studying behavioral aspects of the known approaches to altering risk factors and to making recommendations for increasing the interest and motivation of both clinicians and persons at risk in taking the necessary steps to create successful risk factor reduction programs.'' One year later, in June, 1974, this committee sponsored the first multi-disciplinary conference on Applying Behavioral Science to Cardiovascular Risk (Enelow & Henderson, 1975).

In a research area less than 10-years-old there are few definitive results to report. Valid observations of changes in cardiac morbidity, or even of modification of coronary risk factors, can only be made over time and some of the studies to be described in this chapter still have not completed their data collection. Of necessity, therefore, this chapter cannot even attempt a criticial evaluation of the different approaches to coronary risk reduction. Our aims, instead, will be the much more modest ones of surveying work in progress, and of describing the preliminary results that have been reported.

Coronary risk reduction programs come in a bewildering array of shapes and sizes. Samples vary in number from 20 to 20,000, risk factors treated from one to many, health status of sample from community-at-large to specific high risk, mode of treatment from pharmaceutical to behavioral, and so on. It is possible, nervertheless, to order this diversity. Within the field of primary prevention the most useful division is between the large multi-factorial trials and the typically smaller, more experimental, single-factor interventions. In this chapter we shall first review some of the major multi-factorial trials, stressing the similarities and differences between them, and then examine three of the single-factor studies that are of particular interest.

MULTI-FACTORIAL INTERVENTION PROGRAMS

Multi-factorial intervention programs currently occupy the center of the stage in CHD prevention for reasons linked to the nature of the disease itself. There are multiple factors that contribute to CHD and not only are these multiple risk factors associated with each other, but also their combined effects are multiplicative, rather than additive (Criqui, Barrett-Connor, Holdbrook, Austin, & Turner, 1980). In concrete terms, this means that an individual who is high on one risk factor has an increased probability of being high on other risk factors, and that with the addition of each risk factor above zero the risk increases disproportionately from two-fold to four-fold to eight-fold. (Pooling Project Research Group, 1978). For purposes of intervention, therefore, a modest modification of several risk-related variables can be as important as a more dramatic change in any single variable (Meyer, Nash, McAlister, Maccoby, & Farquhar, 1980a).

A second factor leading to the popularity of multi-factorial programs are the conceptual and methodological difficulties posed by interventions directed toward single risk factors. In a smoking reduction project, for instance, to insure that any improvement observed in coronary risk status results from changes in smoking alone, it would be necessary to control for fluctuations in other risk factors. However, individuals who are receptive to a health education program and are thereby led to stop smoking are also likely to manifest their increased health consciousness via concurrent changes in diet and exercise. Conversely, smoking cessation can lead to weight gain which, in turn, can lead to higher blood pressure. A partial solution might be to allow these changes to occur and then control for them statistically, but even here one would have to go to the effort and expense of measuring the variables to be controlled. There is also the issue of the ethical obligation to treat iatrogenic effects should they occur. Given the multiple problems inherent in a unifactorial coronary risk reduction program, it has seemed more satisfying and more economical to incorporate associated risk behaviors into the initial design.

The first controlled multi-factorial prevention studies were launched in the early 1970s. To date there are at least six underway or completed: the Gothenberg study (Wilhemsen, Tibblin, & Werko, 1972); the Oslo study (Leren, Askevold, Foss, Froili, Grymyr, Helgeland, Hjermann, Holme, Lund-Larsen, & Norum, 1975; Hjermann, 1980); the Multiple Risk Factor Intervention Trial in the United States (Multiple Risk Factor Intervention Trial, 1976); the Belgian Multi-factorial Preventive Program in CVD (De Backer, Kornitzer, Thilly, & Depoorter, 1977); the Stanford Heart Disease Prevention Project (Maccoby, Farquhar, Wood, & Alexander, 1977); and the North Karelia Program in Finland

(Puska, Koskela, Pakatinen, Puumalainen, Soininem, & Tuomilehto, 1976). Another half dozen projects are currently in preparation. For this chapter we have chosen to describe in detail four of the projects completed or in process, selecting them to illustrate the range of treatment approaches being used.

The most obvious resemblance between all these multi-factor programs is the large samples involved. Studies focusing on individuals have samples of 12,000 (Multiple Risk Factor Intervention Trial) to 20,000 (Belgian Multi-factorial Preventive Program), community studies range from 8,000 (Stanford Heart Disease Prevention Project) to an entire county with a population of 180,000 (North Karelia). A second common characteristic are the specific risk factors tackled: Smoking, serum cholesterol and blood pressure are major targets for all the programs. There is a similar unanimity in choosing what risk factors not to treat. None of the multi-factor programs includes interventions directed toward the psychological risk factors, such as life dissatisfaction or type A behavior (Jenkins, 1976). A fourth bond between the studies is their common focus on a middle-aged population, approximately ages 35–60. (The North Karelia project includes individuals as young as 25, but defines this as middle age!)

What most sharply distinguishes the studies from one another is their respective focus on high risk individuals versus the community at large. Interventions directed toward high risk individuals resemble the traditional medical approach of curing illness in that specific individuals are identified as "patients" (because of the presence of one or more designated risk factors) and are "treated" for their "symptoms" by a health practitioner. Interventions directed toward the community at large, in contrast, are based on an educational model of improving health awareness and practices in individuals at all levels of risk. Of the four studies to be described in detail, one (MRFIT) is restricted solely to high risk individuals, one places most of its emphasis on high-risk individuals though including other levels (the Belgian study), while the remaining two (Stanford and North Karelia) are primarily community studies with sub-programs for high risk individuals. The two studies that are entirely or primarily directed toward high risk individuals intervene mainly via professional face-to-face contact, while the two community studies make extensive use of media or lay persons to deliver their programs. Finally, MRFIT and the Belgian study limit their sample to men, while the Stanford and North Karelia studies include women.

The Multiple Risk Factor Intervention Trial (MRFIT)

Of the various intervention programs to be discussed in this chapter, the Multiple Risk Factor Intervention Trial (MRFIT) comes closest to the traditional model of clinic-based health service delivery. The individuals selected for treatment are identified as patients by virtue of their high risk status, the locale of treatment is a medical setting and the intervention is delivered by health professionals. The outcome measure, too, reflects the medical orientation: death from coronary heart disease (Multiple Risk Factor Intervention Trial, 1976).

Twenty clinics across the United States are participating in the 6 year trial attempting to reduce coronary mortality in high risk men between ages 35–57 by reducing cholesterol, blood pressure, and smoking levels. Participants for the program were selected via a three stage screening process designed to identify individuals in the upper 15% of the population distribution for risk of CHD as determined by the Framingham Study predictions of risk. Three factors were used in calculating risk status: serum cholesterol levels, blood pressure and degree of cigarette smoking. Individuals with verified pre-existing clinical coronary heart disease were excluded.

Once through the sceening process, participants were randomly assigned to intervention and usual care groups. Those in the usual care group have no direct contact with the program staff beyond the annual medical examination. However, it is possible that individuals in this category will receive advice from their physicians concerning diet and exercise, and even medication for hypertension, since it was ethically and practically unfeasible to stipulate no intervention. One can also speculate that the screening process itself, the identification of the person as high risk, and the annual reminder via the medical examination, might motivate individuals to actively search out professional help for coronary risk reduction.

The intervention group receives advice re diet and smoking, as well as anti-hypertensive drugs where indicated, directly from the program staff. The usual procedure is to begin intervention with 10 group sessions and to follow this with periodic reinforcement sessions, either in groups or individually. Unfortunately, there is very little information available as to precisely what strategies are being used during these treatment sessions to produce the desired effects. For instance, one of the goals of the intervention is a 10% reduction in serum cholesterol. We are told that, for this purpose, participants "receive dietary counsel emphasizing an overall balanced diet low in saturated fats and appropriate in caloric count". There is also a detailed description of the methods developed for scoring food intake in general, and fat intake in particular, as well as for determining compliance with dietary advice (Remmell & Benfari, 1980; Remmell, Gorder, Hall, & Tillotson, 1980). What is missing from these reports, however, is a description of the specific therapeutic strategies comprised under the term "dietary counsel". Nor is there any indication of what procedures, if any, are used to handle problems of noncompliance. The same complaint of vagueness concerning treatment procedures applies to the other therapeutic goals, such as smoking cessation and weight loss.

Formal screening for this 6-year trial began in November 1973 and was terminated in February 1976. Thus, no outcome data can be expected until 1982. Seven percent of the 370,559 men seen at first screening, that is approximately

25,000 persons, were eligible by risk-factor criteria. Of these, 12,866 were found to be eligible on all the other admission criteria and also were willing to participate. The average levels of the three risk factors for the men enrolled were diastolic blood pressure, 90.5 mm Hg., serum cholesterol, 253 mg per deciliter, and cigarettes, 20 per day. Over 60% of the men eventually enrolled were cigarette smokers at the first screening visit (Farrand & Mojonnier, 1980).

Although intervention efforts in MRFIT are restricted to three risk factors (serum cholesterol, hypertension, and smoking), this study is also being used to test the importance for CHD of another lifestyle risk factor, the type A behavior pattern. For a sub-sample of 3110 men at eight different treatment centers, the Structured Interview for assessing type A behavior was conducted before individuals were assigned to a treatment condition (Multiple Risk Factor Intervention Trial Group, 1979). A four-fold classification system was used ranging from extreme type A (type A_1) to moderate type A (type A_2) to equally mixed A and non A characteristics (type X) to definite non-type A (type B). These ratings will be correlated with the incidence of non fatal coronary events, as well as CHD deaths, during the subsequent 6 years.

The MRFIT data are also being used to investigate the possible adverse consequences, psychological and physiological, that might inadvertently occur in the course of attempting to achieve the over-all beneficial goal. There are now published reports on three of the possible negative side-effects, namely, (1) the psychological stress that might be created by being informed of one's high risk status, (2) the anxiety and hypochondria that might result from being excluded from treatment after being labelled high risk, and (3) the effects of a cholesterol lowering diet on HDL, a form of cholesterol believed to serve as a protection against heart disease.

The issue whether being informed of one's high risk status creates stress was explored with participants in the San Francisco center, a sample of 575 men (Horowitz, Hulley, Alvarez, Billings, Benfari, Blair, Borhani, & Simon, 1980). One third of the men did, in fact, report intrusive or avoidance experiences 1 year after the receipt of the news of increased risk. The special intervention group, with its more frequent reminders, had significantly higher levels of intrusive ideas and feelings about the news of risk than did the usual care group, but also more signs of coping with this stress.

Investigators at the Harvard center were also concerned about the psychological state of individuals informed of their high risk status, but who were, in contrast, not assigned to the treatment group. They hypothesized that persons alerted but not treated might experience increased anxiety and depression, or even increased functional heart pains. Fortunately, examination of the records of the 616 participants at this center proved these fears groundless (Benfari, McIntyre, Eaker, Blumberg, & Oglesby, 1979).

There was also the worry that dietary recommendations directed toward lowering total serum cholesterol might inadvertently also lower HDL. Examination of changes in HDL cholesterol levels during the first two years of the study, with a sample of 2151 participants, showed that conventional risk reduction programs are not likely to lower circulating HDL cholesterol. In fact, program components such as weight reduction and smoking cessation may actually increase the levels (Hulley, Ashman, Kuller, Lasser & Sherwin, 1979).

Even before publishing its results the MRFIT program has been subject to considerable criticism, some of it published, but even more circulating through the rumor channels of the scientific community. This close attention is not surprising since MRFIT is one of the first programs of this type to be mounted in the United States and, therefore, may be viewed as a potential model for intervention programs for a variety of other diseases. Complaints concerning MRFIT have touched all aspects of the program, ranging from overall design considerations to the way the program is being administered in a specific center. Even supporters of the program have expressed concern that treatment results may be misinterpreted either because the length of follow-up was too brief, the difference in risk factor reduction between special intervention and usual care groups was too small, or the population was too high risk and, therefore, participants were already suffering at intake from extensive subclinical atherosclerosis (Kuller, Neaton, Caggiula, & Falvo-Gerard, 1980). Even should the results prove all that was hoped for, it is doubtful whether they could be easily generalized to the population at large, or that most communities would have the resources necessary to introduce programs of this nature (Syme, 1978). Nevertheless, in spite of all these *caveats,* the value of MRFIT remains undisputed. Should the program produce favorable results, it will demonstrate that which still remains to be proven: Risk factor reduction can reduce cardiac mortality and/or morbidity. Following this, one could then focus on the separate issue of developing suitable methods for bringing about risk factor reduction in ordinary community settings.

The Belgian Multi-Factor Preventive Trial in CVD

In the continuum from clinic-based to community-based trials, the Belgian Preventive Trial (or the Belgian Heart Disease Prevention Project as it is sometimes called) falls midway between the clinical MRFIT and the community Stanford and North Karelia projects. In contrast to MRFIT, selection for the Belgian project was not on the basis of individual health risk but, rather, on the basis of membership in an occupational group. The unit of assignment to treatment or control condition, too, was the factory, rather than the person. In this fashion of utilizing the workplace as a miniature community, the Belgian project can be classed as a community study. Within the factories, however, only men aged 40–59 were eligible for the program, and a good part of the intervention efforts were channeled into individual professional consultations with the 20% of the sample designated as high risk. In these characteristics, the Belgian project resembles MRFIT and other clinic-based trials for high risk individuals.

The Belgian Multi-factor Preventive Trial, part of the larger WHO European Collaborative Study (World Health Organization European Collaborative Group, 1974), started in 1972 and was planned as a 6-year follow-up (De Backer et al., 1977). The program was directed toward five risk factors: serum cholesterol, cigarette smoking, hypertension, obesity, and sedentary lifestyle. The sample for the project was drawn from 30 factories scattered throughout the four main regions of Belgium (two Dutch speaking, one French speaking, and one bilingual). These factories were paired by industry and then randomly assigned to treatment and control conditions. There were 15 factories in each condition.

At the time the project was begun, these 30 factories employed 19,390 men aged 40–59 and hence eligible for the program. Of these, 83.7% (16,222 men) accepted an invitation for a risk factor screening examination. For individuals in the factories assigned to the intervention group, all (n = 7398) were examined for systolic blood pressure, weight, height, as well as serum cholesterol level, and all underwent a 12 lead ECG under resting conditions. In addition, the participants completed demographic questionnaires, the Jenkins Activity Survey (Jenkins, Rosenman, & Friedman, 1967), the Bortner test (Bortner 1969), the Sandler-Harazi questionnaire (Sandler & Hazari, 1960) and the Eysenck Personality Inventory (Eysenck & Eysenck, 1971). For individuals in the control factories (n = 8824), 10% of the subjects in each occupational unit were randomly selected to undergo the same complete initial examination as all the subjects in the intervention group; the other 90% were subjected only to an ECG at rest.

The second stage in the screening process consisted of establishing risk scores for all the subjects in the intervention project and for the 10% of the control group that underwent the same initial examination. The risk score was a composite based on age (<50 vs. 50+), degree of job activity (heavy, light, and sedentary), number of cigarettes a day (<5, 5+, 20+), systolic blood pressure (<120, 120+, 140+, 160+) and serum cholesterol level (<210, 210+, 220+, 230+, 240+, 250+, 260+). The range of possible scores was 0 to 11. The subjects who belonged to the top 21% of the risk score distribution were arbitrarily placed in the high risk group (n = 1601), and the others in the low risk group.

Intervention in the Belgian project was primarily via individual face-to-face counselling from the two project physicians, at least for the high risk group, but also involved written and visual material, limited environmental manipulation, and an attempt to mobilize the support of family and occupational physicians. At the beginning of the project, high risk subjects in the intervention group were given written information concerning their personal risk factors. They were then invited to an individual counselling session in which all were given dietary advice designed to reduce serum cholesterol levels. In addition, individuals who smoked five or more cigarettes a day, had mean systolic blood pressures of 160 mm Hg or more, were 15% or more overweight by local standards, and/or who were sedentary at work and at leisure were given specific advice for these conditions. For hypertensive individuals, the advice included the recommendation to consult with their family physicians who had previously been sent instructions on the treatment of choice. This counselling session, accompanied by a medical examination, was repeated twice yearly for high risk subjects in the intervention group. In addition, eight times during the life of the project a random sample of 5% of the total intervention group received a single couselling session and a complete medical examination.

While the criteria for deciding who was to be treated for what risk factor are detailed and precise, the Belgian study shares the vagueness of MRFIT in failing to describe exactly what treatment procedures were used during the counselling sessions. Certainly the limited time devoted to each subject precluded psychotherapy or behavior therapy. Because the aim was to develop an intervention project that could be applied by any occupational medicine service, the total time devoted to each high risk subject in the intervention group (including screening) was 1 hour in the first year and 30 minutes per year there after (Kornitzer, De Backer, Dramaix, & Thilly, 1980a).

Except for those selected for the various random samples, the low risk subjects in the intervention group received only mass counselling via posters, anti-smoking talks, and dietary advice to the factory canteen staff concerning changes in canteen menus. High risk subjects and the random samples in the intervention group were also exposed to this mass counselling program. In summary, all high risk subjects in the intervention group (n = 1597) received both individual and mass counselling, as well as periodic health examinations, about 3000 individuals in the random samples received a single individual counselling session, the mass program, and a single examination,[1] while the remaining 1400± persons in the low risk intervention group received only mass counselling and no examination beyond the initial one.

To date, the only detailed outcome results available from this project are for the first two years of the intervention (De Backer, Kornitzer, Dramaix, Huyghebaert, Verdonk, Vuylsteek, Graffar, Pannier, & Lequime, 1979a; Kornitzer et al., 1980a; Kornitzer, Dramaix, Kittel, & De Backer, 1980b). The complexity of the research design makes it desirable to specify the groups for which the comparisons are being made. Essentially there are two types of comparisons, between treated and untreated high risk individuals, and between treated and untreated randomly selected sub-sample (see Table 8.1).

---

[1]There were eight random samples of approximately 370 persons each. Since they were drawn from the intervention sample at large, they were composed of high risk and low risk subjects. Those designated high risk received more than a single counselling session. Presumably, too, a low risk individual could have been chosen up to eight times for the random sample and in this way received up to eight counselling sessions.

TABLE 8.1
Comparison Groups for Outcome Results

	Intervention (total N = 7398)	Control (total N = 8824)
High risk	N = 1597	N = 90
	21% of intervention sample at highest risk	10% of examined control sample at highest risk
	Full treatment	No treatment
Random samples	N = 370	N = 901
	5% of total intervention group	10% of men in each occupational unit
	Some full treatment; some single session	No treatment

After 2 years of treatment, the high risk intervention group showed improvement on all the risk variables measured (see Table 8.2). The control group, by contrast, improved on two (though significantly less than the treated group) and deteriorated on the other two. At the end of 2 years, the treated group showed a net composite risk factor change of 32.5% compared to the control group. The risk score, it will be recalled, is a composite based on age, degree of job activity, number of cigarette a day, systolic blood pressure and serum cholesterol levels.

Treatment effects for the random samples (see Table 8.3) are smaller than for the high risk subjects. Compared to the control random sample, treated subjects improved more on systolic blood pressure and deteriorated less on serum cholesterol. There is also a slight decline in the intervention group in total risk score, a small improvement but one that becomes highly significant compared to the 25% deterioration shown by the control group. Nevertheless, only for blood pressure is the difference between treated and untreated subjects as large for the random samples as for the high risk ones, and for the smoking variables there is no treatment effect at all in the random samples.

TABLE 8.2
High Risk Subjects: Comparison of Percentage Change in Risk
Factors After Two Years of Intervention

	Systolic Blood Pressure	Serum Cholesterol	% Cigarette Smokers	Cigarettes/day (for continuing smokers)	Total Risk Score
Treated	−7.8***	−3.9***	−18.7*	−18.8**	−20.0***
Control	−3.4	+ 0.4	−12.2	+ 8.6	+12.5

*p < .05 T-C
**p < .01 T-C
***p < .001 T-C

TABLE 8.3
Random Samples: Comparison of Percentage Change in Risk
Factors After Two Years of Intervention

	Systolic Blood Pressure	Serum Cholesterol	Risk Factors % Cigarette Smokers	Cigarettes/day (for continuing smokers)	Total Risk Score
Treated	−4.7***	+1.0***	−12.6	−9.1	−2.26
Control	−0.3	+4.3	−12.5	−3.0	+25.0

***p > .001 T-C

These results of the Belgian study are difficult to interpret because of the ambiguous nature of the random samples. They contain both high risk and low risk individuals (in unknown proportions) who received different degrees of individual counselling according to their risk status. Thus one does not know if individuals in the random sample intervention group showed lesser treatment effects than the high risk treatment group simply because they were initially low risk, or, rather, because their low risk status placed them in the category of those receiving less frequent individual counselling. It should be noted that no outcome results are reported for the low risk individuals who received only mass counselling.

An attempt to evaluate the importance of selected sample characteristics for risk factor improvement was undertaken by the investigators of the Belgian project. The dependent variable in this analysis was the composite risk score, or, as it is sometimes called, the multiple logistic risk function (MLF). In a multi-variate linear regression of the modification of MLF after 2 years of intervention the following variables were used as possible predictors: baseline MLF, age, socioeconomic category (blue collars, white collars, executives), level of education (primary, secondary, university) marital status (married vs. others), place of residence (French-speaking Wallonia vs. other parts of Belgium), changes in eating habits (reduction in fat intake vs. others), Bortner scale (behavior type A or B) and anality, obsessionality, neuroticism and extroversion scores on the Sandler-Hazari and Eysenck inventories. Decline in MLF scores after 2 years was found to be correlated with baseline MLF, age, and place of residence. Subjects with the highest initial risk status showed the greatest drop ($r = 0.52$). In addition, the younger subjects showed a greater drop than the older subjects, and the subjects residing in the French-speaking part of Belgium showed a more significant drop than those residing in the north or Dutch-speaking part of the country. This final finding may be a spurious one resulting from the fact that inhabitants of French-speaking Wallonia have been shown to have the highest CHD risk (Kornitzer, De Backer, Dramaix, & Thilly, 1979), a factor that in itself increased receptivity to the intervention.

In addition to its intervention efforts, the Belgian project is also serving as a test of the relationship between type A behavior and CHD. This epidemiological investigation is extremely important because it constitutes one of the first prospective studies of CHD in type A individuals outside the United States (Kittel, Kornitzer, Zyzanski, Jenkins, Rustin, & Degré, 1978; Rustin, Dramaix, Kittel, Degré, Kornitzer, Thilly, & De Backer, 1976). All subjects in the intervention group completed the Jenkins Activity Survey or JAS (Jenkins et al., 1967) and an adapted version of the Bortner scale (Bortner, 1969). The 10% of the control sample who received the complete medical examination also completed the JAS and Bortner scale, but, in addition, were administered the Structured Interview. To make the use of these scales in Belgium possible, they were translated into French and Flemish.

Both the Interview and the JAS were completed by 524 Flemish-speaking subjects and 202 French speaking ones. Since neither language nor age led to significantly different behavior pattern ratings, persons of both languages and all ages were combined for the subsequent analysis. Compared to the finding of the Western Collaborative Group Study (Rosenman, Friedman, Straus, Wurm, Kositchek, Hahn, & Werthessen, 1964), there were fewer extreme As (A_1) and Bs (B_4) in the Belgian study and a much higher percentage of uncertain (X) ratings (22% vs. 1%). This latter finding, however, can be explained largely by the different instructions given to raters regarding the use to be made of the uncertain category. Indeed, when the percentages of definite As and definite Bs are compared, the proportions in Belgium (38% As vs. 39% Bs) are almost identical to those in California (50% As vs. 49% Bs). On the JAS, however, a measure of self-perception of type A behavior, the Belgians manifested a greater tendency towards B behavior than did the Californians. The JAS was standardized on the WCGS sample to yield a mean of 0 and a S.D. of 10 with positive scores indicating type A behavior and negative ones type B behavior. The mean for the Belgian sample was -3.0, a score in the B category.

The ability of the Bortner and the JAS to predict the Interview rating of behavior type was studied in a sample of 507 persons (Rustin et al., 1976). According to this analysis, the Bortner scale predicted the interview rating in 78% of subjects and the JAS in 70% of subjects. Unfortunately, the composition of this particular sub-sample is not specified and it is impossible to determine how these 507 persons compare to the 726 for whom the interview ratings have been described in the previous paragraphs.

The investigators of the Belgian project have gone beyond the behavior ratings and have sought to verify previous findings of differences in catecholamine excretion in A versus B subjects (De Backer, Kornitzer, Kittel, Bogaert, Van Durme, Vincke, Rustin, Degré, & De Schaepdrijver, 1979b). From the nominal rolls of men participating in the control examination (the 10% of the control sample who received the full medical examination), 80 white collar men were selected and 40 pairs were formed, each pair including one subject classified as type A and one as type B. Both members of the pair were employed by the same factory and both belonged to the same age class. During a given working day, these men were asked to void in the morning and then to collect their urine throughout the day. For this day, they also wore portable one-lead ECG monitors (Avionics or Medilog) to measure cardiac arrythmias and heart rate.

Fifty of the eight men initially selected were available and produced analyzable data; 18 original pairs, 7 As and 7 Bs. There were no significant differences between these As and Bs in cholesterol, systolic blood pressure, relative weight, and number of cigarettes smoked daily. There were also no differences in excretion of urinary catecholamines and heart rate during the working day. This finding differs from the results of a previous study in American men by Friedman and his colleagues which found that type A men secreted significantly greater amounts of urinary catecholamines during the working day than did their type B counterparts (Friedman, Byers, Rosenman, & Elevitch, 1970). One possible explanation for the discrepancy between the findings of the two studies is that the American study selected extreme As and Bs, while the subjects studied in the Belgian project were almost entirely less extreme A_2s and B_3s.

Another innovative use of the data in the Belgian project is the attempt to delineate the psychosocial characteristics associated with the presence of specific risk factors at baseline, and with receptivity to change in these factors. To date, this form of analysis has been carried out for smoking (Kornitzer et al., 1980b; Rustin, Kittel, Dramaix, Kornitzer, & De Backer, 1978). The prevalence of smoking in this Belgian sample of men aged 40-59 appears very high. At baseline, two thirds of the sample examined were cigarette smokers, while the remaining third consisted of almost equal numbers of non-smokers, ex-smokers, or pipe or cigar smokers. Cigarette smoking decreased with age, but other types of smoking increased proportionately. Among men aged 55 or older, only one in ten had never smoked regularly and only a quarter were current non-smokers! Smoking was significantly associated with lower educational and occupational achievement, a job calling for heavy physical work, residence in a Dutch speaking area of Belgium, and not being married.

It did not appear to be associated with traditional risk factors; on the contrary, smokers manifested significantly lower weight, systolic blood pressure and serum cholesterol levels. However, this was a spurious finding based on the smokers' lower weight; at the same relative weight, cigarette smokers presented higher cholesterolemia values than non-smokers. The lower blood pressure, too, can be explained as a function of the smokers' lower weight. Among the personality variables, the most surprising result was a lesser prevalence of type A behavior (Bortner scale) among cigarette smokers, a finding contrary to the positive correlation between type A and cigarette smoking previously reported for American and Canadian samples. When the various discriminating factors were analyzed in a stepwise fashion, the following variables discriminated smokers from non-smokers (in decreasing order of importance): lower relative weight, lower level of education, less marked type A behavior, greater extraversion, higher cholesterolemia, more marked neuroticism, residence in northern Belgium, and greater age.

Two years later, almost 19% of the smokers in the high risk intervention group had quit smoking (the prevalence dropped from 84% to 68%), compared to 12% of the smokers in the comparable control group (the prevalence drop here was from 80% to 70%). A multiple stepwise discriminant function analysis between smokers in the intervention group who had quit and those who had not showed three significanct discriminating factors: lower initial smoking rate, more frequent previous attempts to stop, and residence in the Campine region of Belfium. In the control group, the sigificant discriminating factors between those who had stopped and those who continued were more frequent previous attempts to stop, and higher education.

As is the case for MRFIT, the final results of the Belgian project are not yet in and so no evaluation can be made of its success in meeting its stated objectives. Nevertheless, there are a number of reasons that already make this study important. First of all, it is the only intervention trial that has explored the possibility of reaching people via their place of work, an approach that holds promise of being both effective and economical. Secondly, the limited personnel employed in service delivery (two physicians and a single part-time dietician) means that this type of intervention could easily be replicated elsewhere. Thirdly, the fact that this project is conducted outside the United States and involves two linguistic groups provides the opportunity to examine cultural variations in response to intervention. Fourthly, the investigators of this project have already gone beyond the mere reporting of outcome results and are using their rich mine of data to explore such phenomena as prevalence of type A behavior, predictors of treatment outcome for selected risk variables, and so on. Given these multiple virtues, it may appear peevish to voice two relatively minor criticisms. Nevertheless, this project may not receive the exposure it merits because key data are published in journals with limited distribution. (Only one library in North America carries the Hart Bulletin in which the design of the study is described!). In addition, it is often difficult to interpret the findings of the various sub-studies because data are lacking concerning the characteristics of the particular partial sample being used, and the relationship between this partial sample and the partial samples of other sub-studies.

The Stanford Heart Disease Prevention Program

Proponents of a community-based model of coronary risk reduction, in contrast to the medical or high risk model, cite the multiple advantages of their preferred approach. Community-based intervention is believed to be more effective therapeutically than traditional clinical efforts because it treats the individuals as part of a group, rather than as if he or she existed in a social vaccuum. Changing

community attitudes toward smoking, for instance, increases the natural rein-
forcements and social supports available to individuals who are trying to stop
smoking (Farquhar, 1978b). The practical advantages of the community approach are that the inclusion of more "normal" individuals may make it easier to
show treatment benefits,and the use of groups vs. individuals reduces the sample
size required.

The Stanford Heart Disease Prevention Program (SHDPP), also called the
Three Communities Study, is a major example of the community-based approach
in that its intervention program was directed at entire communities. Corresponding to this community orientation, the evaluation of its effectiveness was also
based on examination of probability samples from the community-at-large. A
third way in which the SHDPP differs from traditional medical care is that some
treatment conditions involved delivery via the media (T.V., radio, billboard,
newspapers), rather than solely by face to face interactions. Where the SHDPP
resembles the medical model programs, was in its sub-program for high risk
individuals, and in its exclusive reliance on professionals to deliver both the
inter-personal and the media programs.

The SHDPP was a three year intervention trial launched in 1972 in three
comparable northern California towns. There were three levels of intervention.
One community (Tracy) served as the control and received no direct intervention, one community (Gilroy) was exposed to a 2 year multimedia campaign,
while in the third community (Watsonville) the same multimedia campaign was
supplemented by an intensive instruction program for high risk subjects (Farquhar, Maccoby, Wood, Alexander, Breitrose, Brown, Haskell, McAlister,
Meyer, Nash, & Stern, 1977; Maccoby et al., 1977). It should be noted that
communities were not randomly allocated to treatment conditions, but were
designated on the basis of convenience in delivery of media messages.

To assess the effects of the interventions, sample surveys were conducted to
gather baseline and yearly follow-up data from a random sample of adults ages
35–59 in all three towns. The first survey took place just prior to the first
campaign year in the autumn of 1972. Follow-up surveys took place at the end of
each of the two campaign years, in autumn 1973 and autumn 1974. Each survey
included a behavioral interview and a medical examination of each subject. The
behavioral interview was designed to measure both knowledge about heart disease and individual behavior related to cardiovascular risk, such as eating and
smoking habits. The physical examination included measures of plasma total
cholesterol and trygliceride concentrations, systolic and diastolic blood-pressure,
relative weight and electrocardiograms. Demographic, behavioral and physical
data were combined to yield an estimate of the risk of developing CHD within
the next 12 years, using the equation developed in the Framingham study (Truett,
Cornfield & Kannel, 1967).

Both the mass media community program and sub-program of counselling for
high risk individuals shared the same aims of increasing knowledge about the

causes of C.H.D., and fostering modifications in quality and quantity of diet, smoking and exercise habits. Specific techniques were suggested for achieving and maintaining the desired changes in behavior. The mass media campaign to deliver these messages consisted of about 50 television spots, three hours of television programming, over 100 radio spots, several hours of radio programming, weekly newspaper columns, newspaper advertisements and stories, billboards, posters, and printed material posted to participants. A campaign was also created for the sizeable population of Spanish speakers.

In addition to this media campaign, groups of high risk subjects (individuals in the top quartile of coronary risk at baseline) were identifed in each of the three communities (Meyer et al., 1980a). In Watsonville, two thirds of those at high risk were randomly assigned to the intensive instruction, in Gilroy all high risk individuals received a media only program, while those in Tracy received no intervention. Counselling was done over a 3 month period, either by nine group sessions for subjects and spouses, or by eight individual home visits (six more for smokers). The SHDPP staff recommended the group format, but were prepared to send counsellors to the home if participants chose this mode of program delivery. Treatment procedures included self-monitoring of the target behavior, modeling and guided practice of alternate behaviors, charting of progress, token rewards, and a gradual fading of therapist reinforcement and contact. Throughout the second year of the program sporadic contact was maintained, but this, too, was faded out in the third year.

The Stanford sup-program with high risk individuals is noteworthy in that it is the first of the interventions examined to date that resembles the type of behavior therapy used in clinical practice. It is the first project, too, to present data on degree of program participation. Of the 113 high risk individuals in Watsonville selected for counselling, 107 actually attended counselling, but only 77 of them and 34 of their spouses completed all three interviews and examination. Moreover, although the SHDPP recommended the group format, 40% of the sample chose instead individual home visits. Unfortunately, no data are reported on the relationship between program format (group vs. individual) and program adherance.

Results can be calculated for the sample as a whole and for the sub-sample of high risk individuals. For the sample as a whole, there are four comparison groups: Tracy (control), Gilroy (media only), Watsonville 1 (media only), and Watsonville II (media and intensive instruction). The most important findings are (1) that all treated groups showed significantly greater improvement than the control group on all variables except relative weight and (2) that a media only intervention was as effective in producing change as a mixture of media and intensive instruction. At the end of 2 years of intervention, there was a net difference of 23–28% in estimated total coronary risk between combined treatment samples (Gilroy, Watsonville I, Watsonville II) and control sample (Tracy). Watsonville II, the sample in which some members received intensive instruction, demonstrated the greatest treatment effect during the first year, but this difference was largely wiped out by the continued improvement shown by the media only groups during the second year.

For high risk subjects, in contrast, intensive instruction appeared to be more effective than a media only program in lowering risk scores. This superiority of intensive instruction for high risk subjects is largely due to its effectiveness in reducing smoking. Half of the high risk smokers exposed to intensive instruction had stopped smoking after 3 years, compared to cessation percentages of .0 and -11.3 in the two media only communities, and $-.14.9$ in the control one. There was a parallel drop in number of cigarettes smoked daily, with intensive instruction smokers reducing their cigarette consumption by half, compared to percentage reductions of $-.16$, -11.8 and -21 in the other communities. While diet and blood pressure also improved in the treated high risk samples, compared to the control one, for these variables there were no differences between treatment methods. Relative weight and physical activity did not change in any treatment group.

The pioneering nature of the SHDPP has elicited published commentary from two other research groups (Kasl, 1980; Leventhal, Safer, Cleary, & Gutman, 1980). Though praising the effort, both have reservations about the methods used. Kasl, for instance, questions whether the Stanford project was, in fact, a real community-based intervention. Although the Stanford intervention was directed to the community at large, rather than restricted to selected high risk individuals, for program delivery it relied exclusively on professionals from outside the community, and made no attempt to involve existing community leaders and organizations. Under these conditions, the wished-for goal of somehow mobilizing community processes may have been more myth than reality. As Kasl tongue in cheek points out, there are no evident differences in the social setting of a small smoking-cessation group, regardless of whether this group forms part of MRFIT or of the Stanford program.

Even more telling is the questioning by the Leventhal group of the appropriateness of the multiple risk logistic as the primary outcome measure. By choosing to evaluate a *behavioral* intervention program via changes in *biological* variables, the SHDPP did not allow for the possibility that behavioral change does not necessarily lead to physiological change, nor is even a necessary condition for it. Thus when change occurs or fails to occur, we are unable to locate what exactly happened or did not happen.

The data of the Stanford project have also been used to make the first comparison of outcome between studies. Undertaken by the Belgian investigators (Kornitzer et al., 1980a), this Belgian versus Stanford comparison involved two different treatment conditions; (1) high risk individuals who received face-to-face intervention and (2) random community samples, some members of whom received face-to-face intervention, and others whose health messages were delivered via meda.

TABLE 8.4
The Stanford vs. the Belgian Project: Outcome Results at 2 Years

	Watsonville vs. Tracy		Belgian Project	
	High risk I vs. C	Random sample I vs. C	High risk I vs. C	Random sample I vs. C
Serum cholesterol (mg/dl)	−5	−5.6	−11.2	−7.6
Systolic Blood Pressure (mm Hg)	−6	−5.6	−7.5	−6
Cigarette smokers (%)	−37	−21	−6.5	+0.1
Cigarettes/day (%)		−27		−12.1
Multiple logistic function %	−28	−20.6	−32.5	−27.3

Abbreviations: I = intervention; C = control

At first glance, (see Table 8.4), the Belgian project appears to have been the more cost effective of the two. The change in overall risk score (MLF) is substantially the same in both communities but, it will be recalled, the intervention was much less extensive and less costly in the Belgian one. More detailed examination, however, shows that the similar changes in global risk scores were achieved by rather different means; for the Stanford project the major impact was on cigarette smoking, while for the Belgian one it was on serum cholesterol level. And while the MLF permits us to calculate the relative weight of cigarette smoking and serum cholesterol in predicting CHD, there is no empirical evidence as yet showing that the same weighing system is valid in the reverse order, i.e., for the removal of previously established risk factors. Only when changes in coronary risk status will have been translated into changes in CHD morbidity/ mortality will it be possible to evaluate the relative benefits of reducing serum cholesterol versus changing smoking habits.

The North Karelia Project

While individuals may see themselves as sick and hence requiring professional attention, it is extremely rare for an entire community to cast itself in the patient role. North Karelia, a rural county in eastern Finland with a population of about 180,000, is one of these rare cases. In January, 1971, members of Parliament and other representatives of the local population signed a petition asking for national help in reducing their high mortality and morbidity for coronary heart disease (Puska, Tuomilehto, Salonen, Neittaanmaki, Maki, Virtamo, Nissinen, Koskela, & Takalo, 1979a). The need was indeed great: North Karelia had the dubious distinction of manifesting the highest incidence of CHD in the entire world.

A baseline survey of risk-factor status was carried out the following year in North Karelia and the demographically comparable county of Kuopio, using samples of 4,500 from Karelia and 6,300 from the reference community. The age range extended from 25–60. Comparison of the results with data from other industrialized nations suggested that as much as two thirds of the excess ischemic heart mortality observed in Karelia could be explained by the heightened risk score in the community at large. For instance, the average serum cholesterol value was 269 mg/dl for men and 265 mg/dl for women. Sixty percent of men aged 45–49 and fully 70% of the women aged 50–54 manifested cholesterol values above the criterion value for hypercholesteremia, (cholesterol ≥ 271 mg/dl). Similarly, the mean casual blood pressure values were 147/91 mm Hg for males and 149/91 mm Hg for females. Even using a relatively high criterion for hypertension (systolic blood pressure ≥ 160 mm Hg), 23% of men and 31% of the women were classifiable as hypertensives. A majority of the hypertensive men and 34% of the women were unaware of their health problem, and even among those who were aware, only 13% of the men and 10% of the women had medically restored normotension. More than 50% of adult men and 15% of women in Karelia smoked in comparison to the United States where slightly more than 25% of adults aged 25–60 are smokers. (Alderman, 1979; Puska, Tuomilehto, Nissinen, & Salonen; 1979b; Tuomilehto, Puska, Virtamo, Salonen, & Koskela, 1979).

Based on these findings, a 5 year intervention project was launched in 1972 (Puska et al., 1976). The main objective was to reduce mortality and morbidity from CHD, particularly among middle-aged men. The program had both preventative and curative aspects. Prevention focused on the familiar triad of coronary risk factors: smoking, blood pressure and serum cholesterol. Considering the high prevalence of these risk factors, primary prevention was seen as an activity directed to the whole population and not only to the individuals who had clinically extreme findings. Individuals within the county already suffering from coronary heart disease were to benefit, as well, via early detection, improved treatment, and rehabilitation.

To provide a complete range of primary, secondary and tertiary prevention services to a population of 180,000 persons obviously requires considerable organizational and personnel resources. Two innovative characteristics of the Karelia Project were an attempt to direct and develop existing health services to meet the needs of the new program, and, secondly, an extensive use of community organizations and lay persons in implementing the program. Health centers, existing smoking programs, the local heart association, and so on, all became part of the community effort to reduce coronary risk. In addition, nearly 300 natural community leaders were trained to detect cardiovascular risk factors (smoking, high cholesterol diet, high blood pressure), and to advise community members of the desirability of lowering these factors (Neittaanmaki, Koskela, Puska, & McAlister, 1980).

A multitude of intervention methods were used, directed both to the environment and to the individual. For instance, dietary change was fostered not only by advice to individuals, but also by making the recommended foods more available. Food producers and distributors were encouraged to provide alternatives to the standard high fat saturated diet; skimmed milk and a sausage made mainly of mushrooms and soybeans were introduced. Among individuals drinking milk in Karelia, the percentage of persons consuming low-fat milk rose between 1972-74 from 20 to 50 for men, and from about 25 to 60 for women.

The approach to blood pressure control involved a vigorous public education compaign and a recruitment of general practitioners, hospitals, industrial health personnel, and public health departments to identify all those with hypertension and to ensure that they enter treatment. Everybody with established high blood pressure levels (160 and/or 95 in three consecutive measures) was registered according to the WHO protocol. Providers were advised of acceptable forms of therapy, and in large communities centralized blood pressure follow-up centers were established where nurses and paraprofessionals offered continuing care in a convenient setting under the aegis of a referring physician. Local physicians referred patients to the center for monitoring and adjustment of medication. They received regular reports of their patients' progress and maintained control over chemotherapy. After 4.5 years of the intervention, the percentage of adults 25–60 under antihypertensive drug treatment increased from 3 to 11 among men and from 9 to 13 among women (Puska et al., 1979b).

The North Karelia Project included a special sub-program for rehabilitation among patients who had already experienced an acute myocardial infarction. The target group for this aspect of the program were persons under the age of 65 who had suffered a myocardial infarction according to the records of community-based MI register, and had survived the acute phase of the disease. The program consisted of systematic long-term medical follow-up at an outpatient clinic, and of decentralized, local, group-rehabilitation units offering health education, exercise testing and training, and vocational and psychosocial counselling. Of the 1,308 persons under the age of 65 who survived an MI between 1973 to 1977, 515 visited the outpatient MI clinic and 575 took part in the rehabilitation groups (Salonen & Puska, 1980).

To evaluate the changes in coronary risk factors over the 5 year life of the program, probability samples of 10,000 persons, similar in demographic characteristics to those of the baseline survey, were drawn from Karelia and the control community of Kuopio (Puska et al., 1979a). Although these samples were independent from the baseline ones, the same cohort was surveyed, that is the individuals tested were now 30–64 years old. The new examinations showed a significant change in coronary risk factors in North Karelia. Whereas North Karelians had a higher global coronary risk score in 1972, compared to residents of Kuopio, during the 5 years of the program this difference was reversed in men and disappeared among women. The net reduction in the estimated CHD risk in North Karelia was 17.4% in men and 11.5% in women. Greatest success was achieved in reducing the prevalence of raised blood pressure values, and in lowering serum cholesterol concentration in men. Men in the oldest and youngest age groups were most likely to show change, while in women the finding was different, with the greatest changes occurring in ages 40–49.

Changes in the mortality and incidence of CHD in North Karelia during 1972-77 were monitored via community-based registers of cases of acute myocardial infarction and stroke, and data on death certificates (Salonen, Puska, & Mustaniemi, 1979). Community-based registers were not established in Kuopio since they were regarded as part of the intervention. Instead, only partial comparison data on morbidity were obtained via a special register set up for 5 months in Kuopio at the end of the program.

In North Karelia itself the incidence of MI in individuals 30–64-years-old fell by 16% among men and 5% among women, while that of stroke fell by 38% among men and 50% among women. Mortality from cardiovascular disease in general decreased by 13% among men and 31% among women. Unfortunately, neither for morbidity nor mortality is this reduction significantly different from that observed in the control community during this time period. The authors suggest, however, that 5 years may be too short a time period to evaluate this dimension. Only in the next few years will it be possible to judge whether the treatment effect observed in risk factor status is eventually translated into a similar effect for morbidity and mortality.

Critics who complain of the artificiality of clinical trials and of their divorce from the real world of service delivery should find the North Karelia Project the answer to their fondest hopes. Rather than being imposed on an arbitrarily chosen sample, this project was initiated by a real clinical need expressed by the target population itself. Instead of selecting program recipients by age or health status, this program attempted to reduce coronary disease in all age groups and at all levels of risk. Instead of importing outside professionals to run the program, and then have them steal away at the termination of research funding, this program made maximum use of existing health organizations and of lay people within the community. Instead of seeking to change personal habits in a social vaccuum, this program also focused on modifying the environment in a way that would facilitate the adoption and maintenace of desirable health habits.

Unfortunately, nirvana for clinical researchers is not yet at hand. The multiplicity of interventions that make the Karelia project so exciting from a clinical viewpoint, unfortunately, also make the task of evaluation extremely difficult. With so many changes occurring simultaneously, it is impossible to separate those interventions that were more effective from those that were less so. Instead, the two outcome studies to date for the community as a whole are limited to global changes in coronary risk factors (Puska et al., 1979a) and morbidity and mortality (Salonen, Puska, & Mustaniemi, 1979). And even here, it is difficult to discriminate between changes that result from the program and those that would have occurred in any case in this community already highly motivated for health change.

SINGLE-FACTOR INTERVENTION PROJECTS

Multi-factorial intervention trials are the Broadway productions of coronary risk reduction. Like their metaphoric counterparts, they are expensive to produce, receive considerable public attention both positive and negative, and are subject to stringent criteria of success and failure. The off-Broadway of preventive cardiology is the single-factor project. Here the productions are usually smaller and less well-mounted, but also more likely to experiment with new targets and methods. Should they succeed, their techniques may eventually become part of the establishment multi-factorial programs.

The three single-factor trials that we have selected for discussion in this section are all noteworthy, each for a difference reason. The first of the triad, The Diet and Coronary Heart Disease Project, is a pioneer among coronary risk reduction efforts. Mounted in 1957, it antedates by at least 14 years the first of the multi-factorial programs and continues to merit attention, if only because it has a much longer follow-up period than any other program presented in this chapter. The second project to be described, a smoking-deterrant program for adolescents, was selected because of its novel target population. To prevent the onset of smoking in teen-agers is very different from helping middle-aged persons kick a habit of 15 or 20 years duration. The final selection concerns the work of my colleagues and myself in seeking to develop a treatment program for the type A behavior pattern. None of the multi-factorial intervention programs includes type A as a therapeutic target, partially because this behavior pattern has only recently received recognition as a risk factor (cf. Roskies, 1980), but also because there is no accepted treatment program for the behavior in question, nor even accepted criteria by which to judge outcome. It is the successes and failures that my colleagues and I have experienced in meeting the challenges of this newest risk factor that will constitute the subject matter of the description.

The Diet and Coronary Heart Disease Project (The Anti-Coronary Club)

To anyone used to the methodological perfection—at least, intended prefection—of the current preventive trials, reading the early reports of the Anti-Coronary Club (cf. Jolliffe, Rinzler, & Archer, 1959; Jolliffe, Baumgartner, Rinzler, Archer, Stephenson, & Christakis, 1963) must inevitably produce an indulgent smile. Instead of being planned by a large expert committee that attempted to foresee every detail of the experimental protocol, the Anti-Coronary Club was generated by the efforts of a single individual and much of the design was improvised in the course of carrying out the experiment. The result makes us smile because there are errors in methodology that first year students in epidemiology could easily spot. The indulgence, on the other hand, is aroused by the courage and humanity of those who undertook this pioneering effort at coronary risk reduction. In contrast to the impersonal publications characteristic of the current trials, these early reports of the Anti-Coronary Club give us a glimpse of research in action, real people making decisions and then modifying them according to changes in circumstances and thinking. Unfortunately, as the Anti-Coronary Club becomes more methodologically sophisticated over the years, so do its publications assume the faceless neutrality common to scientific reports (Christakis, Rinzler, Archer, & Kraus, 1966; Singman, Berman, Cowell, Maslansky, & Archer, 1980).

To place the Anti-coronary Club in historical focus, it belongs to what is known as the "first generation" diet trials. There were four such trials begun in the 1950s to investigate the effects of diet change on serum cholesterol and coronary outcome. Two were with free-living males in Chicago and New York, one with Finnish mental patients, and one with veterans living in a residence in Los Angeles (cf. Stamler, 1978). These constitute the first systematic efforts at coronary risk reduction, as well as the first serious efforts at evaluation. A characteristic of all four studies is that they utilized samples numbering in the hundreds, rather than the thousands or tens of thousands characteristic of current efforts.

On October 15, 1956, Norman Jolliffe, M.D., then Director of the Bureau of Nutrition, submitted to Leona Baumgartner, M.D., Commissioner of Health of the City of New York, a proposal for a study on the prevention of coronary artery disease. Based on his reading of the existing epidemiological and metabolic studies, Dr. Jolliffe, in contrast to many of his colleagues, believed that the time was ripe for a public health test of the "quality-of-fat" hypothesis concerning the etiology of coronary artery disease. The major goals of the project were (1) to develop palatable, nutritionally adequate diets capable of lowering serum cholesterol levels; (2) to induce middle-aged men to adhere to these diets for long periods of time; and (3) to determine if the changes in the serum cholesterol-lipoprotein system produced by such diets were associated with favorable changes in the morbidity and mortality from coronary heart disease.

In the initial conception of the study, the experimental group was to consist of some well-defined population, for example, Department of Health employees, which would possibly be split into experimental and control group on some random basis. It was debated, however, whether this a priori assignment into experimental and control groups was really necessary because if the expected 50% drop-out occurred, subjects who did so could then be utilized as a self-selected control group! In any case, to pilot test the feasibility of such a project, as well as treatment and evaluation procedures, it was decided to run a preliminary study and recruit applicants via a newspaper release and radio announcement. At the end of the first year, however, the decision was taken to abandon the planned recruitment procedure, and, instead, simply to continue the study with the volunteers initially recruited for the pilot project.

The short time period from conception to realization of this project contrasts vividly with the many years required for current intervention trials. Dr. Jolliffe's letter, it will be recalled, was written in October, 1956. The project was activated in February, 1957 and by June of that year the original goal of 200 subjects had been reached. The criteria for the selection of participants in the study were that they be (1) residents of New York City, (2) between 50–59 yrs. of age, (3) male, (4) free of serious disease which might terminate life shortly, and (5) physically capable and with time available during normal working hours to attend the study facilities.

This initial sample continued to grow. After 5 months, it was decided to include 350 more men, some of whom were younger (aged 20–40) and/or had already experienced CHD. Further additions were made subsequently, mainly by word-of-mouth publicity from those already participating. By the end of the fourth year, the treated group had grown to 989 men aged 20–59, 525 of whom had been on the diet more than a year. When the study was terminated in November, 1972, 14 years after initiation, 1113 male subjects had been involved in treatment.

Because of the admission of the treatment sample in stages, there are few descriptive data for the sample as a whole. In the third year of the study there was an examination of the demographic characteristics of the 308 men in the project aged 50 to 59. They were found to be predominantly Jewish, in the upper professional and managerial class, and more health conscious than the general population. It is tempting to speculate concerning the proportion of type As in this sample of eager beavers.[2] Base cholesterol values were determined for the first 400 men enrolled in the treatment group. The mean was 260 mg per 100 ml, but it should be noted that 20% had initial cholesterol values under 220, and 7.7% under 200.

In September, 1959, 2 years after the initial treatment group was constituted, it was decided to recruit a control group from a population of 400 men aged 40–59 attending a Cancer Detection Clinic. These control men were matched with experimental subjects on height, weight, blood pressure and serum cholesterol level. The incentive for their participation was the offer of a free annual cardiovascular examination. They were not informed of either the nature of the intervention, nor of the objectives of the study.

Upon admission to the project, the subjects in the treatment group underwent a 1–3 months observation period. While following their usual diet, serum cholesterol levels were measured bi-weekly. In the course of this observation the subjects also had their diet evaluated by a nutritionist. For this purpose, partici-

---

[2]A paragraph in the final outcome report indicates that the Jenkins Activity Survey (Jenkins et al., 1967) was, in fact, administered to participants at some point during the course of the program. Not surprisingly, active participants were found to be significantly more type A than the inactive or control groups.

pants were asked to keep a 7-day diet record prior to the visit and during it the subject (with the assistance of his wife who was also present) was asked to recall a diet for an average week as far back as he could remember.

When the work-up was completed, the individual was seen by a panel of physicians who reviewed his baseline data with him and introduced him to what came to be known as The Prudent Diet. For individuals of normal weight this involved (1) reducing or eliminating saturated fats and (2) reducing the total fat in the diet to 30 to 33% of calories consumed. For individuals classified as overweight, the instructions were to maintain a diet of 1600 calories, with not more than 19% of these calories in the form of fat. To help maintain the diet and evaluate its effects, there were consultations with the nutritionist and serum cholesterol determinations scheduled every 5 weeks, and a review with the panel of physicians every 10 weeks. There was also an annual examination, complete with medical history, physical, laboratory, electrocardiographic and roentgenographic examinations.

Outcome results have been presented at intervals during the course of the project, but for the sake of brevity we shall restrict our presentation to those contained in the most recent report (Singman et al., 1980). There were 859 participants in the program who were aged 40–59 and free of CHD at time of entry. At the end of the program, the dieticians rated 283 men (approximately one third of the total sample of 859) as manifesting excellent or good adherence, 409 (slightly less than half) as manifesting fair or poor adherance, and the remaining 167 as unratable because of poor attendance. In short, 14 years after initiation at least one third of those recruited were adhering, more or less, to the recommended diet.

In terms of continued participation in the program, 256 men attended regularly until the end of the project, 436 men discontinued regular attendance after an average attendance of 2 years but returned for periodic examinations, and 167 were drop-outs. The degree to which continued active participation was necessary for satisfactory adherence depends on the classification system used. When excellent, good, fair and poor categories were used, active participants showed significantly better adherence compared to those inactive at the time the rating was made. When the classification was collapsed into two categories, however, (excellent and good vs. fair and poor), then there were no significant differences in adherance between active and inactive participants; almost half of the good adherers (134 subjects) were in the inactive category. With this two category system, age at entry began to make a difference in eventual adherence, with older enrollees (50–59 vs. 40–49) more likely to show good adherence.

For the analysis of the prevalence of hypercholesterolemia, hypertension and obesity, the authors of the final outcome report contrast active and inactive participants with the control group, rather than dividing subjects in the treatment group according to their level of dietary adherence. This decision is unfortunate because, as we have seen, participation and adherence were not synonymous. In any case, active participants showed significantly greateer decreases in serum cholesterol than did the inactive and control groups. The older active subjects (men aged 50–59 at entry) also showed a significantly greater drop in obesity compared to men of the same age in the two other groups. Hypertension, in contrast, did not decrease more in the active participants than in the other groups. Finally, active participants had a significantly lower incidence of new CHD events than did inactive or control participants.

The absence of a randomly selected control group makes it impossible to view this study as a critical test of the diet-heart hypothesis. The fact that the sample of active participants was largely composed of type A, New York, Jewish business and professional men also makes it diffiuclt to generalize its findings to the population at large. Nevertheless, this study remains a landmark, if only because it provides invaluable data on the possibility of convincing at least some middle aged men to permanently and substantially modify their diets.

Deterring Smoking in Adolescents

The progression from coronary risk behavior to increase in biological risk variables (e.g., serum cholesterol) to atherosclerosis to overt signs of heart disease is a slow one and may occur over a period of 30 years or longer. Coronary risk reduction programs directed towards middle-aged persons, therefore, are limited in their capacity for impact. Firstly, behavior of long duration is likely to be embedded in a whole network of precipitating stimuli and reinforcing consequences, making it resistant to change. Secondly, even should we succeed in eliminating the risk behavior, we cannot eliminate completely the physical damage already done. Hence the importance of programs that seek to prevent the risk behavior from ever getting established.

Smoking would seem to be an ideal therapeutic target for this form of risk factor prevention not only because it is an extremely difficult habit to change once established (Bernstein & McAlister, 1976; Lichenstein & Danaher, 1976), but also because of its relatively short high risk period for initiation. The critical age of onset is early adolescence, with few persons beginning addictive smoking either before they enter junior high or after they leave senior high (Evans, Rozelle, Maxwell, Raines, Dill, Guthrie, Henderson & Hill, 1980). It is this latter characteristic that led Evans and his colleagues to hypothesize that ''a deterrence-to-smoking program successfully implemented in the junior high school years might be one significant approach to reducing the incidence of active smoking''.

Richard Evans is a social psychologist working in an academic rather than a medical setting (the University of Houston) and his program reflects its academic origins. In contrast to the purely pragmatic outcome orientation that characterizes many of the coronary risk reduction efforts, the work of Evans and his colleagues both originates in social-psychology theory and serves as a test of it. The diagnosis of the problem is derived from Bandura's (1971) social learning theory: Adolescents start to smoke because of the pressure to imitate powerful role models, such as peers, teachers, parents and T.V. heroes. The possible deterrant to this harmful process is suggested by McGuire's (1974) persuasive communication-cognitive inoculation model which propounds that existing attitudes may be strengthened by inoculating individuals against the counter arguments to which they may be exposed at some future time. Building on his belief that most early adolescents consider smoking harmful and don't really want to adopt the habit, Evans hypothesizes that the process of imitation can be interrupted by training adolescents in advance to recognize and cope with the pressures to smoke that they may eventually encounter.

A series of preliminary studies tested various aspects of the theoretical model, as well as methods of implementation. In depth interviews with a sample of seventh-grade students confirmed the role of social pressure in smoking initiation (Evans, 1976). A technique was devised to increase the validity of self-reports of smoking behavior (Evans, Hansen, & Mittelmark 1977). Finally, a pilot study with 750 students entering the seventh grade showed that students exposed to a videotape and poster program based on the conceptual model were significantly less likely to start smoking at the end of a 10 week period (Evans, Rozelle, Mittelmark, Hansen, & Bane, 1978).

The full-scale test of this novel approach to deterring smoking was a 3 year program conducted in 13 of the 36 junior high schools in the Houston Independent School District (Evans et al., 1980). For the first year of the test, the smoking program became part of the regular seventh grade health education instruction and in consecutive years it was promoted, as were the pupils who received it, to the eighth and ninth grades. Measurements were made in the fall and spring of each year, with the same progression from seventh to ninth grade. Sample size at each measurement period varied from 1100 to 3300. Because of mobility in and out of the school district, a particular child may have participated in the program for 1, 2, or 3 years.

The basic treatment consisted of a series of 10 to 15-minute sound color films. Two of these dealt with some immediate physiological effects of smoking, namely, increased nicotine in saliva and a high carbon monoxide level in the breath. Three more films focused on the various social pressures to smoke emanating from peers, media, and parents, while a sixth demonstrated ways of resisting these pressures in simulated incitement-to-smoke situations. To increase credibility, students served as narrators throughout and were employed as actors in the simulated social-pressure-to-smoke scenes. The message of the films was supplemented by posters reproducing individual scenes from the treatment films with appropriate captions (e.g., "You can resist social pressures to smoke."). To avoid the boredom and habituation resulting from seeing the same films each year, film and poster content were varied for eighth and ninth graders.

The dependent measure used was a 15-item computer-scores questionnaire measuring current smoking behavior, future smoking intentions, and information about smoking. The validity of the self-reports of smoking was increased by use of the nicotine-in-saliva analysis procedure. Subjects were encouraged to be truthful in reporting their smoking behavior by being shown a film depicting how saliva can be analyzed for nicotine concentration, and being led to believe that this procedure would be carried out.

There were seven treatment conditions. Three groups received all or part of the intervention efforts. Four others received different frequencies of measurement, some with and some without the nicotine-in-saliva analysis film.

The basic hypothesis of this study was that the intervention program would affect intention to smoke and deter frequent or addictive smoking behavior. Since fewer than 2% of 12–14-year-olds are as yet heavy smokers, the usual criterion of addictive smoking (10 cigarettes or more a day) could not be used with this group. Instead, the investigators selected as the primary outcome measures declared intention to smoke or not to smoke, and present incidence of two or more cigarettes a day.

Because of changes within and movement into and out of the school system, it was difficult to conduct the traditional longtitudinal analysis of the cohort over the 3 year time span. Instead, the investigators chose to examine the data from each year independently, comparing the beginning of the school year to the end. At the beginning of the seventh grade there was no significant difference between groups (pre-experimental equivalence), while at the end of this grade there was the disappointing finding that those exposed to the full treatment package showed the greatest amount of smoking behavior and the highest percentage of frequent smokers (two or more a day). At the end of the eighth grade, however, pupils receiving either full or partial treatment evidenced the lowest amount of smoking behavior, and continued to show this lower incidence at the end of the ninth grade. The full treatment group also had the lowest percentage of frequent smokers at the end of the ninth grade (9.5%), and less declared intention to smoke.

To test whether these differences in smoking behavior and intentions could be attributed to the effects of the intervention program itself, the treatment groups were divided at the median for amount of program information retained and then smoking behavior scores were calculated separately for the high and low information retention sub-groups. The results of this analysis support the view that differences in smoking were attributable to the program. Both smoking and heavy smoking were least frequent among those who retained the most knowledge presented in the films and posters.

The authors are cautious in interpreting the significance of their findings. They remind us of the quasi-experimental nature of the study, the cross-sectional rather than the longtitudinal method of analysis, and the high ''noise level'' resulting from changes in the schools during the course of the program. They consider this study only an encouraging first approximation and emphasize the need for replication. It would be a foolhardy reader who would ignore these appeals to caution. Nevertheless, it would also be an unusual one who would fail to be excited by this innovative approach to a difficult health problem. The work of Richard Evans and his collaborators serves as an excellent illustration of the old adage that there is nothing as practical as a good theory.

Modification of Type A Behavior

Even before smoking, lack of exercise, and a high fat diet were identified as risk factors for CHD, there were numerous other health reasons, not to speak of aesthetic considerations, that propelled some tobacco addicts, some pot-bellied individuals, and some obese persons to seek professional help for improving health and appearance. As a consequence, when investigators became interested in mounting coronary risk reduction programs directed toward these health problems, they could draw on a wealth of previous clinical experience in smoking cessation, exercise programming and obesity treatment. In sharp contrast to this state of affairs, researchers in type A intervention are dealing with a health problem that is so new that the relevant clinical literature is just beginning to be written. The first report of type A intervention was published in 1975 (Suinn, 1975) and, to date, there are fewer than 10 published treatment studies (cf. Roskies, 1982). All are small, methodologically inadequate, and only half even touch on the issue of primary prevention, that is the modification of type A behavior in individuals who do not yet suffer from clinical heart disease.

It is not newness alone, however, that makes the type A behavior pattern a difficult area for intervention. Rather, the major problems in designing a treatment program stem from the ambiguity and complexity of the therapeutic target. Instead of constituting a single, discrete behavior, the label type A applies to a heterogeneous collection of physical, behavioral and emotional characteristics: Type A individuals as a group speak louder, faster and more explosively than their type B counterparts (Schucker & Jacobs, 1977); they show greater cardiovascular and biochemical reactivity to certain types of challenge (Dembroski, MacDougall, & Shields, 1977; Dembroski, MacDougall, Shields, Pettito, & Lushene, 1978; Dembroski, MacDougall, Herd, & Shields, 1979; Friedman, Byers, Diamant, & Rosenman, 1975; Glass, Krakoff, Contrada, Hilton, Kehoe, Mannucci, Collins, Snow, & Elting, 1980); they report less contentment on their jobs, but also feel more able to make a change should they desire it (Howard, Cunningham, & Rechnitzer, 1977); on a treadmill task, they work closer to the limits of their endurance, but, even as they do so, they are more likely to suppress feelings of fatigue (Carver, Coleman, & Glass, 1976); they prefer to wait with others prior to working on a stressful task, but while actually doing the task they prefer to work alone (Dembroski & McDougall, 1978).

What this catalogue of presumed type A characteristics does not do, unfortunately, is to discriminate between those attributes which are simply chance findings in a specific sample, those which are generalizable to most type A people but are irrelevant to increased risk of CHD, and those which are the true pathogenic ones (Roskies, 1980). As a consequence, before he or she can even consider specific treatment techniques, the would-be therapist is faced with defining exactly what in type A pattern requires treatment, and deciding precisely how the success or failure of treatment will be evaluated. This problem can be avoided somewhat by those who choose to work with heart disease patients and can therefore use decreased rate of reccurrence as an indirect measure of successful type A modification (Friedman, 1978, 1979), but for researcher choosing to work in prevention, the challenge of explaining why one is seeking a particular type of change is almost as great as that of effecting the changes desired (Roskies, 1979).

A second dilemma confronting the would-be therapist is the potential conflict between the physiological harm inherent in the type A pattern and its considerable psychological and social value. To be competitive, ambitious and hard working may increase one's chances of suffering a heart attack, but it also augments the likelihood of rapid job promotion (Mettlin, 1976). To exert maximum effort to master a challenging situation not only increases wear and tear on the coronary arteries, but also enhances the person's feelings of self-esteem and self efficacy (Bandura, 1977). Thus, there are obvious ethical constraints on the treatment procedures than can be used to modify type A behavior. For instance, we now have considerable laboratory and field data showing that even in predisposed individuals, environmental factors play an important role in eliciting the pattern (Cohen, Syme, Jenkins, Kaga, & Zyzanski, 1979; Dembroski et al., 1977, 1978, 1979; Manuck, Craft, & Gold, 1978; Glass, 1977; Glass et al., 1980; Van Egeren, 1979). Before advising a type A client in a high pressure job to "drop out", however, there are the counterbalancing considerations that such a radical change in lifestyle might entail material and psychological loss to the individual, disruption of family roles and relationships, and even lowered productivity for society as a whole.

For type A individuals themselves, the widespread social approbation given to this behavior pattern is likely to have a negative effect both on the motivation to seek change and the ability to sustain a modified way of life. By the time most type A individuals reach the age where they become concerned about heart attacks, they have a lifetime of prior learning equating an achievement-oriented, aggressive, and time-pressured existence with psychological satisfaction and social rewards. The process begins with maternal approbation for type A behavior in childhood (Matthews, 1976), continues through the reward of higher grades in college (Waldron, Hickey, McPherson, Butensky, Gruss, Overall, Schmader, & Wohlmuth, 1980), and reaches its peak with rapid job advancement in adulthood (Mettlin, 1976). To seek to change a lifestyle as deeply engrained and richly rewarded as this inevitably raises questions about the costs to be paid for the benefits obtained. It would be the rare type A person who would not wonder whether the attempt to save his life might not be at the cost of the achievements and rewards that make his life worthwhile. Even should he overcome the motivational barrier and take the risk of modifying his characteristics pattern, the type A person may find himself under strong social pressure to revert to his old ways. Given the high prevalence of type A behavior in business and professional circles, the successfully modified type A is likely to find himself in a situation analogous to that of the reformed alcoholic condemned to live in an environment of heavy drinkers.

In spite of these methodological, ethical and motivational obstacles (or maybe because of them; researchers, too, are not immune to type A behavior!), I became involved about 5 years ago in developing intervention programs for healthy type As. The work of my colleagues and myself to date has centred on type As with specific demographic characteristics: middle-aged male managers and professionals. We chose to work with middle-aged males because this group is at greatest risk for premature coronary heart disease, and because the best data linking type A to heart disease comes from the Western Collaborative Group Study which used a sample with these demographic characteristics (Rosenman et al., 1964). We chose to work with managers and professionals both because type A is most prevalent at this occupational level (Zyzanski, 1977), and because this group is likely to experience most acutely the conflict between the physical cost of type A versus its social benefits.

In designing our first intervention program, the main focus was on avoiding the ethical and motivational problems posed by radical lifestyle change. To counsel type A individuals that their path to salvation lay in leaving their high pressure jobs, or even in reducing their emotional investment in occupational achievement, was to tender advice that was both ethically unwarranted in the present state of our knowledge and practically useless in that it was alsmost certain to go unheeded. Instead, the challenge was of finding a way of changing the harmful aspects of type A behavior while respecting the values and needs that had initially given rise to the behavior. In summary, we were searching for a therapeutic procedure that would yield a maximum effect for a minimum amount of behavior change.

David Glass' conceptualization of type A behavior served as the starting point for this search (Glass, 1977; Glass, Snyder, & Hollis, 1974). According to his view, type A behavior is essentially a coping response used to counter the threat of actual or potential loss of control. In contrast to individuals who are unable or unwilling to adapt to social norms, type A individuals have internalized thoroughly Western society's emphasis on the ability to control one's environment. The positive side of this mastery orientation is enhanced self-esteem and increased social reinforcement. The negative side of this adaptive pattern, in contrast, is the threat experienced in any situation in which the individual cannot be sure of complete control. When signs of possible loss of control do occur, as inevitably they must, the initial response is an increased effort to regain control, involving greater mental and physical exertion, stepped up pace, heightened competitiveness, and so on (Glass, 1977; Glass & Carver, 1980). Even in situations where control is not attainable, type A subjects tend to avoid recognition of this fact and continue actively struggling. Only when the cues signifying absence of control are highly salient will the type A individual lapse into a state of learned helplessness (Krantz, Glass, & Snyder, 1974; Glass, 1977). Thus, the usual coping style of the type A person is one of psychological and physiological hyper-responsiveness interspersed with periods of helplesness and hypo-responsiveness.

Assuming this pattern of functioning in type A individuals, it should be possible to leave the basic need for mastery untouched, but, instead, to focus on the behavior that the individual uses to cope with threat. A series of muscular and breathing relaxation exercises, common techniques in behavior therapy, could be used as a substitute coping strategy for the usual pattern of frantic activity. Once he had learned the basic techniques, the type A individual could be given instructions in monitoring his level of tension during his daily activities and in using relaxation to reduce tension whenever necessary. Even if he could not control the situation, the type A individual could control his reactions to it.

The advantage of this treatment approach was its potential appeal to healthy, occupationally successful, type A managers and professionals. Rather than repeating the same tired arguments concerning the physical harmfulness of their hyper-active lifestyle, we would approach the men in an area where they were unused to reproach and, therefore, highly vulnerable: Type A behavior was an ineffective way of coping with the stresses of daily life. The individual who responded to all stress situations with an automatic four-alarm mobilization was clearly showing his inability to exert control, as well as placing a great deal of wear and tear on his coronary arteries.

Our solution to this hyper-reactivity was, once again, very different from the usual advice to "take it easy". Instead, we suggested that a more healthful coping pattern involved active effort, but effort directed as much toward control of self as toward control of the outside world. By following our treatment program, type As would be trained to become aware of their level of muscular tension and to attribute importance to bodily cues of loss of self-control (i.e., heightened tension). When confronted with a challenging situation (a tense business meeting, a difficult project with a tight deadline), the usual coping pattern of frenzied activity could be replaced, or at least supplemented, by efforts at tension regulation. In this way the previous stereotyped response would be replaced by a more differentiated one, and the person would probably be able to accomplish more with less strain.

To test the feasibility and utility of tension regulation for healthy type A men, we decided to recruit 30 type A individuals. Criteria for entry into the program were stringent: extreme type A characteristics (type A_1), ages 39–59, non-smoker, full-time managerial or professional position, salary $25,000+, commitment to attend at least 12 of the 14 treatment sessions, and willingness to deposit $100 as a guarantee of attendance. The method of recruitment was via a newspaper article describing the program and the criteria for entry. The nature of the recruitement appeal and/or the stringent criteria for entry obviously appealed to the type of sample we wished to attract for we were deluged by over 150 applicants.

The Structured Interview was used to screen for type A characteristics: The interview process and the resulting classification are described in chapter three of this volume (c.f. Dembroski, Mac Dougall, Herd, & Shields). All individuals selected for the pilot program were fully developed As (type A_1).

Of the 27 individuals who passed the physical examination (6 of the 33 men initially selected as A_1 were later placed in a separate group because of cardiac abnormalities revealed on an exercise ECG), 13 were randomly assigned to a 14-week tension regulation program. In this program individuals were first taught how to quantify their level of tension using a 0–10 scale and then instructed for a period of a week to record hourly the activity currently in progress and the level of tension experienced. This self-observation permitted participants to become more aware of variations in their level of arousal and the situations assoicated with these changes. At the same time, a sequence of relaxation exercices designed to foster physiological self-control was introduced. A 15-minute modified version of Jacobsonian muscle relaxation (Jacobson, 1938) was presented and participants were asked to practice this exercice twice daily following recorded instructions and noting tension levels before and after each practice session. After a few weeks of this regime, the muscle relaxation exercice was shortened to 5 minutes and specific neck and shoulder and breathing exercices were added.

Eventually, participants reached a level of proficiency where they could both detect early warning signs of physical tension and relax upon command. The task now became one of using these skills to maintain a comfortably low level of tension. Regularly occuring events in the daily routine (e.g., shaving, opening one's agenda book, driving the car) became signals to check tension level and adjust it if necessary. Even when unexpected or strong arousal did occur (e.g., a discourteous driver cutting in, an argument with one's superior), relaxation techniques could be used to lower the tension level.

Although we had previously rejected the possibility of psychotherapy for non-clinical subjects, the necessity of finding a control condition that would be credible to these type A men led us to turn to the psychotherapy unit of the hospital in which the program was carried out. But instead of simply serving as an attention-placebo condition, the therapists concerned, experienced and enthusiastic practitioners of brief psychotherapy, utilized their 14 sessions to run an active treatment program. Based on their view of type A behavior as an initially useful solution to a conflictual family constellation in childhood, the aim of therapy became one of showing these men how their childhood perceptions and responses distorted their current behavior. The assumption here was that once the individual understood why he was behaving in a certain way then he would be free to change this automatic pattern. While there was no explicit instruction in behavior change, the male and female co-therapists did serve as role models for a more relaxed, less competitive, behavior style.

The weakest part of this pilot study was the evaluation procedures used. There is no self-evident criterion for measuring clinically significant change in the type A pattern. Neither of the two methods currently in use for diagnosing the presence of the pattern, the Structured Interview and the questionnaire Jenkins Activity Survey, is sufficiently accurate to measure intra-individual change over time. While reduction in cardiac morbidity and mortality constitute acceptable substitute criteria from the clinical standpoint, these indices are only likely to show significant change when very large or very high risk samples are followed over long periods of time. For the purposes of the pilot study, therefore, we simply measured change in standard physiological and psychological risk factors.

The results of this study were encouraging in that without apparent change of their diet or exercise habits, and while continuing to work the same hours per week and to carry the same type of responsibility, men in the behavior therapy group showed significant decreases on physiological (serum cholesterol, systolic blood pressure) and psychological (time pressure, life dissatisfaction) risk factors (Roskies, Spevack, Surkis, Cohen, & Gilman, 1978). Even more important, 6 months later most of these changes had been maintained (Roskies, Kearney, Spevack, Surkis, Cohen, & Gilman, 1979). However, contrary to our expectations, men in the psychotherapy group showed almost as good treatment effects immediately after treatment; although the drop in serum cholesterol was larger and more consistent for the relaxation group, differences between the two treatment conditions were not statistically significant. They only became so at the follow-up (Roskies et al., 1979).

The fact that participants in the pilot program were motivated to stay in treatment and seemed to derive benefits from it encouraged us to attempt a more ambitious intervention effort. For this new, improved version, significant changes were made in sample constitution, program content, and evaluation procedures. In terms of sample, we wanted to see if the results obtained with a very select group of extreme type As could be broadened to a less carefully chosen, but probably more representative, group of managers. With the cooperation of medical and personnel officers of three large Canadian companies, letters were sent to all men at a designated middle-management level inviting them to participate in a research stress management program. Entry criteria were much less stringent than for the previous program: All men at the designated occupational level who did not manifest overt signs of heart disease would be accepted. The degree to which participants had to commit themselves to the program was also considerably less. In contrast to the first study, there was no deposit and both the initial screening interview and the treatment program were held at the worksite.

Sixty six men volunteered during the 2 week recruitment period in December 1978. Unlike the men in the first sample, all of whom had been English-speaking, 44% of this group was Francophone. Because these men were chosen at the middle-manager level rather than the senior managers and professionals of the first study, they were also considerably younger ($\bar{x} = 41.33$ vs. $\bar{x} = 47.6$). In this study smokers were not excluded and, in fact, 30% of the sample were currently smokers. Most important of all, however, was the difference in type A status. In contrast to the first study where all participants had been classified as extreme type As (A_1), here only 47% of the sample (31 men) were placed in that category. An additional 40% were less extreme As, while 14% were classified as non-As (B and X).

Forty of these 66 men were randomly assigned to a 13 week immediate treatment program, while 26 constituted a waiting list control. The men in the immediate treatment condition met weekly in groups of 10 (there were 2 Anglophone and 2 Francophone groups) for thirteen 1½ hrs sessions between February and June 1979. Participants in the waiting list control condition were offered the same treatment between October 1979–February 1980.

For this second project, we also made major changes in the treatment program (Roskies, 1982; Roskies & Avard, 1982). Rather than simply seeking to modify the physiological response to a given stressor, we wanted to change as well the mental set with which the person approached a potential stress situation and the ways in which he sought to manage both the tension and the situation (Roskies & Lazarus, 1980). For this purpose, we increased the number of coping strategies taught to include muscle relaxation (Bernstein & Borkovec, 1973), rational-emotive thinking (Ellis & Grieger, 1977, Maultsby & Ellis, 1978), communication skills training (Stuart, 1974), problem-solving (D'Zurilla & Goldfried, 1971) and, in a special role, an adaptation of stress inoculation (Meichenbaum, 1977).

The third change was in the measures used to evaluate outcome. Based on our belief that it was the frequency, intensity, and duration of sympathetic arousal that constituted the pathogenic elements in the type A pattern, we attempted to measure change by charting a number of indices of this arousal, both in a laboratory and a field situation (Roskies, 1979). Prior to and immediately following the intervention, all participants were exposed to a standard stress situation in the laboratory and fluctuations in systolic blood pressure, diastolic blood pressure, heart rate, plasma epinephrine, and plasma norepinephrine before, during and after the task were recorded.

In the field situation, one working day every fortnight during the course of the project was designated as a monitoring day (nine days in all). During this day four types of measures were tracked: psychological state, blood pressure, urinary catecholamines, and serum cholesterol and testosterone. Participants were asked to record hourly levels of muscular tension, irritability, time pressure and performance (using a 0-10 scale) and follow this by a blood pressure reading using an electronic machine—Labtronix 4000—designed for home use. Urine for analysis of catecholamine levels was collected for 24 hrs. divided into three time periods: the night before the working day, the working day itself, and the evening after.

The data analysis for this second project is still not complete, but based on our initial findings the results are mixed. While not quite as high as for the initial project, attendance continued to be good (29 of the 40 men in the initial treatment group attended at least 8 of the 13 sessions) and only 5 men completely abandoned the program. There were also significant increases in reported life satisfaction and significant decreases in reported psychophysiological symptoms for men in the treated group compared to those in the control group. Where no clear treatment effects were shown, was in measures of physiological reactivity. Most of these measures did show a significant decline over time, but the changes were not significantly different for men in the treatment condition than for the controls.

The fact that we did not produce the desired changes in physiological reactivity has left us disappointed, but far from discouraged. Before concluding that the treatment program itself is ineffective, there are reasons for subjecting both our data collection and our sample selection procedures to critical scrutiny. The complexity of the measures we sought, coupled with deficiencies in equipment and personnel, led to considerable missing and/or invalid data. For instance, we were unable to include in the statistical analysis the urinary catecholamine data of more than half the sample, either because a given day's collection was incomplete, or there was an insufficient number of measuring days (We required a minimum of six for analysis, two at the beginning of treatment, two in the middle, and two at the end), or because of problems in transportation, storage and handling. Blood pressure measures during the working day had the additional handicap of invasiveness, i.e., the fact that the subject had to pull out his apparatus to measure his blood pressure meant that he was unlikely to do so at the moments of greatest upset, precisely those time periods we most wished to record. To the degree that we learn to overcome some of these methodological problems, we are likely to provide a better test of treatment effectiveness.

A second unanticipated problem was the heterogeneity of the sample in terms of the principal dependent measures—physiological reactivity. Type As as a group are more reactive than type Bs, but not *all* type As are reactive. (Not all type As have heart attacks either, and it is possible that physiological reactivity is one of the discriminating indices). In our future intervention efforts, we should probably select men who are physiologically reactive, as well as being type A. It is these possibilities that we are currently examining in designing our next project.

CONCLUDING COMMENTS

To draw up a balance sheet of the successes and failures of coronary risk reduction efforts to date, is to record one major plus and one major minus. The plus comes, of course, from the positive results of several of the intervention projects (Belgian, Stanford, North Karelia) in significantly modifying the statistical risk status of the populations towards which they were directed. The minus lies in the fact that, as yet, no intervention effort has succeeded in translating *statistical* improvements in risk status into *clinical* lowering of disease incidence. In fact, the only study to date which has reported on changes in disease incidence, North Karelia, found that the treatment community did not differ significantly from the control one.

If one shares the optimism of the North Karelia investigators, then it is simply a question of time until improved risk status is reflected in improved mortality/ morbidity. This optimism, however, depends on the assumption that the mathematical equation linking risk factors to heart disease works backwards as well as forwards, that is, in exactly the same way that the presence of risk factors leads to increased incidence of CHD, so will the removal of these risk factors lead to reduced incidence. Given the current absence of evidence supporting or contradicting this possibility, such an assumption is no more than an expression of faith. Only when the various intervention projects begin to publish outcome results relating to mortality/morbidity can we have an empirical answer to this question.

But even the publication of outcome results is unlikely to end the debate between true believers and sceptics concerning the value of coronary risk reduction efforts. For one thing, no study has yet succeeded in choosing either a sample, therapeutic targets, or even intervention strategies, that would render its findings-positive or negative-immune to contradictory interpretations. The fact that MRFIT has chosen to work with carefully selected high risk men makes it almost inevitable that non-believers will cast doubt on the value of any improvement observed. Should the treated men show a significantly lower incidence of coronary mortality, this finding can be explained away as a function of these mens' pre-existing readiness for change. Similarly, any good results observed in Karelia can be attributed more to the characteristics of this self-selected patient, than to the nature of the treatment applied. Paradoxically, the use of a high risk sample can also be used for the opposite purpose of excusing therapeutic failure. Believers can claim that no changes in morbidity/mortality are observable because the men already had sub-clinical CHD at program entry.

Another possible point of controversy concerns the appropriateness of the risk factors that have been targeted for intervention. As we have seen, the various multi-factorial projects have been unanimous in choosing to focus on blood pressure, serum cholesterol, and smoking, and equally unanimous in ignoring psychological stress, type A behavior, overwork, life dissatisfaction, and so on. While the three risk factors selected for intervention account for half the variance in CHD incidence, the psychological factors not being treated account for a good part of the other half. Moreover, it is possible that emotional factors not only act independently to increase risk, but also influence smoking, blood pressure and cholesterol, as well as the ability to modify existing smoking and eating habits. Should intervention efforts fail, therefore, it can be argued that this apparent lack of success is attributable more to the inappropriateness or incompleteness of the therapeutic targets selected, rather than to any fundamental weakness in intervention per se.

A final source of controversy concerns the validity of the various intervention strategies used in the different projects. There is considerable difference between projects in the importance placed on the mechanisms of change. Stanford, for instance, seems to have given considerable thought and attention to the therapeutic strategies to be employed, and report their intervention techniques in considerable detail. MRFIT and the Belgian project, in contrast, are very vague in describing what exactly went on during treatment sessions. One does not know if there was a standard therapy procedure, nor even the qualifications of the therapists. Should these projects produce less than ideal results, one could question whether the therapists and therapy techniques used were good enough to give intervention a fair trial.

These multiple problems in producing unequivocal results demonstrating the efficacy of coronary risk reduction efforts do not seem to have discouraged prospective investigators. On the contrary, coronary risk reduction at this time can be compared to a mountain where no one has yet succeeded in scaling the summit, but many are racing toward it. Funding agencies, too, appear to be sufficiently impressed by progress to date, as well as by the importance of the problem, to continue to invest the large sums of money necessary to mount multi-factorial programs. Even before the first generation of multi-factorial programs has issued its final reports, there is already a new group of studies being launched (Minnesota, Oslo, Pawtucket, Stanford Five Communities).

What form is this new wave of multi-factorial prevention programs likely to take? To some degree, it will be more of the same. Current indications are that the programs now in preparation will continue to focus on blood pressure, smoking and cholesterol as primary targets, and none will seek to treat directly emotional risk factors. The current division between projects directed toward high risk individuals versus those directed toward the community at large is also likely to continue. The intervention currently taking shape as part of the ongoing (Oslo study (Bjartveit, Foss, Gjervig, & Lund-Larsen, 1979) is very similar to MRFIT in its selection of a sample of high risk middle-aged men, while the Stanford Five Communities Program (Farquhar, 1978b) and the Pawtucket Heart Health Project (Carleton, 1979) exemplify the community-based approach.

The area where most of the innovation is likely to occur is in the techniques used to achieve behavior change. In particular, we are likely to see much greater emphasis on the use of indigenous community resources. The Stanford group has been receptive to the criticism that its initial effort did not really use community structures, and this time it will devote considerable attention to enhancing the participation of existing community organizations, as well as that of professionals and lay workers from within the community. Going even further in its emphasis on social setting, the Pawtucket Heart Health program has declared that it will seek to change not only individuals, but also the health *mores* of the culture in which they live.

Our discussion of problems and prospects in coronary risk reduction has focused exclusively on the multi-factorial programs. This pre-occupation can be defended on the grounds that primary prevention studies large enough to use coronary morbidity and mortality as end points are almost inevitably going to be directed toward more than one risk factor. Pioneering as the Anti-Coronary Club may have been in its time, this attempt to test the diet-heart hypothesis marked the end of an era as well as its beginning. Faced with the methodological inadequacies of these first diet intervention studies, the funding agencies had to decide between seeking to promote a diet study that would constitute a critical test or whether, instead, to choose an alternative approach. The Inter-Society Commission for Heart Disease Resources was formed to study this issue in 1970 (cf. Report of the Diet-Heart Review Panel of the National Heart Institute, 1969; Report of the Inter-Society Commission for Heart Disease Resources, 1970; Stamler, 1978) and decided upon the multi-factorial approach exemplified by MRFIT. There has never been a definitive test of the coronary effects of diet intervention alone, and it is now unlikely that one will ever be mounted.

Nevertheless, there still continues to exist a role for intervention projects that seek to develop new treatment approaches for specific risk factors. Richard Evans' work in preventing the intiation of smoking in teenagers has not only generated a great deal of interest (cf. Fisher, 1980), but has also led, within a very short time period, to other attempts to explore this avenue of approach (McAlister, Perry, Killen, Slinkard, & Maccoby, 1980; Perry, Killen, Telch, Slinkard, & Danaher, 1980). Progress in type A modification in non-clinical subjects is likely to be slower, if only because there is still no acceptable measure of outcome, but even here it is encouraging that one of the current multi-factorial programs (Pawtucket) has expressed interest in adding a treatment program for this risk factor.

Perhaps the best sign of the current ferment in coronary risk reduction efforts is the virtual impossibility of writing an up to date review. This chapter could not have been written even a year or two earlier because a good portion of the data cited here only became available within the past year. By the time it is published, however, its material is likely to be considerably behind the current state of the art. The inability of reviews to keep pace with the rapid changes in a subject area makes for frustrated reviewers, not to speak of equally frustrated readers. Fortunately, it also makes for exciting science.

ACKNOWLEDGMENTS

The work on type A intervention reported in this chapter was supported by grants to the author from Health and Welfare, Ottawa and Conseil de la Recherche en Santé de Québec.

REFERENCES

Ahrens, E. H., Jr. The management of hyperlipidemia: whether, rather than how. *Annals of Internal Medicine,* 1976, *85,* 87–93.

Alderman, M. H. Communities with unusually short life-spans: The effects of life-style modification. *Bulletin of the New York Academy of Medicine,* 1979, *55,* 357–366.

Bandura, A. *Social learning theory.* New York: General Learning Press, 1971.

Bandura, A. Self-efficacy: Toward a unifying theory of behavioral change. *Psychological Review,* 1977, *84,* 191–215.

Benfari, R. C., McIntyre, K., Eaker, E., Blumberg, S., & Oglesby, P. The psychological effects of differential treatment of a high risk sample in a randomized clinical trial. *American Journal of Public Health,* 1979, *69,* 996–1000.

Bernstein, D. A., & Borkovec, T. D. *Progressive relaxation training.* Champaign: Research Press, 1973.

Bernstein, D. A., & McAlister, A. The modification of smoking behavior: Progress and problems. *Addictive Behaviors,* 1976, *1,* 89–102.

Bjartveit, K., Foss, O. P., Gjervig, T., & Lund-Larsen, P. G. The cardiovascular disease study in Norweigan counties. *Acta Medica Scandinavica,* 1979, *634,* (Suppl.), 1–79.

Borhani, N. O. Primary prevention of coronary heart disease: a critique. *American Journal of Cardiology,* 1977, *40,* 251–259.

Bortner, R. J. A short rating scale as a potential measure of pattern A behavior. *Journal of Chronic Diseases,* 1969, *22,* 87–91.

Carleton, R. Pawtucket Heart Health Program: Cardiovascular Disease Prevention by Community Activation, Grant application to the U.S. Public Health Service, Dept. of Health, Education and Welfare, 1979.

Carver, C. S., Coleman, A. E., & Glass, D. C. The coronary-prone behavior pattern and suppression of fatigue on a treadmill test. *Journal of Personality and Social Psychology,* 1976, *33,* 460–66.

Christakis, G., Rinzler, H., Archer, M., & Kraus, A. Effect of the anti-coronary club program on coronary heart disease risk factor status. *Journal of the American Medical Association,* 1966, *198,* 597–604.

Cohen, J. B., Syme, S. L., Jenkins, C. D., Kagan, A., & Zyzanski, S. J. Cultural context of type A behavior and risk for CHD: A study of Japanese-American males. *Journal of Behavioral Medicine,* 1979, *2,* 375–384.

Cooper, R., Dyer, A., Moss, D., Stamler, R., Soltero, I., Liu, K., & Stamler, J. A continuing decline in cardiovascular mortality, U.S.A., 1968–1975: Why? *Preventive Medicine,* 1978, *7,* 53 (Abstract).

Corday, E., & Corday, R. Editorial Prevention of heart disease by control of risk factors: the time has come to face the facts. *American Journal of Cardiology,* 1975, *35,* 330–333.

Corday, E. Can we reverse or retard an obstructive coronary lesion by risk factor intervention? *Cleveland Clinic Quarterly,* 1978, *45,* 5–8.

Criqui, M. H., Barrett-Connor, E., Holdbrook, M. J., Austin, M., & Turner, J. D. Clustering of cardiovascular disease risk factors. *Preventive Medicine,* 1980. *9,* 525–533.

De Backer, G., Kornitzer, M., Thilly, C., & Depoorter, A. M. The Belgian Multifactor Preventive Trial in CVD: Design and methodology. *Hart Bulletin.* 1977, *8,* 143–146.

De Backer, G., Kornitzer, M., Dramaix, M., Huyghebaert, M., Verdonk, G. Vuylsteek, K., Graffar, M., Pannier, R., & Lequime, J. Risk factor changes in the Belgian Heart Disease Prevention Project. *Acta Cardiology,* 1979a, *23,* (Suppl.), 125–132.

De Backer, G., Kornitzer, M., Kittel, F., Bogaert, M., Van Durme, J. P., Vincke, J., Rustin, R. M., Degré C., & De Schaepdrijver, A. Relation between coronary-prone behavior pattern, excretion of urinary catecholamines, heart rate and heart rhythm. *Preventive Medicine,* 1979b, *8,* 14–22.

Dembroski, T. M., & MacDougall, J. M. Stress effects on affiliation preferences among subjects possessing the type A coronary-prone behavior pattern. *Journal of Personality and Social Psychology,* 1978, *36,* 23–33.

Dembroski, T. M., MacDougall, J. M., & Shields, J. L. Physiologic reactions to social challenge in persons evidencing the Type A coronary-prone behavior pattern. *Journal of Human Stress,* 1977, *3,* 2–10.

Dembroski, T. M., MacDougall, J. M., Shields, J. L., Petitto, J., & Lushene, R. Components of the Type A coronary-prone behavior pattern and cardiovascular responses to psychomotor performance challenge. *Journal of Behavioral Medicine,* 1978, *1,* 159–176.

Dembroski, T. M., MacDougall, J. M., Herd, J. A., & Shields, J. L. Effect of level of challenge on pressor and heart rate responses in Type A and B subjects. *Journal of Applied Social Psychology,* 1979, *9,* 209–228.

Dwyer, T., & Hetzel, B. S. A comparison of trends of coronary heart disease mortality in Australia, U.S.A. and England and Wales with reference to three major risk factors–hypertension, cigarette smoking and diet. *International Journal of Epidemiology,* 1980, *9,* 65–72.

D'Zurilla, T. J., & Goldfried, M. R. Problem solving and behavior modification. *Journal of Abnormal Psychology,* 1971, *78,* 107–126.

Ellis, A., & Greiger, R. (Eds.) *Handbook of rational-emotive therapy.* New York: Springer, 1977.

Enelow, A. J., & Henderson, J. B. (Eds.). Introduction. *Applying behavioral science to cardiovascular risk: Proceedings of a conference.* New York: American Heart Association, 1975.

Evans, R. I. Smoking in children: Developing a social psychological strategy of deterrence. *Preventive Medicine,* 1976, *5,* 122–127.

Evans, R. I., Hansen, W. B., & Mittelmark, M. B. Increasing the validity of self-reports of behavior in a smoking in children investigation. *Journal of Applied Psychology,* 1977, *62,* 521–523.

Evans, R. I., Rozelle, R. M., Maxwell, S. E., Raines, B. E., Dill, C. A., Guthrie, T. J., Henderson, A. H., & Hill, P. C. Social modeling films to deter smoking in adolescents: Results of a three year field investigation. Paper presented at the annual meeting of the American Psychological Association. Montreal, September, 1980.

Evans, R. I., Rozelle, R. M., Mittelmark, M. B., Hansen, W. B., Bane, A. L., & Havis, J. Deterring the ouset of smoking in children: Knowledge of immediate physiological effects and coping with peer pressure, media pressure, and parent modeling. *Journal of Applied Social Psychology,* 1978, *8,* 126–135.

Eysenck, H. J., & Eysenck, S. B. *Inventaire de la personnalité d' Eysenck.* (Manuel) Paris: Les éditions du Centre de Psychologie appliquée, 1971.

Farrand, M. E., & Mojonnier, L. Nutrition in the Multiple Risk Factor Intervention Trial (MRFIT): Background and general description. *Journal of the American Dietetic Association,* 1980, *76,* 347–351.

Farquhar, J. W. *The American way of life need not be hazardous to your health.* New York: Norton, 1978a.

Farquhar, J. W. The community-based model of life style intervention trials. *American Journal of Epidemiology,* 1978b, *108,* 103–111.

Farquhar, J. W., Maccoby, M., Wood, P., Alexander, J., Breitrose, H., Brown, B. W., Haskell, W. L., McAlister, A. L., Meyer, A. J., Nash, J. D., & Stern, M. P. Community education for cardiovascular health. *The Lancet,* June 4, 1977, 1192–1195.

Fisher, E. B. Progress in reducing adolescent smoking. Editorial, *American Journal of Public Health, 70,* 1980, 678–679.

Friedman, M. Modifying "type A" behavior in heart attack patients. *Primary Cardiology,* 1978, *4,* 9–13.

Friedman, M. The modification of type A behavior in post-infarction patients. *American Heart Journal,* 1979, *97,* 551–560.

Friedman, M., Byers, S. L., Rosenman, R. H., & Elevitch, F. R. Coronary-prone individuals (type A) behavior pattern: Some biochemical characteristics. *Journal of the American Medical Association,* 1970, *212,* 1030–1037.

Friedman, M., Byers, S. O., Diamant, J., & Rosenman, R. H. Plasma catecholamine response of coronary-prone subjects (Type A) to a specific challenge. *Metabolism,* 1975, *24,* 205–210.

Glass, D. C. *Behavior patterns, stress and coronary disease.* Hillsdale, N.J.: Lawrence Erlbaum Associates, 1977.

Glass, D. C., & Carver, C. S. Environmental stress and the type A response. In A. Baum & J. E. Singer (Eds.), *Advances in environmental psychology vol. 2: Applications of personal control,* Hillsdale N.J.: Lawrence Erlbaum Associates, 1980.

Glass, D. C., Snyder, M. L., & Hollis, J. F. Time urgency and the type A coronary-prone behavior pattern. *Journal of Applied Social Psychology,* 1974, *4,* 125–140.

Glass, D. C., Krakoff, L. R., Contrada, R., Hilton, W. F., Kehoe, K., Mannucci, E. G., Collins, C., Snow, B., & Elting, E. Effect of harassment and competition upon cardiovascular and catecholamines responses in type A and type B individuals. *Psychophysiology,* 1980, *17,* 453–463.

Hjermann, I. Coronary heart disease prevention: the Oslo study. *Journal of the Oslo City Hospital,* 1980, *30,* 21–36.

Horowitz, M., Hulley, S., Alvarez, W., Billings, J., Benfari, R., Blair, S., Borhani, N., & Simon, N. News of risk for early heart disease as a stressful event. *Psychosomatic Medicine,* 1980, *42,* 37–46.

Howard, J. H., Cunningham, D. A., & Rechnitzer, P. A. Work patterns associated with type A behavior: A managerial population. *Human Relations,* 1977, *30,* 825–836.

Hulley, S., Ashman, P., Kuller, L., Lasser, N., & Sherwin, R., HDL Cholesterol Levels in the Multiple Risk Factor Intervention Trial (MRFIT) by the MRFIT Research Group. *Lipids,* 1979, *14,* 119–124.

Jacobson, E. *Progressive relaxation.* 2nd ed. Chicago: University of Chicago Press, 1938.

Jenkins, C. D. Recent evidence supporting psychological and social risk factors for coronary disease. *New England Journal of Medicine,* 1976, *294,* 987–994, 1033–103

Jenkins, C. D., Rosenman, R. H., & Friedman, M. Development of an objective psychological test for the determination of the coronary-prone behavior pattern in employed men. *Journal of Chronic Disease,* 1967, *26,* 371–79.

Jolliffe, M., Rinzler, S. H., & Archer, M. The anti-coronary club; including a discussion of the effects of a prudent diet on the serum cholesterol level of middle aged men. *American Journal of Clinical Nutrition,* 1959, *7,* 451–462.

Jolliffe, H., Baumgarten, L., Rinzler, S. H., Archer, M., Stephenson, J. H., & Christakis, G. J. The Anti-Coronary Club: The first four years. *New York State Journal of Medicine*, 1963, *63*, 69–79.

Kasl, S. W. Cardiovascular risk reduction in a community setting: Some comments. *Journal of Consulting and Clinical Psychology*, 1980, *48*, 143–149.

Kittel, F., Kornitzer, M., Zyzanski, S. J., Jenkins, C. D., Rustin, R. M. & Degré, C. Two methods of assessing the type A coronary-prone behavior pattern in Belgium. *Journal of Chronic Diseases*, 1978, *31*, 147–155.

Kornitzer, M., De Backer, G., Dramaix, M., & Thilly, C. Regional differences in risk factor distributions, food habits and coronary heart disease mortality and morbidity in Belgium. *International Journal of Epidemiology*, 1979, *8*, 23–31.

Kornitzer, M., De Backer, G., Dramaix, M., & Thilly, C. The Belgian Heart Disease Prevention Project: Modification of the coronary risk profile in an industrial population. *Circulation*, 1980a, *61*, 18–25.

Kornitzer, M., Dramaix, M., Kittel, F., & De Backer, G. The Belgian Heart Disease Prevention Project: Changes in smoking habits after two years of intervention. *Preventive Medicine*, 1980b, *9*, 496–504.

Krantz, D. S., Glass, D. C., & Snyder, M. L. Helplessness, stress level and the coronary-prone behavior pattern. *Journal of Experimental Social Psychology*, 1974, 19, 284–300.

Kuller, L., Neaton, J., Caggiula, A., & Falvo-Gerard, L. Primary prevention of heart attacks: The Multiple Risk Factor Intervention Trial. *American Journal of Epidemiology*, 1980, *112*, 185–199.

Leren, P., Askevold, E. M., Foss, O. P., Froili, A., Grymyr, D., Helgeland, A., Hjermann, I., Holme, I., Lund-Larsen, P. G. and Norum, K. R. The Oslo Study: Cardiovascular disease in middle-aged and young Oslo men. *Acta Medica Scandinavica*, 1975, *588*, (Suppl.), 1–38.

Leventhal, H., Safer, M. A., Cleary, P. D., & Gutmann, M. Cardiovascular risk modification by community-based programs for life style change: comments on the Stanford study. *Journal of Consulting and Clinical Psychology*, 1980, *48*, 150–158.

Levy, R. I. Progress in prevention of cardiovascular disease. *Preventive Medicine*, 1978, *7*, 464–475.

Lichenstein, E., & Danaher, B. G. Modification of smoking behavior: A critical analysis of theory research and practice. In M. Hersen, R. M. Eisler & P. M. Miller (Eds.) *Progress in behavior modification*, vol. III, New York: Academic Press, 1976.

McAlister, A., Perry, C., Killen, J., Slinkard, L. A., & Maccoby, N. Pilot study on alcohol and drug abuse prevention. *American Journal of Public Health*, 1980, *70*, 719–722.

Maccoby, N., Farquhar, J. W., Wood, P. D., & Alexander, J. Reducing the risk of cardiovascular disease: Effects of a community-based campaign on knowledge and behavior. *Journal of Community Health*, 1977, *3*, 100–114.

McGuire, W. J. Communication-persuasion models for drug education: experimental findings. In M. Goodstat (Ed.) *Research on methods and programs of drug education*. Toronto, Addiction Research Foundation, 1974.

Manuck, S. B., Craft, S. A., & Gold, K. J. Coronary-prone behavior pattern and cardiovascular response. *Psychophysiology*, 1978, *15*, 403–411.

Matthews, K. A. Mother-child interactions as a determinant of Type A -Type B behavior. Unpublished doctoral dissertation, University of Texas, Austin, 1976.

Maultsby, M., & Ellis, A. Techniques for using rational-emotive imagery. In A. Ellis, & E. Abraham (Eds.) *Brief psychotherapy in medical and health practice*. New York: Springer, 1978.

Meichenbaum, D. *Cognitive behavior modification: An integrative approach*. New York: Plenum, 1977.

Mettlin, C. Occupational careers and the prevention of coronary-prone behavior. *Social Science and Medicine*, 1976, *10*, 367–373.

Meyer, A. J., Nash, J. D., McAlister, A. L., Maccoby, N., & Farquhar, J. W. Skills training in a cardiovascular health education campaign. *Journal of Consulting and Clinical Psychology,* 1980a, *48,* 129–142.

Multiple Risk Factor Intervention Trial. A national study of primary prevention of coronary heart disease. *Journal of the American Medical Association,* 1976, *235,* 825–827.

Multiple Risk Factor Intervention Trial Group. The MRFIT Behavior Pattern Study-1. *Journal of Chronic Diseases,* 1979, *32,* 293–305.

National Heart and Lung Institute Task Force on Arteriosclerosis. *Arteriosclerosis: A Report.* Washington D.C.: Dept. of Health, Education and Welfare. Publication No. (NIH) 72–137, 1971.

Neittaanmaki, L., Koskela, K., Puska, P., & McAlister, A. L. The role of lay workers in community health education: Experiences of the North Karelia Project. *Scandanavian Journal of Social Medicine,* 1980, *8,* 1–7.

Perry, C., Killen, J., Telch, M., Slinkard, L., & Danaher, B. S. Modifying smoking behavior of teenagers: A school-based intervention. *American Journal of Public Health,* 1980, *70,* 722–724.

Pooling Project Research Group. Relationship of blood pressure, serum cholesterol, smoking habit, relative weight and ECG abnormalities to incidence of major coronary events: Final report of the Pooling Project. *Journal of Chronic Diseases,* 1978, *31,* 201–306.

Puska, P., Koskela, K., Pakatinen, H., Puumalainen, P., Soininem, V., & Tuomilehto, J. The North Karelia Project: a programme for community control of cardiovascular diseases. Scandanavian Journal of Social Medicine, 1976, *4, 57–60.*

Puska, P., Tuomilehto, J., Salonen, J., Neittaanmaki, L., Maki, J., Virtamo, J., Nissinen, A., Koskela, K., & Takalo, T. Changes in coronary risk factors during comprehensive five-year community programme to control cardiovascular diseases (North Karelia project). *British Medical Journal,* 1979a, *2,* (6199), 1173–78.

Puska, P., Tuomilehto, J., Nissinen, A., & Salonen, J. Principles and experiences of a community control programme for hypertension as part of the North Karelia Project. *Acta Medica Scandinavica,* 1979b, *626* (Suppl.), 22–24.

Remmell, P. S., & Benfari, R. C. Assessing dietary adherence in the Multiple Risk Factor Intervention Trial (MRFIT) II: Food record rating as an indicator of compliance. *Journal of the American Dietetic Association,* 1980, *76,* 357–360.

Remmell, P. S., Gorder, D. G., Hall, Y., & Tillotson, J. Assessing dietary adherance in the Multiple Risk Factor Intervention Trial (MRFIT): I Use of a dietary monitoring tool. *Journal of the American Dietetic Association,* 1980, *76,* 351–356.

Report of the Diet-Heart Review Panel of the National Heart Institute. Mass field trials of the diet-heart question: their significance, timeliness, feasibility and applicability. *American Heart Association Monographs,* 1969, *28.*

Report of the Inter-Society Commission for Heart Disease Resources. Primary prevention of the atherosclerotic diseases. *Circulation,* 1970, *42,* 55–95.

Rosenmann, R. H., Friedman, M., Straus, R., Wurm, M., Kositchek, R., Hahn, W., & Werthessen, N. T. A predictive study of coronary heart disease: The Western Collaborative Group Study. *Journal of the American Medical Association,* 1964, *189,* 15–22.

Roskies, E. Evaluating improvement in the coronary-prone (type A) behavior pattern. In D. J. Osborne, M. N. Gruneberg, & J. R. Eiser (Eds.) *Research in psychology and medicine, Vol. 1,* New York: Academic Press, 1979.

Roskies, E. Considerations in developing a treatment program for the coronary-prone (type A) behavior pattern. In P. Davidson & S. M. Davidson (Eds.), *Behavioral medicine: Changing health lifestyles.* New York: Brunner/Mazel, 1980.

Roskies, E. Stress management for type A individuals. In D. Meichenbaum & M. Jaremko (Eds.), *Stress prevention and management: A cognitive-behavioral approach.* New York: Plenum, 1982.

Roskies, E., & Avard, J. Teaching healthy managers to control their coronary-prone (type A) behavior. In K. Blankstein & J. Polivy (Eds.), *Self-control and self-modification of emotional behaviors*. New York: Plenum, 1982.

Roskies, E., & Lazarus, R. S. Coping theory and the teaching of coping skills. *In* P. O. Davidson and S. M. DAvidson (Eds.) *Behavioral medicine: Changing. health lifestyles*. New York: Brunner/Mazel, 1980.

Roskies, E., Spevack, M., Surkis, A., Cohen, C., & Gilman, S. Changing the coronary-prone (type A) behavior pattern in a non-clinical population. *Journal of Behavioral Medicine*, 1978, *1*, 201–215.

Roskies, E., Kearney, H., Spevack, M., Surkis, A., Cohen, C., & Gilman, S. Generalizability and durability of treatment effects in an intervention program for coronary-prone (type A) managers. *Journal of Behavioral Medicine*, 1979, *2*, 195–207.

Rustin, R. M., Dramaix, M., Kittel, J., Degré, C., Kornitzer, M., Thilly, C., & De Backer, G. Validation des techniques d'évaluation du profil comportementa "A" utilisées dans le "Projet Belge de Prévention des affections cardiovasculaires" (P.B.P.) *Revue Epidémiologie et Santé Publique*, 1976, *24*, 497–507.

Rustin, R. M., Kittel, F., Dramaix, M., Kornitzer, M., & De Backer, G. Smoking habits and psycho-socio-biological factors. *Journal of Psychosomatic Research*, 1978, *22*, 89–99.

Salonen, J. T., & Puska, P. A community programme for rehabilitation and secondary prevention for patients with acute myocardial infarction as part of a comprehensive community programme for control of cardiovascular diseases (North Karelia Project). *Scandanavian Journal of Rehabilitation Medicine*, 1980, *12*, 33–42.

Salonen, J. T., Puska, P., Mustaniemi, H. Changes in morbidity and mortality during comprehensive community programme to control cardiovascular diseases during 1972–7 in North Karelia. *British Medical Journal*, 1979, *2* (6199), 1178–83.

Sandler, Y., & Hazari, A. The obsessional: on the psychological classification of obsessional character traits and symptoms. *British Journal of Medical Psychology*, 1960, *33*, 113–132.

Schucker, B., & Jacobs, D. R. Assessment of behavioral risk for coronary disease by voice characteristics. *Psychosomatic Medicine*, 1977, *39*, 229–240.

Singman, H. S., Berman, S. N., Cowell, C., Maslansky, E., & Archer, M. The Anti-Coronary Club: 1957 to 1972. *The American Journal of Clinical Nutrition*, 1980, *33*, 1183–1191.

Stamler, J. Lifestyles, major risk factors, proof and public policy. *Circulation*, 1978, *58*, 3–19.

Stern, M. P. The recent decline in ischemic heart disease mortality. *Annals of Internal Medicine*, 1979, *91*, 630–640.

Stuart, R. B. Paper presented at the annual meeting of the Association des Spécialistes en Modification du Comportement. Moncton, New Brunswick, June, 1974.

Suinn, R. M. The cardiac stress management program for Type A patients. *Cardiac Rehabilitation*, 1975, *5*, 13–15.

Syme, S. L. Life style intervention in clinic-based trials. *American Journal of Epidemiology*, 1978, *108*, 87–91.

Truett, H. J., Cornfield, J., & Kannel, W. A multi-variate analysis of the risk of coronary heart disease in Framingham. *Journal of Chronic Diseases*, 1967, *20*, 511–524.

Tuomilehto, J., Puska, P., Virtamo, J., Salonen, J., & Koskela, K. The levels of the major risk indicators of cardiovascular diseases in Eastern Finland prior to a community-based intervention programme (The North Karelia Project) *Acta Cardiologica*, 1979, *34*, 359–374.

Vaisrub, S. Changing life-styles and ischemic heart diseases. Editorial. *Journal of the American Medical Association*, 1980, *244*, 700.

Van Egeren, L. Social interactions, communications and the coronary-prone behavior pattern: A psychophysiological study. *Psychosomatic Medicine*, 1979, *41*, 2–18.

Waldron, I., Hickey, A., McPherson, C., Butensky, A., Gruss, L., Overall, K., Schmader, A., & Wohlmuth, D. Relationships of the coronary-prone behavior pattern to blood pressure variation, psychological characteristics, and academic and social activities of students. *Journal of Human Stress,* 1980, *6,* 16–27.

Walker, W. J. Changing United States life-style and declining vascular mortality: Cause or coincidence? *New England Journal of Medicine,* 1977, *297,* 163–165.

Wilhelmsen, L., Tibblin, G., & Werko, L. A primary preventive study in Gothenberg, Sweden. *Preventive Medicine, 1,* 1972, *153–160.*

World Health Organization European Collaborative Group. An international controlled trial in the multi-factorial prevention of coronary heart disease. *International Jouranl of Epidemiology,* 1974, *3,* 219–224.

Zyzanski, S. J. Associations of the coronary-prone behavior pattern. *In* T. M. Dembroski, S. M. Weiss, J. L. Shields (Eds.), *Proceedings of the forum on coronary-prone behavior.* Washington, D.C.: Dept. of Health, Education and Welfare, Publication No (NIH) 78-1451, 1977.

9 The Non-Pharmacologic Treatment of Hypertension

Alvin P. Shapiro
Department of Medicine, University of Pittsburgh School of Medicine

Progress in the elucidation and management of cardiovascular diseases provides a major illustration of the advances during the past quarter century in medical science and medical care. Perhaps the most outstanding in these achievements has been the knowledge which has accumulated about hypertensive disease. Although examples of major accomplishments are evident in many aspects of cardiovascular disease, the growth of information concerning hypertension has several striking reasons for deserving the accolade. First, hypertension is the most common cardiovascular ailment, affecting in varying degrees upwards of 10 to 15% of our population. Second, the knowledge gained about hypertension during this last 25 years comprises contributions from virtually all subdivisions of medical science, ranging from basic physiological, pharmacological, hormonal, neurological and psychological insights concerning mechanisms, to clinical applications and patient care by medical, surgical, endocrinological, psychiatric, and nutritional techniques. Third, hypertension is a risk factor involved in the development of many other ailments, non-cardiac as well as cardiac, and since its control is now possible, it represents a risk factor which lends itself to treatment more readily than most other threats to man's cardiovascular health, such as his cholesterol levels and his smoking habits.

The progress which has been made in hypertension control is the product of this growth of information about the mechanisms involved in the elevation of blood pressure plus the rapid proliferation of pharmacologic agents which lower blood pressure by affecting one or more of these mechanisms. The melding of these two accomplishments, so as to match the pharmacologic action of the drug to the distorted mechanism, represents a striking demonstration of basic and

277

applied science at work in the development of ways to achieve better patient care.

Our capacity to intervene pharmacologically in the management of hypertension and its complications is perhaps nowhere illustrated as well as in the medical history of Franklin D Roosevelt, our four-time President who most would agree was the most influential and powerful man of at least the first half of this century. FDR was first noted to have mild hypertension in the midst of his first term in office, during 1932 to 1936. In early 1944, then towards the end of his third term and at the height of W.W. II, he first experienced the symptoms and signs of congestive heart failure, with blood pressures in the range of 180–210/100–120 mmHg. He was treated in the best fashion then available, namely with digitalis, mercurial diuretics, and a mild sedative. No specific antihypertensive agents were administered for the very simple reason that there were none. His heart failure was brought under control but his blood pressure remained elevated and in April of 1945, at the age of 63, he suffered a massive and fatal cerebral hemorrhage, then a most common cause of demise in hypertensive patients.

The salient point of this story is that whereas in 1945, no specific therapeutic agent was available for controlling FDR's hypertension, within the next 10 years drugs were developed that were readily and inexpensively available to the "common man," which have made a considerable dent in the incidence of death from hypertensive cerebral hemorrhages and virtually eliminated hypertensive congestive heart failure in the treated patient. It requires no great stretch of imagination and conjecture, therefore, to agree with the suggestion of Dr. Howard Bruenn, who was FDR's physician and has made the above data available, that the course of world history might well have been changed if present day drugs for the pharmacologic management of hypertension had been available only a few years earlier (Bruenn, 1970; Rogers, 1975).

The empirical evidence that lowering of blood pressure by certain newly developed pharmacologic agents was beneficial first began to accumulate in the early 1950s. It became rapidly apparent that in so-called malignant hypertension, an accelerated form of the disease associated with virtually 100% mortality within 2 to 3 years, progression could be halted even with the only modest blood pressure decline achieved by the then rather crude drugs available. In the 1960s, a landmark study done in a male population at Veterans Administration Hospitals by Freis and his colleagues convincingly demonstrated the prevention of cerebrovascular events and hyptertensive heart failure in patients with moderately severe hypertension (i.e. those with diastolic blood pressures greater than 105 mmHg) (Freis, 1970). However, these studies still left unanswered the question of the value of pharmacologic therapy, as compared to its risk, in the mildly hypertensive patients (i.e. those with diastolic blood pressures in the 90 to 105 mmHg range), a classification which includes the vast majority (approximately two-thirds) of the 20 to 30 million individuals with hypertension in this country.

The recent publication of the data from the Hypertension Detection and Follow-up Program (HDFP) has provided major answers to the value of of treatment in these mild hypertensives (HDFP, 1979,a,b). This study was performed on a sample of 10,000 hypertensive subjects assembled by house-to-house screening of approximately 150,000 persons between the ages of 30 to 69. After the presence of hypertension was confirmed at several clinic visits and the status of their hypertension was established, one half of the subjects were returned to their usual and regular source of care (RC group); the other half were treated in a quite specific fashion in special community clinics set up solely for this purpose (SC group). The key aspects of the treatment plan for the SC group was the setting of a goal for lowering the blood pressure, the addition of drugs to their regimen by a strict protocol until this goal was achieved, meticulous followup of the patients at intervals of at least four times per year, free drugs and counseling, and often provision of overall medical care.

The results of this comparison clearly indicate a significant decrease in all cause mortality in the SC group (6.7%) as compared to the RC group (7.7%). The difference was present in the mild hypertensive group (5.9 vs. 7.4%) as well as the entire sample of 10,000 patients, but applied primarily to those subjects 50 years of age or older. In the sample of subjects with mild hypertension below the age of 50 years, among whom overall death rates are low, the difference was not at a statistically significant level (3.3% in SC vs. 3.5% in RC). The favorable effect of the intensive therapy in the SC group also was most predominant in the black patients in the sample (10.6% vs. 13.0% in black men; 5.2% vs. 7.2% in black women).

In view of these impressive results with pharmacologic therapy, it is appropriate to ask why we should even consider non-pharmacologic approaches. One obvious reason is the concern about harmful effects of pharmacologic agents—materials foreign to the organism—taken over a prolonged period of time, a concern which has particular meaning in hypertension, a "lanthanic syndrome" (i.e. a disorder without symptoms) that is rarely cured but rather is only "controlled" by therapy. Although the mass studies such as the HDFP experience demonstrated that side effects were minor in degree, minimal in number, and far outweighed by the benefits of therapy, nevertheless, the desire for a more "natural" form of therapy is held by many, patients and physicians alike. The lack of evidence for a decrease in mortality in the younger aged patient with mild hypertension provides a possible argument for delay in initiation of pharmacologic treatment. Some evidence is available that treatment even in young subjects decreases the development of cardiac strain, but these morbid endpoints are reversible (Smith, 1977). Most importantly, non-pharmacologic methods of treating high blood pressure need not be considered as *alternatives* to pharmacologic therapy, but rather as *adjuncts* which can supplement drug treatment throughout the patient's life. Such an approach is in keeping with the modern day management of hypertension which recognizes that this chronic ailment is one with a multifactorial etiology and as such requires multiple approaches to its treatment.

In summary, the asymptomatic nature of hypertension, its prolonged course, its relative mildness in the majority of patients, the slowness of the development of target organ damage, the reluctance of patients to take potentially harmful, or at least inconvenient, medication, and the multifaceted nature of the ailment which requires simultaneous or consecutive treatments of different types, all constitute adequate reasons for studying and using non-pharmacologic therapies. The three major modalities of non-pharmacologic therapy are *diet*—with particular attention to sodium intake and weight control—,*physical exercise,* and *behavioral modification.*

DIET

1. Sodium

That sodium intake, as common salt, is a significant factor in the pathogenesis of hypertension has intrigued investigators for years and many studies in animals and man have provided evidence of its importance. Sodium intake can be considered a behavior of man; in fact, Denton has argued that the salt-seeking behavior of man has had major evolutionary effects (Denton, 1965). In any case, some of the most potent adaptations in man are directed at salt conservation and one can cite evidence that the development of the renin-angiotensin system (RAS) was primarily related to salt conservation (Cappeli, Wesson, & Aponte, 1970). Salt is essential to human life, yet its intake can vary in man within exceedingly broad limits, ranging from as low as 2 mequiv/day to as high as 400 and even 800 mequiv/day, while the organism still maintains normal health and function.

It is not the purpose of this review to discuss in detail the evidence for the importance of the role of sodium. However, some of the epidemiologic data concerning the effects of sodium in man, as they apply to social and cultural influences on hypertension, deserve mention. Studies of various cultural groups have indicated that sodium intake in closed primitive societies correlates with differences in levels of blood pressure among such societies. Sodium intake in the most primitive tribes is quite low as is the prevalence of hypertension among them (Page, Danion, & Moellering, 1970). Henry (Henry & Stephens, 1977) and Cassel (1974) have discussed the process of acculturation in terms of the increasing stress which particular societies experience but Lot Page (Page et al, 1970) has argued that acculturation is also associated with increased sodium intake which plays at least an equally important role in the development of hypertension. A recent presentation by Waldron has shown that both factors independently affect blood pressure. When social acculturation is defined as development of a money economy and salt consumption is controlled, a positive correlation to blood pressure elevation is noted, whereas if the economic factor is controlled, salt consumption is a positive correlate (Waldron, 1980). The high sodium intake of civilized people (approximately 150–200 mequiv/day in Americans) can be considered "unnatural" or unnecessary since primitive groups often subsist quite adequately even in hot climates with intakes of less than 40 mequiv/day. The Yanomano Indians of South America are particularly striking. For instance, they have intakes averaging less than 5 mequiv/day and there is literally no hypertension among them. They do not show the usual rise in blood pressure with advancing age and of interest in view of what we have mentioned earlier about the evolutionary development of the RAS as a sodium conserving mechanism, these people maintain their normal blood pressure despite PRA values that are two to three times normal values (Oliver, Cohen, & Neel, 1975).

The evidence that decreasing sodium intake in the diet will lower blood pressure in man derives mainly from the effectiveness of the diuretics and from the results of drastic sodium restriction with such regimens as the Kempner rice diet of years ago, in which sodium intake was decreased to approximately 10 mequiv/day. Direct evidence that lesser degrees of sodium restriction (on the order of 75 to 100 mequiv/day which can be achieved by avoidance of added salt and well-known high sodium foods) can have a measureable effect on blood pressure in man is only now becoming available.

In the past few years, a study by Parijs et al. has demonstrated that a reduction of sodium in the diet from the usual 200 mequiv/day to approximately 100 mequiv lowered blood pressure about 10/5 mmHg and supplemented the effects of diuretics (Parijs, Joosens, Van der Linden, Verstreken, & Amer, 1973). Similarly, Morgan et al. have demonstrated a diastolic decline averaging 7.3 mmHg in a group of patients with a modest reduction of sodium intake from approximately 191 mequiv to an average of 157 mequiv. There was a wide variation in the success in reducing sodium intake in Morgan's patients; those with values approaching 100 mequiv/day had the better blood pressure results. These results developed and persisted over a two-year period (Morgan, Gillies, Morgan, Adam, Wilson & Carney, 1978).

Luft and his colleagues have derived the reverse data, namely that in healthy people put on progressively greater intakes of sodium starting at low levels and rising to as high as 800 mequiv/day, blood pressure will show a proportional rise (Luft, Bloch, Weyman, Murray, & Weinberger, 1978). This certainly would be expected from animal data like those of Meneely and Dahl who have shown this phenomenon in numerous experiments in rats (Dahl, 1961; Meneely & Ball, 1958). In Dahl's studies he demonstrated that there are salt-sensitive and sal-resistant strains of rats, and recently, studies of increasing sodium intake in man, reported by Kawasaki et al., noted that mild hypertensive patients divided themselves into a group who were quite sensitive to increased salt intake and a group who were relatively insensitive (Kawasaki, Delea, Bartter, & Smith, 1978).

What does all of this mean as a risk factor for hypertension? First of all, we do not really understand man's craving for salt intake in excess of his physiologic need and his ability to conserve it. It seems at least in part to be a learned habit. There is evidence that infants have little or no taste for salt, a fact which finally has persuaded baby food manufacturers to remove sodium from their products since they primarily were adding it for the "tasting mothers" rather than the "consuming infants." Avoidance of salt can be learned (or perhaps salt taste can be "unlearned") as have been our experience in treating hypertensives; patients who observe their behavior for a significant period of time develop a sensitive sodium taste-threshold and can taste salt in situations where others do not.

On the other hand, there seems to be some evidence of an increased salt avidity in hypertensives. The classic question "Do you salt your food before you taste it?" is said to be answered in the positive by hypertensive patients although I do not know of any adequately controlled study of this phenomenon which includes normotensives. Interestingly enough, Langford has shown that patients put on diuretics can develop an increased salt intake if they are not closely watched in that regard (Langford, Watson, & Thomas, 1977).

We suggest that what all this means is that man has developed a powerful tool to maintain the sodium content and concentration in his body at appropriate levels for maintenance of life and this has played a significant evolutionary role in development from marine to terrestrial animals. Because of food preservation, cooking habits and other cultural influences on taste in modern day society, man currently consumes considerably more sodium than he needs for his vital functions and it is probable that this increase in sodium intake, at least in particularly prone individuals, plays a significant role in the development of hypertension.

The origin of the sensitivity to sodium is a subject of considerable study. Bianchi has developed a strain of rats in whom ability of the kidneys to handle salt load seems to determine the sensitivity to hypertension after sodium feeding. Cross-transplantation of kidneys from salt-sensitive to salt-resistant rats, and vice versa, results in appearance of hypertension in the previously salt-resistant group, and its disappearance in the counterparts receiving kidneys from the salt-resistant group (Bianchi, Fox, Francisco, Giovanetti, & Pagetti, 1974). Differences in accumulation of sodium in arterial walls in hypertensive animals, and changes in the Na:K gradients affecting arterial responsivity, have been advocated as providing the pressor effects by Tobian and his colleagues (Tobian, 1972), and by Friedman (Friedman & Friedman, 1976), respectively.

In any case, reduction of sodium intake in man to a more physiologic amount (e.g. 100 mequiv/day of sodium or about 4 to 5 grams of salt) would require major social and cultural behavioral changes. Data to support such a mass attempt at re-education, particularly in view of other dietary onslaughts on our hopeful but skeptical public, are not available at present. Freis has suggested editorially that reduction of salt intake to low levels owuld "wipe out hypertension in several generations'' (Freis, 1976), but this statement comes into the category of a provocative suggestion rather than a pragmatic proposal.

Although we may not easily achieve reduction of sodium intake in normals, we do have enough data for its use as part of first step management of the hypertensive patient. Diminished sodium intake is an important part of the non-pharmacological approach to the management of hypertension and is a behaviorally oriented therapy. In addition to being a first step in management, it applies perhaps even more particularly when the patient is then put on a diuretic, since reduction of sodium intake does result in a lesser incidence of hypo-kalemia, which is one of the side effects of diuretics.

2. Weight Control

Obesity is another cultural and behavioral phenomenon which plays a role in hypertension. No one knows why the prevalence of hypertension is higher in the obese patient. Some have thought it is merely related to the excess sodium intake which occurs in such patients but several recent studies have demonstrated that weight loss without sodium restriction will result in significant decrease in blood pressure (Ramsay, Ramsay, Hettiarachchi, Davies, & Winchester, 1978; Reisen, Abel, Modan, Silverberg, Eliahow, & Modan, 1978). Again weight reduction is an important behavioral method of managing high blood pressure representing a non-pharmacological approach to at least the mild hypertensive and certainly a supplemental way of managing all hypertensives.

PHYSICAL EXERCISE

The effects of exercise on the cardiovascular system constitute a huge literature but relatively little of it is concerned with the specific therapeutic benefits of exercise in hypertensive patients. From the standpoint of their hemodrynamic patterns, there are basically two types of exercise, *isometric* and *isotonic*.

Exercise that causes skeletal muscles to change in length with little change in tension is termed isotonic (dynamic), whereas isometric (static) exercise involves change in muscle tension with little change in length. Both types have been suggested for controlling hypertension, although their short-term hemodynamic effects are sharply different. Isotonic exercise increases heart rate and cariac output and can produce peripheral vasodilation because of the large increase in muscle flow. Systolic blood pressure rises but diastolic usually does not, and may in fact, decline, and consequently mean blood pressure is only slightly elevated. On the other hand, isometric exercise, even involving a small number of muscles, results in small increases in cardiac output but may cause large increases in peripheral resistance and mean blood pressure. Most exercise is not purely isotonic or isometric but a mixture of both. Such activities as walking, running, cycling, swimming, and rhythmic calisthenics are primarily dynamic, whereas lifting or pushing heavy weights and contracting muscles against fixed objects are static (Mitchell & Wildenthal, 1974).

In view of these different patterns, it is clear that theoretically isometric exercises are not likely to be of long-term value to the hypertensive while the sudden surge of blood pressure acutely can be potentially harmful. On the other hand, a few investigations of the long-term effects of isotonic exercise have suggested a significant fall in blood pressure in hypertensives (Mitchell & Wildenthal, 1974, Boyer & Kasch, 1970; Sannerstedt, Wasir, Henning, & Werko, 1973). Certainly in mild to moderate hypertensives, isotonic exercise is unlikely to be harmful and can be encouraged. However, controlled studies of supervised and graded isotonic exercise in various types of hypertensives in different age groups are necessary. Moreover, the effects of pharmacologic agents on exercise response, particularly in the fixed and more severe hypertensives, need further evaluation. A recent study by Lee et al. has looked at this pattern in fifteen moderate hypertensives, five of whom had cardiac hypertrophy, and demonstrated some dampening of the acute systolic response to running on a treadmill when the patients were on hydrochlorothiazide or alpha methyl dopa, without impairment of exercise capacity (Lee, Fox, & Slotkoff, 1979). These are encouraging data but obviously do not answer questions about long-term effects.

It should also be pointed out that regardless of its hemodynamic effects, exercise is an important factor in weight control and needs to be part of any successful program to achieve this goal in the hypertensive patient. Moreover, most individuals who exercise regularly achieve a general sense of well-being which may impart certain of the beneficial aspects of relaxation or other behavioral therapies. For example, Blumenthal and co-workers have recently shown a decrease of Type A behavioral scores in a group of individuals undertaking a supervised exercise program (Blumenthal, Williams, Williams, & Wallace, 1980).

BEHAVIORAL MODIFICATION

The use of behavioral techniques to lower blood pressure in hypertensive patients derives from the hypothesis that emotional and behavioral stimuli stemming from the individual's environment have been factors in the development and/or maintenance of the hypertensive state. That such stimuli stress the organism in a variety of ways is clearly evident and the concept that hypertension is one of a number of "diseases of stress" has been argued about for many years. The concept of stress diseases, however, has ceased to have scientific or even heuristic value but the word "stress" in its original engineering meaning of the reaction of a substrate to a stimulus, does have some value and is a convenient term to use. We employ it from time to time in our further discussion, both as a verb and a noun, to specifically mean those reactions of the blood pressure which are induced by stimuli of behavioral origin.

The validity of the concept that stress plays a role in hypertension is supported by anecdotal clinical experiences and by experimental studies in animals and man which we have reviewed in previous publications (Shapiro, 1960, 1972, 1982). However, the precise and quantitative nature of the impact of stress and the manner which it integrates with other stimuli, in the production and maintenance of hypertension, remains elusive. Reasons include problems in quantifying the effect of behavioral stimuli, the retrospective nature of most case analyses, and the difficulty in preventing such stimuli or controlling them in an experimental context. Moreover, because of its individualistic nature, a given stimulus to a subject may seem ephemeral to the observer, while acute changes observed in blood pressure fail to establish whether chronic disease can be produced. Nevertheless, although stress, in common with most other causal mechanisms in hypertension, rarely provides a single explanation for the disease, the available evidence has increasingly documented that the effects of behavioral change must be considered seriously among the variables which combine to explain the pathogenesis of this multifactorial disorder.

It should be understood that the primary mechanism involved in production of an effect on blood pressure by noxious stimuli of behavioral origin is neural and that the brain and central nervous sytem (CNS) play the role of the perceptive organs in mediating their impact. Yet is should also be clear that the CNS in turn operates through peripheral mechanisms which include renal, hormonal, and cardiovascular pathways. Similarly, the peripheral mechanisms can influence the brain and behavior so that in a very literal sense the behavioral components in hypertension are not unique, but parts of a finely tuned system whose disharmonies evoke hypertensive disease.

Behavioral modification as a therapeutic modality to alleviate the stress-induced components of hypertension has been a practice of therapists dating to well before the era of pharmacologically active antihypertensive agents. We treated the disease often with "a pill and a prayer," the *pill* being usually a mild sedative such as phenobarbital, and the *prayer,* the reassurance, to patient and physician, that the disease was asymptomatic and only slowly progressive. More specific psychotherapeutic techniques were used as well, but in the past decade, there has been a considerable resurgence of interest following the development of more specific ways to get at the aforementioned perceptive organs, i.e. the brain and the CNS. Among these are the application of instrumental or operant conditioning procedures which has demonstrated that animals and humans can learn to voluntarily regulate their pressure when provided with appropriate biofeedback and rewards for blood pressure change. Studies by DiCara and Miller (1968), Benson, Herd, Morse, and Kelleher (1969), and Harris, Gilliam, Findley, and Brady (1973) in animals demonstrated that selective regulation of various cardiovascular parameters can be achieved with operant conditioning precedures. The conditioning procedures can produce learned increases and decreases in blood pressure.

Animals can be taught to generate acute elevations of pressure in the hypertensive range using appropriate schedules of feedback and reward for increases in pressure (Benson et al., 1969; DiCara & Miller, 1968). When procedures are applied to decreases in pressure, return of blood pressure to normotensive values can be achieved (Benson et al., 1969). Although some of the basic data in animals is in dispute, they provide a foundation for the potential use of biofeedback and reward procedures in the treatment of hypertension, but many questions regarding optimal behavioral procedures for producing the effects, central and peripheral mechanisms by which they are mediated, and individual differences in response remain (Shapiro, Schwartz, Ferguson, Redmond, & Weiss, 1977).

Human subjects can be trained to voluntarily increase or decrease their systolic blood pressure with biofeedback and reward (Schwartz, 1972, 1977) and under appropriate conditions of feedback and instructions, changes in blood pressure can be produced without corresponding changes in heart rate (Schwartz, 1972). Conversely, selective increase or decrease in heart rate with feedback and reward, without corresponding changes in pressure can be produced (Schwartz, 1972; D. Shapiro, Mainardi, & Surwit, 1977).

The clinical utility of biofeedback/conditioning procedures in developing a therapeutic plan for management of hypertension will be discussed later. For the present discussion, the application of these procedures to elucidate the CNS and peripheral mechanisms by which behavioral stimuli influence the regulation of blood pressures deserves comment. Schwartz (1977) has described how biofeedback interacts with the specific instructions given to subjects, leading to regulation of different patterns of CNS processes in the control of heart rate. The application of patterned biofeedback procedures for training subjects to regulate combinations of CNS and cardiovascular processes provides a research strategy for uncovering linkages or disharmonies between physiological systems.

We have recently reviewed the literature on methods of behavioral modification, including the older observations of psychotherapy, suggestion, the use of placebos, and environmental modification, as well as recent attempts at biofeedback and relaxation therapies (Shapiro et al., 1977). These data need not be repeated here but will be summarized and brought up to date. For many years, psychotherapy, both supportive and analytic, has been used both formally and informally in the management of hypertension and is capable of producing modest changes in blood pressure. As mentioned earlier, it was in fact the mainstay in treating hypertension prior to the present drug era. Patients were reassured and levels of blood pressure per se were deemphasized, and when relaxation could be achieved by sedatives, these frequently were utilized. Placebo effects of pharmacologically non-specific agents were frequently evident; these are readily recognized whenever new drugs are introduced in the management of hypertension and their control by the use of double-blind techniques has been one of the accomplishments of the modern clinical pharmacologist. Environmental modification,—including job change, domestic and marital rearrangements, hospitalization, rest therapy, etc.—has been applied for years by clinicians who can provide considerable anecdotal data as to their value.

In this context, the recent work with *biofeedback* and *relaxation* techniques represented a methodological rather than a theoretical advance. *Biofeedback* uses instrumentation to provide moment-to-moment information to a patient about a specific physiologic process that is under control of the nervous system but is not clearly or accurately otherwise perceived by the patient. *Relaxation* therapies are techniques to elicit physical and emotional calmness in order to decrease sympathetic arousal and so lower blood pressure. Through 1977, the reported data for each of these methods, when carefully examined in our review by the same standard that one would use for clinical pharmacologic study of a new drug for hypertension, were mostly of the Phase I type (i.e. small numbers of subjects studied in relatively short-term treatment situations). Phase II studies (controlled trials with comparison with known effective agents) were sparse. The Phase I studies indicated blood pressure effects with all techniques that are relatively similar, namely, declines ranging from 5 to 25 mmHg of mean blood pressure (MBP) with minimal data about the duration of these effects and their relationships to the use of pharmacologic agents. There was considerable variability among individual patients and any apparent difference in the effects resulting from the different approaches could not be assessed because of the paucity of Phase II trials. The major differences between the methods are the ease with which they can be utilized by particular individuals.

Biofeedback and relaxation techniques are of special interest because they represent fresh approaches to phenomena previously not subject to precise measurement. They have provided valuable paradigms stimulating investigators and clinicians to look more seriously at the behavioral influences of hypertension, to develop methods of utilizing these treatment possibilities more precisely and more consistently, and to teach them to health professionals and to patients. The common theme that runs through all of the non-pharmacologic behavioral approaches is that most of the disordered mechanisms of blood pressure regulation in hypertension are to some extent under the control of the central nervous system and thus subject to influence of behavioral stimuli. To the extent that the various behavioral treatments counteract pressor stimuli operating through these various mechanisms, particularly the autonomic nervous system, blood pressure can be lowered, which is why the apparently different types of behavioral treatment produce essentially similar results. In brief, they all try to ameliorate the psychic stress factors, thereby lowering blood pressure. (Fig. 9.1).

In our review we emphasized that Phase II studies comparing the effects of biofeedback and relaxation to each other, as well as to placebo and to pharmacologic modes of therapy, were necessary. Such studies need not be aimed at

RANGES OF REPORTED DEPRESSOR EFFECTS

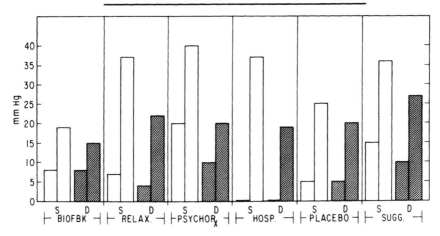

FIG. 9.1 Indicates the range of reported depressor effects on blood pressure of different behavioral methods of therapy of hypertension: BIOFBK, biofeedback, RELAX, relaxation; PSYCHORX, psychotherapy; HOSP, hospitalization; PLACEBO, placebo; SUGG, suggestion. The white bars indicate the lowest and highest falls in systolic, and the striped bars the lowest and highest falls in diastolic for each method. These data have been gathered from reports in the literature (Shapiro et al., 1977).

"either - or" hypotheses, but should look at the abilities of different therapies to complement and/or supplement each other. This is in keeping with the concept we have mentioned earlier that rational therapy of hypertension often requires several treatment modalities simultaneously to get at the different mechanisms involved in the ailment. We urged the pursuit of further information on the carry-over effects of behavioral treatment once the patient had left the laboratory as well as study of the ultimate outcomes up to a year or more after institution of the procedures in this lifelong disorder. Compliance with behavioral therapy is another unexplored issue; such therapies involve more patient involvement than merely taking a pill and motivation for the long haul needs study. Side effects of behavioral therapy can also occur; failure to achieve results can be frustrating and depressing and possible neglect of pharmacological therapies of known effectiveness in an effort to produce results by non-pharmacologic means must be avoided. Finally, we can only speculate about the central and peripheral mechanisms involved in self-regulation of blood pressure. Data suggest that changes in muscle tension and respiration may contribute, but these are not believed to be the sole mechanisms (Schwartz & D. Shapiro, 1973). Since blood pressure is the outcome of the relationship between cardiac output and peripheral resistance, it is apparent that in both biofeedback and relaxation, changes in heart rate, stroke volume, and peripheral resistance may be differentially involved, with the exact details as yet to be specified.

Since our review was prepared, a number of comparative studies have appeared which provide answers to some of the above questions. Surwit and D. Shapiro compared cardiovascular feedback, muscular feedback and relaxation in three groups of eight patients each with borderline hypertension. They showed a modest decline in blood pressure in all three groups, but no significant differences between the three techniques (Surwit, D. Shapiro, & Good, 1978). Taylor et al. studied 31 patients with well-established hypertension, receiving medical therapy which continued throughout the study, and divided them into three groups receiving relaxation therapy, non-specific supportive phychotherapy, and medical therapy only, respectively. At the end of 8 weeks the group receiving relaxation declined an additional 12/5 mmHg, while the medical treatment group was unchanged and the non-specific therapy group fell only 3/2 mmHg. At the end of 6 months, the relaxation group had maintained their decline, but the other two groups had "caught up" to them and significant differences were no longer present (Taylor, Farquhar, Nelson, & Agras, 1977). Frankel and co-workers conducted a 16-week trial in 22 patients divided into three groups; (1) diastolic blood pressure feedback accompanied by EMG feedback and verbal relaxation; (2) sham blood pressure feedback; (3) no treatment; after 16 weeks, 7 patients from groups 2 and 3 crossed over to active treatment as in group 1. Little or no change in blood pressure which carried over outside the laboratory was shown in any of these three groups (Frankel, Patel, Horovitz, Friedewald, & Bardner, 1978). Franklin et al. have recently provided a review of the literature specifically comparing feedback methods to various types of relaxation techniques and conclude that the latter show considerably more promise. However, these authors too suggest their use only as additions to "traditional pharmacologic therapy," except perhaps in borderline hypertensives "reluctant to accept an indefinite course of pharmacologic therapy" (Franklin, Nathan, Prout, & Cohen, 1978).

In brief then, behavioral techniques for therapy *should not* be presented to patients as alternatives to pharmacologic therapy, just as the development of potent antihypertensive drugs did not eliminate the need for understanding and managing the psychologic problems of patients. Primarily, they should be regarded as *supplements* to other therapy, although, as with reduced sodium intake, their use sometimes can delay the institution of drugs if goals are being achieved, as long as the patient is under the supervision of knowledgeable health care providers. All patients should be introduced to some type of behavioral therapy; for most of them, the behavioral approach will continue to consist of support and reassurance in the traditional sense, although guided by the new insights of recent studies. Specific patients can be taught relaxation techniques. Transcendental meditation and some of the more exotic relaxation techniques are not easily accepted by most people or physicians, but simple relaxation methods have been described that can be taught by most practitioners (Benson, 1975). Biofeedback methods are less readily available to most practicing physicians. Biofeedback may have its major application in research strategies directed at eliciting specific pathways of CNS response to stress.

To sum up, reassurance and supportive psychotherapy to assist the patient to adjust his life style are valuable adjuncts to the management of hypertension. The development of biofeedback and relaxation techniques offer the opportunity to achieve amelioration of psychic stress by methods in some ways more applicable to certain patients than conventional psychotherapy. However, none of the techniques is sufficiently advanced to recommend its widespread and uncritical application to the treatment of high blood pressure. Nevertheless, continuing study of long-term effects and careful comparison in cooperative studies of behavioral and pharmacologic influences in essential hypertension continue to be worthwhile.

COMPLIANCE

Behavioral therapies also have application to the difficult task of persuading the patient without symptoms to undertake therapy, perhaps for a lifetime, and remain subject to potential side effects, or at least considerable inconvenience, expense, and anxiety. This problem has led to a new area of investigation, that of *compliance* with physician recommendations. A number of studies have been performed that indicate that compliance is not accomplished simply by educating the patient to the evils of hypertension, but it is best achieved when the patient has been made a participant in his management and exposed to reward systems (Haynes, Gibson, Hackett, Sackett, Taylor, Roberts, Johnson, 1976; Sackett, Gibson, Taylor, Haynes, Hackett, Roberts & Johnson, 1975). In some patients, this includes instruction as to how to take blood pressure, but in others this procedure can be a source of considerable anxiety and unnecessary compulsiveness. The danger of the patient manipulating his own drugs or his own overall therapy are also possibilities in this situation and we hesitate to recommend it as a general procedure.

Our own practice is to try to educate a patient about what elevated blood pressure means, what potential there is for complications, and what he needs to do to lessen these possibilities by taking appropriate drugs as well as instituting other life style manipulations. At the same time, one should offer reassurance that life will by and large be normal for the patient and, particularly for the young hypertensive, that time is on his side, since secondary changes take many years to develop. Most of all, we emphasize that treating hypertension is practicing preventive medicine rather than crisis medicine; it is important for the patient to recognize that treatment is to ''prevent his getting sick,'' not because he is sick. Current widespread dissemination of information about hypertension and its potential threats is double-edged. On one hand, it has made the public considerably more aware of the disease and the need for its management; on the other hand, in some individuals it has caused considerable anxiety and feelings of doom. In fact, in some studies, labeling a patient as hypertensive without introducing a support system has led to increased job absenteism. It is an important task to accomplish our goals without potentiating such discomfort and "disease" in the patient and in this context the behavioral considerations may have their most important application.

REFERENCES

Benson, H. *The relaxation response.* New York: William Morrow, 1975.

Benson, H., Herd, J. A., Morse, W. H., & Kelleher, R. T. Behavioral induction of arterial hypertension and its reversal. *American Journal of Physiology,* 1969, *217,* 30–34.

Bianchi, G., Fox, V., Francesco, G. F., Giovanetti, A. M., & Pagetti, D. Blood pressure changes produced by kidney cross-transplantation between spontaneously hypertensive rats and normotensive rats. *Clinical Science and Molecular Medicine,* 1974, *47,* 435–441.

Blumenthal, J. A., Williams, R. S., Williams, R. B., & Wallace, A. G. Effects of exercise on the Type A (coronary prone) behavior patterns. *Psychosomatic Medicine,* 1980, *41,* 583A.

Boyer, J. L. & Kasch, F. S. Exercise therapy in hypertensive men. *Journal of American Medical Association,* 1970, *211,* 1668–1671.

Bruenn, H. Clinical notes on the illness and death of President Franklin D. Roosevelt. *Annals of Internal Medicine,* 1970, *72,* 579–585.

Capelli, J. P., Wesson, L. G., & Aponte, G. E. A phylogenetic study of the renin-angiotensin system. *American Journal of Physiology,* 1970, *218,* 1171–1178.

Cassel, J. Hypertension and cardiovascular disease in migrants: A potential source of clues? *International Journal of Epidemiology,* 1974, *3,* 204–210.

Dahl, L. K. Effects of chronic excess salt feeding: Induction of self-sustaining hypertension in rats. *Journal of Experimental Medicine,* 1961, *114,* 231–237.

Denton, D. A. Evolutionary aspects of the emergence of aldosterone secretion and salt appetite. *Physiological Reviews,* 1965, *45,* 245–260.

DiCara, L. B. & Miller, N. E. Instrumental learning of SBP responses by curarized rats: Dissociation of cardiac and vascular changes. *Psychosomatic Medicine,* 1968, *30,* 489–494.

Frankel, B. L., Patel, D. J., Horowitz, D., Friedewald, W. T., & Bardner, K. Treatment of hypertension with biofeedback and relaxation techniques. *Psychosomatic Medicine,* 1978, *40,* 276–293.

Franklin, K., Nathan, R. J., Prout, M. F., & Cohen, M. Non-pharmacologic control of essential hypertension in man: a critical review of the experimental literature. *Psychosomatic Medicine,* 1978, *40,* 294–320.

Freis, E. Salt volume and the prevention of hypertension. *Circulation,* 1976, *53,* 541–589.

Freis, E. (Chairman) et al. Veterans Administration Cooperative Study Group on Antihypertensive Agents. Effects of treatment on mobidity in hypertension. II. Results in patients with diastolic blood pressure of 90 through 114 mmHg. *Journal of American Medical Association,* 1970, *242,* 1143–1152.

Friedman, S. M. & Friedman, C. L. Cell permeability, sodium transport and the hypertensive process in the rat. *Circulation Research,* 1976, *39,* 433–437.

Harris, A. H., Gilliam, W. J., Findley, J. D., & Brady, J. Instrumental conditioning of large-magnitude daily 12-hour blood pressure evaluations in the baboon. *Science,* 1973, *182,* 175–177.

Haynes, R. B., Gibson, E. S., Hackett, B. C., Sackett, D. L., Taylor, D. W., Roberts, R. S., & Johnson, A. L. Improvement of medication compliance in uncontrolled hypertension. *Lancet,* 1976, *1,* 1265–1268.

Henry, J. P. & Stephens, P. M. *Stress, health and the social environment.* New York: Springer-Verlag, 1977.

Hypertension Detection and Follow-up Program Cooperative Group. Five-year findings of the Hypertension Detection and Follow-up Program. I. Reduction in mortality of persons with high blood pressure, including mild hypertension. *Journal of American Medical Association,* 1979(a), *242,* 2562–2571.

Hypertension Detection and Follow-up Program Cooperative Group. Five-year findings of the Hypertension Detection and Follow-up Program. II. Mortality by race-sex and age. *Journal of American Medical Association,* 1979(b), *242,* 2572–2477.

Kawasaki, T., Delea, C., Bartter, F., & Smith, H. The effect of high-sodium and low-sodium intakes on blood pressure and other related variables in human subjects with idiopathic hypertension. *American Journal of Medicine,* 1978, *64,* 193–198.

Langford, H. G., Watson, R. L., & Thomas, J. G. Salt intake and the treatment of hypertension. *American Heart Journal,* 1977, *93,* 531–535.

Lee, W. R., Fox, L., & Slotkoff, L. M. Effects of anti-hypertensive therapy on cardiovascular response to exercise. *American Journal of Cardiology,* 1979, *44,* 325–328.

Luft, F., Bloch, R., Weyman, A., Murray, Z., & Weinberger, M. Cardiovascular responses to extremes of salt intake in man. *Clinical Research,* 1978, *26,* 265A.

Meneely, G. R. & Ball, C. O. Experimental epidemiology of chronic toxicity and the protective effect of potassium chloride. *American Journal of Medicine,* 1958, *25,* 713–725.

Mitchell, J. H. & Wildenthal, L. Static (isometric) exercise and the heart: Physiological and clinical considerations. *Annual Review of Medicine,* 1974, *25,* 369–381.

Morgan, T., Gillies, A., Morgan, G., Adam, W., Wilson, M., & Carney, S. Hypertension treated by salt restriction. *Lancet,* 1978, *1,* 227–230.

Oliver, W. J., Cohen, E. L., & Neel, J. V. Blood pressure, sodium intake and sodium related hormones in the Yanomano Indians. *Circulation,* 1975, *52,* 146–150.

Page, L., Danion, A., & Moellering, R. C., Jr. Antecedents of cardiovascular disease in six Solomon Island societies. *Circulation,* 1970, *49,* 1132–1140.

Parijs, J., Joossens, J. V., Van der Linden, L., Verstreken, G., & Amer, A. K. Moderate sodium restriction and diuretics in the treatment of hypertension. *American Heart Journal,* 1973, *85,* 22–25.

Ramsay, L. E., Ramsay, M. H., Hettiarachchi, J., Davies, D. L., & Winchester, J. Weight reduction in a blood pressure clinic. *British Medical Journal,* 1978, *2,* 244–246.

Reisin, E., Abel, R., Modan, M., Silverberg, D. S., Eliahow, H. E., & Modan, B. Effect of weight loss without salt restriction on the reduction of blood pressure. *New England Journal of Medicine.* 1978, *298,* 1–4.

Rogers, D. Presidential Address: On technologic restraint. *Transactions of the Association of American Physicans,* 1975, *88,* 1–9.

Sackett, D. L., Gibson, E. S., Taylor, D. W., Haynes, R. B., Hackett, B. C. Roberts, R. S., & Johnson, A. L. Randomised clinical trial of strategies for improving medication compliance in primary hypertension. *Lancet,* 1975, *1,* 1205–1207.

Sannerstedt, R., Wasir, H., Henning, R., & Werko, L. Systemic haemodynamics in mild arterial hypertension before and after physical training. *Clinical Science and Molecular Medicine,* 1973, *45,* 145–149.

Schwartz, G. E. Biofeedback and patterning of autonomic and central processes: CNS-cardiovascular interactions. In G. E. Schwartz & J. Beatty (Eds.), *Biofeedback: Theory and research.* New York: Academic Press, 1977.

Schwartz, G. E. Voluntary control of human cardiovascular integration and differentiation through feedback and reward. *Science*, 1972, *175*, 90–93.

Schwartz, G. E. & Shapiro, D. Biofeedback and essential hypertension: Current findings and theoretical concerns. In L. Birk (Ed.), *Biofeedback: Behavioral medicine*. New York: Grune and Stratton, 1973.

Shapiro, A. P. Stress and hypertension. In H. Gavras & H. R. Brunner (Eds.), *Clinical hypertension and hypotension*. New York: Marcell Dekker, pp. 367–386, 1982.

Shapiro, A. P. Behavioral approach to the study of cardiovascular disease in man: in neural and psychological mechanisms in cardiovascular disease. In A. Zanchetti (Ed.), *Symposium of the International Society of Cardiology and the WHO*, Stressa, Italy, July, 1971). Milan: Casa Editrice, 1972.

Shapiro, A. P. Psychophysiologic pressor mechanisms in hypertensive vascular disease. *Annals of Internal Medicine*, 1960, *53*, 64–83.

Shapiro, A. P., Schwartz, G. E., Ferguson, D. C. E., Redmond, D. P., & Weiss, S. M. Behavioral methods in the treatment of hypertension. I. Review of their clinical status. *Annals of Internal Medicine*. 1977, *86*, 626–636.

Shapiro, D., Mainardi, J. A., & Surwit, R. S. Biofeedback and self-regulation in essential hypertension. In G. E. Schwartz & J. Beatty (Eds.), *Biofeedback: Theory and research*. New York: Academic Press, 1977.

Smith, W. Mc. Treatment of mild hypertension. Results of a 10-year intervention trial. U.S.P.H.S. Cooperative Study Group. *Circulation Research*, 1977, *40*, 98–105.

Surwit, R. S., Shapiro, D., & Good, M. I. Cardiovascular biofeedback, muscular activity biofeedback, and meditation-relaxation in border-line essential hypertensives. *Journal of Consulting and Clinical Psychology*, 1978, *46*, 252–263.

Taylor, C. B., Farquhar, J. N., Nelson, E., & Agras, S. Relaxation therapy and high blood pressure. *Archives of Clinical Psychology*, 1977, *34*, 339–342.

Tobian, L. A viewpoint concerning the enigma of hypertension. *American Journal of Medicine*, 1972, *52*, 595–609.

Waldron, I. A quantative analysis of cross cultural variation in blood pressure and serum cholesterol. *Psychosomatic Medicine*, 1980, *41*, 582A.

10 Recovery and Rehabilitation of Heart Patients: Psychosocial Aspects

Sydney H. Croog
University of Connecticut Health Center

> *My heart attack of 1955 seemed well behind me, but I was conscious that it was part of the background of my life—just as I was conscious of my family's history of stroke and heart disease. I did not fear death so much as I feared disability. Whenever I walked through the Red Room and saw the portrait of Woodrow Wilson hanging there, I thought of him stretched out upstairs in the White House, powerless to move, with the machinery of the American Government in disarray around him. And I remembered Grandmother Johnson who had had a stroke and stayed in a wheelchair throughout my childhood, unable even to move her hands or to speak so that she could be understood.*
>
> —Lyndon B. Johnson,
> *The Vantage Point: Perspectives of the Presidency, 1963–1969, 1971.*

This quotation from a former President sets forth some of the troubling issues which are common to heart patients from many segments of society. Many are familiar with similar concerns implicit in President Johnson's words: a pressing uncertainty about the future, awareness that the heart attack may happen again, anxiety about the degenerative and disabling process, and possibly feelings of helplessness before the elements of genetic predisposition and of environmental and internal factors beyond one's personal control.

As heart disease is pervasive throughout the world, persons who have experienced heart attacks are legion, particularly in industrialized, western societies.

295

Yet until recently the social and psychological components which help determine the recovery and rehabilitation experience of heart patients have received comparatively little systematic research attention, as compared with the emphasis on the etiology of the illness, its physical process, and on biochemical and surgical therapies.

This chapter reviews some directions of research and principal issues relating to psychosocial aspects of long-term recovery and rehabilitation. Our focus is primarily upon the post-hospital experience of the heart patient, following treatment for myocardial infarction. It centers on a series of life areas: work, family, the doctor-patient relationship, community organizations and facilities, as well as upon some of the social and emotional processes of adjustment. As numerous reviews of the literature on psychosocial factors in cardiac rehabilitation have appeared in recent years, there seems little need for a resummation at present. (See for example, Croog, 1978; Croog, Levine & Lurie, 1968; Doehrman, 1977; Garrity, 1979; Gulledge, 1979; Hackett & Rosenbaum, 1980; and Krantz, 1980). Our purpose is to point up features of some principal, interrelated elements influencing long-term outcomes and living with chronic heart disease. Our secondary aim is to review some gaps in information on primary topics and to underline areas which require further research.

Recovery and Living with Chronic Illness: Frame of Reference

As one means of focusing on issues in long-term recovery and rehabilitation, we employ the notion of "armory of resources" as a framework for organizing the approach (Croog & Levine, 1977, 1982). This armory may be visualized as the total array of available social, psychological, institutional and community resources upon which the individual may draw to cope with problems. Its scope may be illustrated in terms of three levels: (1) *individual* resources, such as personality defense mechanisms and physical status; (2) resources that derive from *larger social or institutional structures,* such as family, church, work and friendship networks; and (3) community resources which consist of such *formal organizational systems* as hospitals, rehabilitation clinics, the physician-medical care network, and federal and local agencies that provide income maintenance programs and other services.

These resources may be used in ways which promote recovery and adaptation to living with the heart disease, and some have variously been described in their constructive applications as social supports, psychosocial assets, coping mechanisms, defenses and coping aids (Caplan & Killilea, 1976; Dunbar, 1948; Kaplan, Cassel, & Gore, 1977; Nuckolls, Cassel & Kaplan, 1972; Smith, 1979). In our use here, we refer to them as resources, potentially available, potentially constructive—but not necessarily so. Our analytic approach is directed (1) to review ways in which they operate, both positively and negatively, and (2) to examine the complex ways in which they serve as supports and/or barriers—an open empirical issue as far as recovery from heart disease is concerned.

For purpose of illustration, some of the various resources can be visualized in terms of simple models, showing their inter-relationships at differing time points in the illness career of the patient. For the post-hospital patient in the chronic phase of the illness, the model of the organization of the resources differs from that often employed in discussion of the critical acute period of myocardial infarction. In the first stages of the illness, particularly in western industrialized societies, the patient and the physician are often conceived of as a "team", working together in dealing with the illness. The physician has resources for making referrals and/or calling upon other personnel, such as nurses, social workers, clergy, agencies, family members, and employers in aiding the patient in initial adjustments. This classic model, reflected in textbooks on coronary care and in medical school instruction, is depicted in Figure 10.1. It is widely accepted by patients as appropriate.

While the model is simplified for our illustrative purposes, it points up the central role of patient and physician in relation to treatment and recovery in the acute phase.

Figure 10.2 portrays the model more commonly characteristic of the long-term post-hospital career of the heart patient in the recovery and chronic stages of the illness. Here the patient is at the center, surrounded by an array of potential resources, as illustrated in some selected examples. The physician is but one component of the array, and the individual may be typically engaged in a complex series of inter-relationships with individuals, groups, and/organizations in each resource area. Further, the resource areas themselves interact, and such interactions ultimately influence the patient in one way or another in this model. For the sake of clarity, we have largely omitted the many arrows indicating this interaction of resource areas.

The model serves to illustrate here the complexity of the interacting systems and resources. It also provides some cues to the difficulties of research in this area—particularly that which attempts to link morbidity or mortality outcomes with the various sets of interaction systems with which the patient is involved.

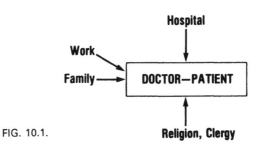

FIG. 10.1.

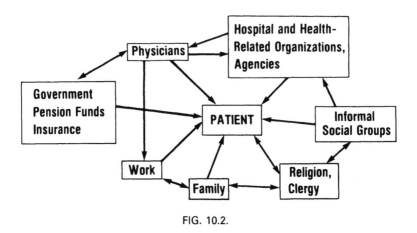

FIG. 10.2.

With this second model as guide, we can proceed to examine selected elements within some principal resource areas.

WORK AND THE HEART PATIENT

Return to Work

As a principal human activity, the multiple functions and meanings of work have long been recognized in terms of their economic, psychological, social status, and emotional aspects. For the heart patient, however, work has special meanings, symbolizing a degree of functional capacity and competence.

For many patients, "return to work" after a heart attack represents return to normal activity after serious illness. In the research literature on recovery of male coronary patients, the single variable "return to work" serves often also as an important measure of rehabilitation. In fact, in recent years this variable has often been used as a more general measure of "quality of life" in related areas of recovery after cardiac surgery. In such studies, the operational assumption is that "return to work" is correlated with a series of positive ratings in other important areas of life.

In regard to work return after myocardial infarction, a broad series of variables have been identified as associated with such aspects as rate of return, proportion of patients changing their place of employment, or altering the work load and responsibilities. The array of studies which contribute to this general picture has been often reviewed, and they need not be recapitulated here in detail. (See Croog, Levine, & Lurie, 1968; Doehrman, 1977; Garrity, 1973, 1979, among others.)

Among these varied studies, there is general agreement that a high proportion of men return to work after a heart attack although the percentages differ according to such factors as geographic setting, characteristics of the study population, and methods of the research. Occupational type, educational level, age, health status, and psychological factors are among the variables which have been frequently found to be associated with rates of work return (Nagle, Gangola, & Picton-Robinson, 1971; Shapiro, Weinblatt, & Frank, 1972). In general, men with higher educational status, in professional and executive occupations, with more favorable cardiac status, and high morale, have a more favorable record in rate of return than do men with minimal education, blue-collar occupations, unfavorable cardiac status, and low morale. The age differential is also important, particularly for older workers. As might be expected, older men nearing retirement age are more likely to leave the work force, reduce their hours, or make other adaptations in their jobs after a heart attack.

Work Activity, Stress, and Health

In contrast to the substantial empirical effort devoted to work return, strikingly little attention has been given to systematic examination of the relationship of work activity and long-term recovery and rehabilitation of the heart patient. The day-to-day experiences in differing types of work and their effects in various physical, social, and psychological dimensions have important influences on the health and the adjustment of heart patients (Hackett & Cassem, 1976; Naughton, 1978; Paffenbarger, Laughlin, Gima, & Black, 1970). But the relationship of work activities to both physical status and psychosocial adjustment remains documented mainly by clinical reports and anecdotal accounts, rather than by more systematic research efforts.

The recent efflorescence of research on stress and health presents a new array of methods and conceptual tools for assessing key issues in this important area in the life of the heart patient. For example, the role of work stress in etiology of heart disease remains unresolved, although some studies report suggestive relationships (Caplan, Cobb, French, Harrison, & Pinneau, 1975; House, 1975). How work stress may relate to recurrences of the acute phase of myocardial infarction is even less clear. Of course, it cannot be assumed that the factors important in the initial development of heart disease are the same as those responsible for recurrences of heart attacks. Nevertheless, numerous clues concerning the role of work stress can be forthcoming with properly designed research on the recovering, rehabilitating heart patient in the work place.

The issue of work stress has practical importance and policy implications, of course, extending beyond its contributions to theories of stress and health. Discriminatory policies of some employers, both overt and covert, are predicated on beliefs and assumptions regarding work stress and heart disease, and the issue persists in workmen's compensation questions (American Jurisprudence, 1966; Hellmuth, 1970; National Commission on State Workmen's Compensation Laws, 1973). One study points out that as many as 86 percent of heart patients blamed emotional and/or physical stress at work as a cause of their heart disease, one year after a first heart attack. Seven years later, 76 percent of the employed survivors continued to hold such beliefs (Croog & Levine, 1977, 1982). "Heart Laws" in a series of states assume that heart disease in policemen and firemen is the product of job stresses (Brush, 1981). The diffusion of such regulations has important economic implications, adding to the costs of pension funds and damage awards.

Other issues relate to the more positive influences of work on health. For example, in what ways does work promote long-term recovery after the acute phases of the illness? Under what conditions do different types of peer relationships, or physical and emotional demands enhance the health status of patients? Among men with equal degree of cardiac damage, does more satisfying and challenging work experience improve survival chances and reduce morbidity? In what ways do creative and satisfying occupational demands offset the physical limitations which may be associated with coronary disease in some patients? Or, obversely, does work dissatisfaction among heart patients serve to exacerbate the negative effects of the illness and increase morbidity, impair functioning, and reduce survival chances?

In considerations of the positive role of work in relation to recovery and rehabilitation of heart patients, such variables as work satisfaction, occupational adjustment, morale at work and similar elements have been shown to be important. Some underlying features of the work situation have relevance also, though they are perhaps more characteristic of social systems in general than of the particular work setting in which the patient is employed. These include the degree of social integration of the patient into the informal system, degree of power and authority, the emotional tone of the work setting, the valuation of the person's occupational skills and current demand for them in the economic system. Such elements as these may be powerful factors in determining the kind of support for—or the barriers against—continuing his or her career in the work setting. They may not be reflected in indices of work satisfaction or work adjustment which are commonly used.

The effects on health of subtle barriers and supports at work may be difficult to assess. Consider one example from the case history of a 55-year-old clerical worker in a small company who had a heart attack several months previously.

The physician instructed the patient that he could carry out all usual activities, except, "Avoid lifting". "Don't pick up heavy boxes at the office." In the first weeks of work return, he finds a sympathetic attitude among co-workers and pleasant relationships. As the occasion arises, he calls upon one or another to lift heavy boxes for him. Co-workers assist him, most willingly, in the first days after his return to work. Eventually, the tone in the office changes, and resentment stirs among those who are called upon to interrupt their own work and lift the occasional heavy boxes. The character of his informal associations alters, and he begins to have the feeling of becoming an outsider. Yet he has received doctor's orders on lifting, and he is unwilling to risk his health or his life by picking up boxes.

Occasional mild chest pain and shortness of breath remind him that he is not the man he used to be. One day he asks a fellow worker to lift a box for him. The response comes, "Why don't you go ahead and drop dead, you lazy son-of-a bitch!"

The solutions are limited for this 55-year-old man. Transferring to another department is not possible, as the company is a small one. Leaving for another job is not possible for many reasons: limited employment opportunities in the marketplace during recession; a record of years of personal attachment to the company; the strains of job hunting, relocating, and adjusting to a new work situation. Trying to win understanding and cooperation from fellow workers is a fruitless task, since the intermesh of personalities, resentments, and personal rivalries common to many offices continue to interfere.

So picking up the heavy boxes seems the easiest solution—but for how long can he continue? What will be the eventual effects on his heart? Anxiety about health, death, and family colors his life.

This brief illustration of work-related stress does not refer, of course, to the larger consequences for emotional state, associated depression, anxiety, feeling of devaluation, nor the influence on interpersonal and family relationships. However, while centering on a particular task, it mirrors in many ways the problems of those heart patients for whom performance of tasks involving physical or emotional stress constitutes a pervasive and continuing threat to health on the job. The work situation, while serving as support and resource contributing to the long-term well-being of the patient is also exerting other, possibly negative effects upon both the biophysical system as well as emotional and social adjustment.

The analysis of this type of work situation in relation to recovery might call upon a variety of theoretical approaches, considering social stress, integration to the informal social system, character of role relationships, locus of control, and social supports. In the current literature, a primary way of dealing with these sociological-psychological factors involving work stress and the heart patient has been through the clinical report and case analysis. Given the importance of work as a resource and its role in the recovery and rehabilitation of heart patients, it seems clear that we need to find better conceptual and methodological ways to clarify their complex interplay.

The Female Worker, the Retired, and the Unemployed

The relationship between work experience and long-term recovery presents some particularly intriguing questions in the case of the female worker. Ironically, the main thrust of research on work adjustment and heart disease appears generally to ignore the fact that half of the women in the United States over age 16 are in the work force and that in their elder years many such women have heart attacks. We know little about the ways in which heart disease impacts upon their fate in the work force, their work careers, and the quality of their lives. How work activity, for example, acts as a support or as a barrier in their psychosocial adaptation to the illness remains largely a pioneer territory, and we cannot assume that duplicate processes operate in women as in men, given their differential roles and statuses in society at large and in the work environment in particular.

Clinicians have often observed that retired persons of similar age, degree of cardiac impairment and other comparable characteristics may respond very differently in living with their heart disease. How the retirement experience affects physical and emotional health, particularly among heart patients, has been examined in only limited ways in empirical research, and the interaction between problems of aging, cardiac status, and other non-cardiac illness conditions for the most part remains to be explored. The condition of retirement and its social, psychological, and economic implications require special attention.

Similarly, if we assume that work itself can be a major resource in promoting recovery and rehabilitation, what are the effects of non-employment among persons who have potential for re-entry into the work force? The social and psychological debilitating effects of being out of work were graphically outlined long ago by Bakke (1934) and others, with primary focus on the employable person in "normal" health. Being unemployed as well as ill implies stresses in many areas including emotional status, social roles, and economic status, and their manifestations may differ among heart patients of varying occupational types. Within each of such groups, these stresses may impact upon cardiac physical status as well as upon psychosocial adaptations to heart disease. We know little about the consequences of non-employment for heart patients, and the patterns of adjustment to their situations.

FAMILY

After a Heart Attack: The Family

As is well known, the family is a key resource and support in times of illness as well as in other types of personal stress situations (Kaplan, Cassel, & Gore, 1977; Litman, 1974; Pratt, 1976). As we have noted, it can also function as an impediment and barrier to recovery (Croog, 1970). In the case of heart patients in the post-hospital phase, these multiple functions of the family have only partially been explored, though knowledge in this area clearly has great potential application in clinical practice and in planning rehabilitation programs (Gulledge, 1979).

Some recent research has focused on the family or home setting as a factor in recovery and rehabilitation after heart attacks, with particular emphasis on the physical aspects. These studies compare the relative efficacy of the Coronary Care Unit and the home environment in affecting recovery among uncomplicated infarct patients (Mather et al, 1971, 1976; Hill, Hampton, & Mitchell, 1978). They report that in general the mortality rates were similar for patients in the home group and those in the hospitalized group. Such studies center mainly on survival and morbidity as linked to treatment setting, rather than on issues of psychosocial adjustment and rehabilitation. Because of its importance, this whole matter deserves further inquiry and documentation.

Many clinicians presenting principles of coronary care specify the dictum that it is important to enlist the support of the spouse and children of patients in rehabilitation (Adsett & Bruhn, 1968; Davidson, 1979; Hackett & Rosenbaum, 1980; Ruskin, Stein, Shelsky, & Bailey, 1970; Wenger, 1975). But given the lack of systematic data from the research literature as guides, in practice it is often possible to draw only on clinical impressions and simple generalizations concerning family relationships. For example, varying degrees of family solidarity and quality of emotional tone in the household have rarely been examined in a systematic manner in relation to cardiac rehabilitation. The possible deeper effects of such elements within the family as stresses, rivalries, power struggles, and conflicting goals are frequently overlooked.

In fact, the research literature on the family and heart patients typically appears to deal in terms of limited stereotypes concerning structure as well as process. Few studies approach the relationship between recovery and various types of family composition, such as (a) the unmarried, divorced or widowed living alone; (b) combinations of husband, wife, and children ranging in size of household; or (c) the patient living with one or more elderly parents. Rather, emphasis is primarily on the nuclear family in terms of the marital pair alone—or husband, wife and children.

As illness often occurs in a family context, the quality of family life may influence how the patient and other family members deal with that illness. Despite many negative aspects, an illness such as heart disease can serve as a challenge which brings spouses together, rallies children, and encourages love, mutual support, and aid. In discussions of coping process, Caplan and others have underlined the generalizability of coping skills to other contexts and with other diseases and life crisis situations (Caplan, 1964, 1974). Over the long term, as some heart patients pointed out in our own study (Croog & Levine, 1982), the illness can become an enriching, ennobling experience, changing the lives of family members and providing them with an even greater resource for coping in the future. It may bring a reaffirmation of religious values among family members and feelings of solidarity based on perception of new closeness with God. In systematic consideration of the impact of heart disease, these positive aspects deserve more ample analysis than they have received.

Social Supports

One approach to this aspect of the family as a resource is through the concept of social supports. As a multi-dimensional phenomenon, the concept of support itself implies a number of component elements, some of which have usefully been outlined in a general framework by Kaplan, Cassel, and Gore (1977). They describe support as "'the metness' or gratification of a person's basic social needs. . . . through environmental supplies of social support," as furnished through social interaction and relationships. "Support is defined by the relative presence or absence of psychosocial support resources from significant others."

In the family of the heart patient, the presence of a confidant such as a spouse or other close relative can have many positive effects—providing emotional support, approval, tension release, and guidance. The family can also provide resources in the form of services, financial aid and other types of practical assistance (Croog, Lipson, & Levine, 1972). In other contexts some researchers have pointed up the importance of the family by suggesting that a minimally supportive role has particularly negative effects, contributing to the etiology of mental illness, suicide, social disintegration, and various psychosomatic ailments (Gore, 1973; Leighton, 1959).

The patterning of services and supports in time of illness may be related to the nature and quality of relationships before the illness. Thus, on the basis of empirical examination of family help patterns, Croog, Lipson and Levine (1972) have reported that the notion of pre-illness social integration may be useful in explaining some support behavior after a heart attack. Heart patients who were part of a network of mutual aid from family members, for example, were more likely to receive aid than those who were comparative social isolates. While there is much suggestive evidence, further research is needed to determine empirically the relationships between (a) health status and personal adjustment, and (b) differing levels of social supports among heart patients with varying social and psychological characteristics.

Stresses and Family Life

Other disintegrative effects, however, are also part of the larger picture of heart disease and its implications for the family. Much empirical data points to severe internal stresses and tensions in families in the country as a whole—as evident in part in high divorce rates, desertion, separation, and proliferation of single parent families. While not specific to families of heart patients, of course, these data imply that the condition of heart attack in a patient often occurs in families already troubled and with precarious interpersonal relationships (Croog & Fitzgerald, 1978). Family stresses clearly can have great potential influence on the character of response to illness by patients and family members as well, as noted in many studies and anecdotal clinical reports. Though we have limited empirical data specifically on the effects of family stresses on cardiac health and long-term adjustment of heart patients, the powerful quality of many case reports indicate their pervasive influence (Halberstam & Lesher, 1978; Lear, 1980).

Some evidence from a few statistical studies points up problems which often appear in the family relationships of heart patients. These include quarreling, feelings of inadequacy, depression, and sexual problems (Finlayson & McEwen, 1977; Hellerstein & Friedman, 1970; Mayou, Foster, & Williamson, 1978; Stern & Pascale, 1979). Often these may exist prior to the illness and are exacerbated by it.

Data from our own study of 345 heart patients and their wives suggest a cycle of guilt and blame, one which inevitably becomes part of the stresses with which the heart patient must cope in coming to terms with his illness. In the year after a first heart attack, one fifth of married male patients cited problems with their wives as factors in its onset. One quarter of fathers cited problems with their children as factors. Among the men surviving 8 years later, nearly 20 percent blamed wives and 16 percent cited children. Many of these were the same men who had earlier pointed to their wives and/or children as contributing to their first heart attack. Another facet of these data was the responses of wives, indicating self-blame for the illness of husbands. In fact, 22 percent of these women mentioned their husbands' problems with them as important in causing the men's heart attacks. Other studies as well point to patterns of guilt and blame in the family as possible handicaps and barriers for the recovering heart patient (Skelton & Dominian, 1973).

Long-term, chronic illness and the threat of recurrence of the heart attack have impact as well on the practical, organizational aspects of family life; this in turn bears on how the patient can deal with his condition. Common issues are: loss of income; the need to change eating habits or living arrangements to conform with physician advice; changes in role relationships among family members; changes in decision-making patterns and shifts in power and authority involving spouses or children; need to change patterns of expenditures and to alter life style; and pragmatic adaptations to the prospect of future invalidism, impairment and death of the patient, such as clarifying matters of ownership, pension rights and property succession.

Even less clear is the relationship between the course of the recovery and how problems and stresses are faced over the years in families differing in structure, socio-economic status, and other features. In an illness such as heart disease—given the sensitivity of the cardiovascular system to stress—the reactive effects of such factors on the patient can be significant (Bove, 1977; Chambers & Reiser, 1953; Eliot & Buell, 1979; Engel, 1971; Klein, Garrity, & Gelein, 1974; Lown, Verrier, & Rabinowitz, 1977). However, we need more than anecdotal evidence on the circular reactions involving illness, family response, and the recovery process.

Risk Factors, Life Style Intervention, and the Family

One major development in recent years involving both the family and the heart patient has been the formulation of programs for life style intervention—reducing cardiovascular risks through various changes in diet, smoking, exercise, stress, and other factors. Large scale clinical trials have been sponsored by the National Heart, Lung and Blood Institute to test the methods and principles of risk reduction (Levy & Feinleib, 1980; Maccoby, Farquhar, Wood, & Alexander, 1977; MRFIT, 1976; Syme, 1978). As other chapters point out, the possibility of change in coronary prone behavior pattern is being tested as well (Roskies, Spevack, Surkis, Cohen, & Gilman, 1978). The critical role of the family, in particular, in changing behavior of Type A heart patients has been emphasized by Jenkins: "While it is important to enlist the cooperation of family members and colleagues in the recovery process of every heart patient, it is essential to Type A patients" (Jenkins, 1979, p. 23).

Physician recommendations for risk reduction through life style change may constitute innovations for the patient which inevitably may redound in many ways on family life, and on relationships between spouses and among other family members. Altering traditional diet may not be easy—or economically feasible—in many families. The prospects of change in attitude, belief, and psychological orientation—while recommended by a physician as therapeutic for the patient—can have less salutary effects on relationships between husbands and wives, upsetting well-established sets of mutual assumptions and expectations in their respective roles. Transformation of the formerly active, aggressive man— admired and loved by his wife for many years—can have profound effects on the sexual and emotional basis of a marriage as well.

Thus, how the life style intervention impacts on the family—and in turn affects the patient—may be important elements in determining the success of the intervention. For clinicians, the ethical questions of inducing such change in the lives of persons other than the patient may not be easy to resolve. Where marriages are shaky, or a family is already troubled by internal stresses, the effects of these new interventions can eventually be destructive and ultimately act against the long-term health interests of the patient. Such issues, while gaining importance in preventive programs, stand as difficult questions for research. They are made more complex by the fact of variation among heart patients in terms of culture, economic resources, and the character of family life.

THE PHYSICIAN AS RESOURCE

The Physician and the Heart Patient: The Post-Hospital Period

Among all the external resources typically available to heart patients, the physician is perhaps the most important. In treatment of patients in the acute phase while in the hospital, the main medical issues primarily concern basic problems of survival and restoration of function. Many heart patients believe—and often with good reason—that their physicians saved them from death. For the long-term patient after hospitalization, however, the illness problems develop another type of complexity, involving such matters as work return, physical capacity, emotional status, motivation for rehabilitation, and other issues noted earlier. After the acute phase of the illness has passed, the role of physicians continues to be important, with provision of supervision, referrals, health maintenance, advice and education. Among their many functions, they may serve as determiners and certifiers of disability, eligibility for pensions, need for hospitalization and further rehabilitative care. They may sometimes act as counselors in regard to matters of work or family life, as related to health. Given the prominent and well-recognized role of physicians historically in the total care of heart patients, the limited research on doctor-patient relationships and on the nature of the course of long-term recovery, rehabilitation, and adjustment to the illness is surprising.

In the post-hospital care of the coronary patient, in what ways do differing patterns of patient management by physicians affect survival and morbidity? In what ways does having one particular doctor rather than another really make a difference in the life, health, and adjustment of the chronic heart patient? Many such questions remain to be answered through empirical study of the physician-patient relationship and the fate of heart patients in the post-hospital period.

Numerous variables involving physicians as resource have been identified as influencing long-term outcomes. These include components of the physician-patient interaction; the nature of physician-patient personal characteristics, including social and psychological factors; the nature of the practice setting or the organization of care.

For example, some theorists have proposed models of doctor-patient interaction, such as those involving the physician as leader or authoritarian figure, or those characterized by joint, cooperative participation between doctor and patient (Bloom & Wilson, 1979; Szasz & Hollender, 1956). In addition, it has often been suggested that a particular mix involving physician and patient personality is important in patient management. Some physician personality types have been noted as more effective than others in eliciting patient cooperation and compliance (Dunbar & Stunkard, 1979; Hollender, 1958).

Current controversies about medical practice suggest that organizations such as prepaid and fee-for-service systems may have differing consequences in patient care. Given current trends in solo practice, and the development of group practice and HMOs, questions have been raised in regard to the larger issues of effectiveness as well as cost in long-term patient management. How these matters relate to the long-term care of chronic heart patients must mainly be conjectured at present, since direct empirical research concerning these variables is rare.

Some empirical data underline the major potential of the physician as a central resource in the long-term careers and life styles of patients with heart disease. In our own longitudinal study of heart patients (Croog & Levine, 1982), many patients showed high long-term commitment to their physicians. For example, after 8 years two thirds of the patients receiving medical care were still seeing the same regular physician who treated them for their heart disease during the year after their first heart attack. Among those who changed, most did so in order to obtain more specialized care, turning from a general practitioner to an internist or cardiologist. Some were forced to change doctors by circumstances such as retirement, or death of their physician, or their own movement to another community.

Structural factors may limit in many ways how well the physician may actually carry out roles in dealing with medical, social and psychological issues related to long-term management of the cardiac patient. For example, the requirements of the practice situation, the demands of numerous patients for the skills of the physician in office practice, and the requirement of maintaining adequate income may combine to limit the amount of time and the kinds of tasks performed. In a national study of ambulatory care, physicians responded in regard to the amount of time they spent in face-to-face contact with their patients in office visits (USDHEW, 1978). They reported that among patients with ischemic heart disease, two thirds were seen for 15 minutes or less. In fact, a substantial percentage of the total group (31.2 percent) were seen for 10 minutes or less. Few had long visits with their doctors; only 5.4 percent of visits lasted 31 minutes or more.

Of course, such data provide no information in regard to patient needs, the purpose of the visit, or the appropriateness, the effectiveness and the quality of the medical care. But they serve here to illustrate possible limitations to the exploration by physicians of complex social, psychological, or occupational factors exacerbating the illness or complicating recovery. Typically, brief encounters in the press of office practice by a busy physician allow little opportunity for this exploration. The patient himself may feel it inappropriate to raise questions, recognizing the limits on physician time.

Compliance with the Medical Regimen: Physician as Resource and Influence

For many patients, an important component in their long-term care may be the degree to which they comply with the medical regimen set forth by their physicians. In seeking to induce patient adherence to their instructions, the tasks of physicians in long-term care of the heart patient may be more formidable than those of the acute phase when immediacy of threat to life is often easily apparent. However, physicians working with chronically ill patients may wish to induce them to follow a regimen that involves complex, repeated behavior, which may require deprivation and discomfort, and whose benefits are not easily apparent. Thus, restrictions on diet, use of alcoholic beverages, or smoking reduction, and exercise may be difficult for patients to follow over an extended, possibly indefinite period. Advice on such matters as avoiding stress, reducing conflicts at home, and "taking it easy" with sexual activity may be so ambiguous that it may arouse anxieties and threat in conscientious patients. Although numerous relevant variables have been suggested as possible influences, methods for inducing compliance with the medical regimen are still being explored and tested (Becker, 1979; Dunbar & Stunkard, 1979; Marston, 1970; Sackett & Haynes, 1976).

One complication in inducing compliance is often the lack of clear relationship between long-term outcome or benefit and level of compliance with the medical regimen. The specific question of the efficacy of particular drugs, degree of compliance, and the long-term benefits of taking the medications is one type of issue. The efficacy of conformity with behavioral recommendations is even more difficult to evaluate. When patients follow physician's advice in regard to work change, family relationships, exercise programs, or stress reduction, is their general coping with the illness improved? Do they have more favorable prognoses for survival and prevention of recurrence of heart attacks? The answers to such questions are of high pragmatic importance to those many heart patients who are called upon by their physicians to make changes in work behavior, style of life, and daily pleasures.

While willingness to comply with the doctor's advice may be one of the essential elements of the doctor-patient relationship, we need to know more about the association between the advice provided the chronically ill heart patient, the degree of compliance, and the efficacy of compliance on the advice items. In particular, the areas of compliance with social, behavioral, and economic recommendations deserve further scrutiny through controlled studies. What indeed happens to the non-compliers or poor compliers over a period of years? The annals of iatrogenic illness present a litany of cases of patients who dutifully followed the doctor's advice but who suffered in regard to medications in particular, then died of conditions strongly suspected of being related to the medications. The cases of reserpine and clofibrate are among the most recent. But the evidence is far less clear in regard to the long-term effects of behavior change, advice and alterations of life style.

Doctor-Patient Communication: Channels and Barriers

In long-term care of the heart patient, the quality of doctor-patient communication has long been recognized as an essential element. Some of the barriers to doctor-patient communication have been outlined in research on illnesses other than heart disease, but their conclusions may be applicable to this illness as well (Bloom & Wilson, 1979). Studies have shown that when physician and patient come from disparate social backgrounds or sub-cultural groups, problems of communication, semantics, and incongruent mutual expectations may arise. In recent years some notable problems of the heart patient in the doctor-patient relationship have been outlined in personal histories of patients, as noted earlier (Halberstam & Lesher, 1978; Lear, 1980).

As many case histories note, what is of great concern to the patient may not be that which the doctor is prepared or inclined to discuss. For example, it has often been reported that communications concerning sexual issues may be particularly difficult between physician and patient (McLane, Krop & Mehta, 1980; Scalzi & Dracup, 1979). In part, this may be due to a general lack of good data on sexuality and the heart patient (Hellerstein & Friedman, 1970). In part, however, the issue continues as one part of minimal training in medical school and residency programs. Despite the openness in discussion of the "new sexuality" of recent decades, both doctor and patient may be restricted by their own anxieties and troubled sensibilities in discussing the matter.

A similar case holds in regard to the emotional problems of heart patients associated with the illness. Problems of communication on such matters may lead to use of standardized format treatment, to routine prescription of palliatives and tranquilizers, rather than to more time-consuming methods of counseling and personal support. In severe cases patients may appreciate referral—but many do not, believing that to see a psychiatrist brings an unbearable stigma and expression of failure.

Another type of complication in doctor-patient communication is the confusion of messages involving physicians, media, and the nature of empirical evidence on benefits of preventive actions. A common theme among patients is the hope that their compliance with the medical regimen will bring rewards of health and extended life. They wish to regard the doctor's advice on smoking, exercise, diet, and stress as a rational scientific formula which can bring happy results. Troubling the doctor-patient relationship, however, is the intrusion of conflicting evidence in the media, folklore, and scientific literature. In a popular article (Lesher, 1974), one particularly expressive heart patient has noted the confusion raised for patients by a variety of theories and research reports.

> Unfortunately, it was difficult for us [heart patients] and for medical scientists to know precisely what they [medical scientists] were finding out. For instance, while [a prominent doctor of our own] University Hospital was convinced that regular and reasonable postcoronary exercise kept patients alive longer and more happily, doctors in San Francisco said they found that joggers seemed to drop dead to an alarming degree. And while there is nearly universal condemnation of smoking, along comes a Harvard scientist who insists smoking will not increase the chances of a heart failure—at least not for people over 65. And while the outdoor life in moderation is extolled widely by heart specialists, a team of doctors have found that Finnish loggers have the highest heart attack rate in the world. And while a West Coast doctor holds a theory that highly competitive people are more prone to heart attacks, he has not explained why a Henry Kissinger, who seemingly will be unsatisfied until he wins *two* Nobel peace prizes, stays healthy. (pp. 9–10).

Though further explanations in recent years have been offered by medical researchers to explain such apparent discrepancies, among many heart patients, the dilemmas and quests for rational answers and reduced confusion persist and are troubling.

Physician and Patient Roles

One emerging problem of the doctor-patient relationship and long-term care is the degree of ambiguity and variation in perceived roles of doctor and patient. Given the press of large numbers of patients, many physicians cannot choose to take the time to review the entire range of issues—social, psychological, economic—which may be an integral part of the patient's current illness experience. Some believe indeed that this is not within their role, that they should best serve through application of the high technology in which they have been trained, utilizing their specialized medical skills for the many patients who specifically need those skills. They consider that their effectiveness is in treating diseases of the heart, not adjustment to the consequences of heart disease.

In line with the popular use of the phrase in the media, "Ask your doctor," many patients bring expectations to the medical office which their physicians may find unrealistic, uncomfortable, or unduly time-consuming. It is not surprising that a busy physician may ask of himself, "What have these questions got to do with medicine? Am I a human relations counselor or a physician?"

If patients have problems at work or at home which might be related to the course of their heart disease, symptoms and underlying condition, the limits of physician responsibility are often not clear. If a man believes that he is being pressured out of his job because of his heart condition, is this problem a medical responsibility? Should a physician counsel him or make a referral? Should a physician take time from a busy practice to hear a succession of social, economic, and emotional problems from one patient after another?

One traditional, often stereotyped answer to such questions is that the physician should make a referral. But such procedures imply that the physician must draw out enough information to decide on the desirability of a referral. Further dilemmas are raised concerning referral to services which may be non-existent, not readily available, overloaded, and/or seen as socially stigmatizing. The information on referral sources may not be known to the physician, or it may take much time to determine the appropriate source. Agencies and institutions have their own needs and may be selective in regard to their client load (Levine, White & Paul, 1963).

Other matters of conflicting ideologies and interests in regard to the physician-patient role also come into play. For example, once a patient has progressed beyond the acute phase of the illness and is doing reasonably well in recovery, some physicians are wary of developing a relationship which encourages dependency of the patient for advice and aid on life problems. Taken to an extreme, particularly in the growing trends in bureaucratization of medicine and the intrusion of government, such dependency in chronically ill patients may have long-term, negative effects contrary to traditional American values of individualism, independence, and self-reliance. At the same time, there are patients who want no intrusion by physicians into matters in their lives which are not clearly medical. They want only a care program and a physician concerned solely with their physical needs.

This brief sketching of ambiguities and conflicting conceptions in regard to physician-patient roles touches in only a limited way on the complex of factors which relate to the physician as resource in the chronic phase of heart disease. The dimensions of these phenomena, their variations, and their sequelae for patient, physician, and the health care process, remain for the most part as matters which have not yet engaged researchers. As noted, we know all too little about such variations and ideologies within the doctor-patient relationship; we know still less about their patterning within social class, ethnic and other sub-groups of our society. We have even fewer empirical data on their consequences for the post-hospital heart patient, the physician, the care process, health care costs, and the health care system.

FORMAL ORGANIZATIONS: INSTITUTIONS AND AGENCIES

After leaving the hospital, a heart patient may turn for further care and support to an array of institutions and agencies in the community designed to serve the disabled, the ill, and the troubled. In many communities, particularly large metropolitan centers, such organizations may be numerous, constituting an important segment of the total set of formal and informal resources which patients may use. Ranging in type, they include cardiac rehabilitation units, work classification centers, social service agencies, exercise rehabilitation programs, vocational rehabilitation services, and counseling and referral services of various kinds. In some communities, group therapy and self-help groups may be found, including Heart Clubs, "Sharing and Caring," and other mutual support or therapy groups.

Despite their importance, the role of these institutions and agencies has not yet been adequately examined in relation to many of the basic issues pertaining to cardiac rehabilitation. Which resources are the most effective and with which sub-populations of cardiac patients? In what ways do the use of such services integrate with use of other resources? What are the appropriate criteria for measuring outcome and effectiveness of these resources over time in the case of chronically ill patients? There are few empirical data concerning even more elementary issues, including documentation of number and types of resources in communities, their relative use, and the needs they meet (Acker, 1979; Gentry, 1979b).

Services as Resources: Availability and Use

Considering data from various sources, it would appear that over recent years most heart patients have not made use of formal agencies and institutional services during their post-hospital recovery. Data from a survey by the Social Security Administration in 1972 (Treitel, 1977) showed that an estimated 3.2 million persons were identified as disabled due to cardiovascular diseases. Within this group, an estimated 60 percent were classified as severely disabled— unable to work regularly or at all. Within the total group of heart disease disabled, however, only 13 percent reported that they had received formal rehabilitation services of some type. Services included job training and placement assistance, employment counseling and guidance, and physical therapy. Degree of severity of disability was not related to use of services (Smith, 1979).

These national data on limited use of services are reflected in other studies as well. For example, Croog and Levine (1977) reported that among 300 patients in the year after a first heart attack, most (72 percent) had no contact with agencies or services other than the hospital. Among the remainder, the majority made use of employment services for job placement or relocation. Similarly, 8 years later, the surviving population reported minimal use of cardiac rehabilitation and related services, either during the previous year or during the full 8-year period of the study. This apparent pattern occurred even though many had been rehospitalized for heart disease or continued to suffer physical, social, and economic problems associated with their illnesses (Croog & Levine, 1982). Other studies seem to portray the same pattern of minimal use of formal resources in the United States and in other countries (Finlayson & McEwen, 1977; Smith, 1979). Despite methodological differences between studies, there seem little evidence of substantial use of such services by heart patients after hospitalization.

Some data point to structural limitations on use of such services after hospitalization. For example, the limited capacity of cardiac rehabilitation units for providing service to large numbers of potential clients is reflected in part by data on the numbers and type of rehabilitation services. As recently as 1975–76, the American Heart Association (1976) listed 148 facilities in its Directory of Rehabilitation Units in the United States. These were located in 35 states; for 15 others, no units were listed. Further, about 60 percent of the units were located in six states, and most were in large metropolitan areas. Taking into account the possibility of incomplete listings and classification, such data imply that at the time heart patients in many sections of the country had limited access to services. Although the number and type of the units has increased in recent years, discrepancies between geographic areas in availability of services persist throughout the country.

Other estimates suggest the current number of potential clients for rehabilitative services may be growing larger, as further improvements occur in acute care and in survival rates (Smith, 1979). Aside from the millions with clear functional cardiac disability, many persons with heart disease are not disabled, but at various times might have need for social supportive or advisory services, such as those provided by formal agencies and professionals in the community.

Why do some heart patients use the services, while most do not? The answers are perhaps more complex in the case of the chronically ill patient surveyed over a series of years, as compared with the patient with acute illness in a limited time period. Aside from issues of access and availability, various factors may play a role in non-utilization. One is need. Many patients, as rated by their physicians and other qualified professionals, do not require these services. They cope well on the basis of their own personal resources and those informal supports already available to them. In fact, some cardiologist-epidemiologists have suggested that assumptions about need for services may be unrealistic, proposing that minimal utilization may reflect cardiac patients' perception of a real lack of need (Dawber, 1982). Another basis for non-utilization is non-referral by the physicians. This may be influenced in part by negative attitudes toward such services, lack of awareness or interest, and doubts about their cost-effectiveness.

Other factors may be patient-centered. Some patients are unaware of services, while others consider them irrelevant to their own cases. Some are reluctant to ask their physicians about resources, assuming that the doctor knows best. It has been suggested that heart patients may resist use of such services as part of a general denial of the illness (Gentry, 1979a). Having passed the acute phase, such patients may wish to regain as normal a life as possible, and prevent further labeling as ''heart patients.'' Those with emotional problems may be particularly sensitive to seeking psychiatric aid because of perceived stigma associated with such services.

Of course, many of these same possible influences are not specific to post-coronary patients, and they have been identified as related to use of services in general. However, research on patients with other types of chronic illness provides little additional insight on health services utilization over time. The key points or stages at which decisions are made, the triggering factors, and the network of change and stability among the interrelated influential variables have rarely been studied. Further, many factors remain to be explored in regard to service usage among sub-groups varying in social, psychological, and health characteristics, and in belief and value systems.

Evaluation and Effectiveness

What of heart patients who do make use of services? We also have inadequate data on the relative efficacy of various types of formal services and agencies in producing desirable ''outcomes'' in heart patients in the post-hospital period. In making judgments, it is important, of course, to consider the services by individual types, rather than as broad, generic categories. The employment counseling service which gives advice once to a patient cannot be evaluated by the same criteria as a cardiac rehabilitation unit, with a continuing program of contacts and multiple services.

In recent years, more systematic effort is being devoted to the development of services such as exercise training programs, counseling services, and rehabilitation units. Some of the problems involved in testing their effectiveness have been detailed in the *Proceedings of the Workshop on Physical Conditioning and Training* (National Heart, Lung and Blood Institute, 1979). Important issues of measurement, sampling, case loss, patient motivation and criteria of "outcome" complicate assessment and evaluation of services and their role as resources (Cromwell, Butterfield, Brayfield, & Curry, 1977; DeBusk, Houston, Haskell, Fry, & Parker, 1979; Naughton & Hellerstein, 1973). Considering the full range of rehabilitative services and their influence on long-term recovery and rehabilitation, the paucity of information in the research literature is a major hindrance to making valid generalizations.

Numerous reports point up the merits of various formal methods of rehabilitation and training, while the larger issues of their efficacy are still under investigation. For example, therapeutic and constructive effects have been noted as a consequence of participation in Heart Clubs, "Sharing and Caring," and other types of mutual support groups (Deegan, 1977; Hackett, 1978; Ibrahim et al., 1974; Rahe, Ward & Hayes, 1979). These programs may enlist only select populations, and those who continue to participate may be different from those who drop out or never enroll. However, program managers cite benefits for those who participate, often maintaining that some degree of help and aid for even select population groups is better than none.

More negative general findings on rehabilitation services are reported by Smith (1979) in a study of adult disabled persons who made use of services of the Vocational Rehabilitation agency. Though the study is not concerned with cardiac patients alone, the findings may be especially pertinent here. Smith reports that use of services was not associated with level of rehabilitation or recovery. Disabled adults using no rehabilitation services had a rate of recovery similar to those who did use these resources. One hypothesis to explain the lack of difference may be that the non-users of formal services had other types of informal aids and supports, and thus they were able to manage as well on the whole as the disabled who used formal services. Such findings point to the need for looking beyond descriptors of use of formal services alone, and to the desirability of centering on the total "armory of resources" and its role in long-term recovery and rehabilitation.

Related Formal Resources: The Self-Help Movement and Mass Media

Improvements in technology, mass communication, and educational level help expand the total social and organizational framework bearing on cardiac rehabilitation. New developments in recent years point to more direct involvement of the patient in responsibility for illness management, during both the acute and chronic phases (Dumont, 1974; Krantz, Baum, & Wideman, 1980; Levin, Katz

& Holst, 1979). For example, the self-help movement is designed to help guide the patient as participant in the care process and as manager and monitor of his or her own health.

The decline of rates of heart disease mortality might suggest as well that mass education efforts by the media may be having an effect on diet, life style, and smoking behavior, which in turn may be reflected in reduction of coronary risk (Levy & Feinleib, 1980). Insofar as the agencies and institutions which promote such behavioral and attitudinal change affect heart patients, they constitute another segment of the formal organizations in the community which are part of the rehabilitation process—though they do not deal directly with patients and are not supported by individual patient fees. While some evidence suggests that such movements may be more effective with better educated patients and those who are most "inner-directed," the extent of their impact still remains to be reliably measured.

RELIGION AND THE CLERGY AS RESOURCES

The religious institution is another type of resource relevant here, although it is not often examined as part of the array of formal resources and services relevant for cardiac rehabilitation. Heart disease, like other life-threatening illnesses, brings persons face-to-face with fundamental issues of death, survival, and the meaning of love and human existence. How chronically ill people confront these issues may be closely related to how well they deal with their illness.

Response to conditions of chronic illness may be crucially molded by faith and beliefs concerning the meaning of life, man's relationship to God, the significance of illness burdens, and conceptions of an after-life. The informal network of interpersonal support available to members of an organized religious group can itself also be a factor in recovery and rehabilitation (Dyer, 1976).

Although many clinicians attest to the importance of faith and religion as powerful supports, it is notable how rarely these resources are mentioned in medical texts as part of the therapeutic armory. Few empirical studies provide information on how factors of faith and religious supports operate among heart patients in differing religious groups in our society. This issue has been even less explored in regard to heart patients from non-Western religions though heart disease is pervasive worldwide.

The influence of religious faith on the course of illness has been largely documented through anecdotal reports and case studies, although rarely in regard to the recovery of the heart patient (Comstock & Partridge, 1972; Vaux, 1976). In fact, most of the data have been provided through studies of sects, faith healers in western society, and of native healers in non-western cultures (Pattison, Lapins, & Doerr, 1973). In laboratory studies, however, emotional responses such as those in the religious experience have been shown to have physiological effects—as measured in catecholamines, blood pressure, and brain activity (Surwillo & Hobson, 1978).

In the case of heart patients, few indications of even minimal changes in religiosity and religious observance over time have been reported. For example, one year after a first heart attack, Croog and Levine (1972, 1977) found that men did not report significant change in church attendance and in their valuation of religion. As in the case of use of other services, virtually none reported that they had contact with clergy in regard to problems of their illness, whether of spiritual or practical nature. Similar patterns were evident among survivors in the same study group after 8 years (Croog & Levine, 1982).

Among cardiac patients, do religious beliefs and closeness to formal religious institutions and the clergy make a difference in survival and morbidity? Are those with religious beliefs more free of physical symptoms than those without such faith? As we have noted, answers are not easily forthcoming from previous research. Virtually no studies have been done which meet the classic requirements of control groups, sampling, or matched populations. Of course, the subtle positive effects of religious attitudes on morale, quality of life, and peace of mind are particularly difficult to measure in empirical studies. Nevertheless, as clinicians are aware, patients do experience such positive effects.

The possible detrimental effects on the recovery and rehabilitation of heart patients must also be noted here. However, we also have little documentation of the more negative effects of religious beliefs on patient lives, as manifest in terms of generalized guilt, feelings of being punished for sins, fear of the afterlife and of the wrath of God (Ness, 1980; Radcliffe-Brown, 1952). In the main, there are a few anecdotal accounts. The early descriptions by Cannon of Voodoo death, for example, have not appeared to trigger substantial empirical exploration of non-therapeutic effects of faith and religious belief in Western societies (Cannon, 1932).

If a series of devoutly religious heart patients have the belief that they are doomed, that their illness is a judgment on their sins, what is their long-term course and their prospect for adaptation and rehabilitation? Few researchers in the field of heart disease have as yet systematically focused on such questions.

EMOTIONAL AND PSYCHOLOGICAL FACTORS

Other important sets of influences upon the course of heart disease are emotional and psychological factors, including such elements as ego structure, defense mechanisms, coping capacity, and other components which are often identified as part of "personality." The model cited earlier in Figure 10.2 refers mainly to the patient in relation to external resources in his social environment. We now turn to a brief review of additional areas of resources, those internal to the patient, the core *persona* of Figure 10.2.

Most of the research on psychological factors in coronary disease thus far has centered on (a) their role in the etiology of the illness or (b) their influence within the immediate, acute phase of the illness. While they are not generally specified as "resources" in the research literature, some studies point up the correlation between particular types of psychological elements whose presence and functioning may influence the long-term course of cardiac disease.

Psychological Status and Behavior Pattern: Mortality and Morbidity

After a person has experienced a first heart attack, is his subsequent illness career influenced by the kind of person he was before the acute episode? Much research on patients who have already experienced myocardial infarction has shown that underlying *biological* process places such patients at greater risk for future heart attacks and cardiac mortality than those persons with no history of heart attack (Humphries, 1977; Kannel, Sorlie, & McNamara, 1979; Kuller, 1979). For example, reviewing "the most important factors in the prognosis of coronary artery disease," Proudfit, Bruschke, and Sones (1978) cite such conditions as "the number of arteries severely obstructed; significant involvement of the left main coronary artery, and generalized impairment of left ventricular function." Given this sort of medical and epidemiological evidence on the matter, what is the role of psychological factors in the illness careers of heart patients?

Some recent evidence offers suggestive indications that physical course after a first infarction may be related to psychosocial and behavioral variables. For example, Jenkins points out that in a study of men with established coronary disease, those with Type A behavior pattern were at significantly greater risk for subsequent coronary events than men who were Type B (Jenkins, Zyzanski, & Rosenman, 1976). Or to put it another way, being a Type B patient in a sense had a "protective" effect, putting such patients at lower statistical risk of heart attack than their Type A cohorts.

Other studies of etiological issues imply that the nature of psychological response among heart patients may trigger physical changes—in blood pressure, catecholamines, or cholesterol (Eliot & Buell, 1979). These issues have been comprehensively summarized by Jenkins in two important papers (1971, 1976). Double-blind studies of coronary vessel obstruction have reported association between Type A behavior pattern and condition of the arteries (Blumenthal, Williams, Kong, Schanberg & Thompson, 1978; Frank, Heller, Kornfeld, Sporn & Weiss, 1978).

In addition, as Levy and Feinleib point out, Type A behavior pattern may notably augment other risk factors associated with coronary disease. In a recent review paper they present a table based on Framingham Study data, reporting on the probability of developing coronary disease in 8 years, given the presence of standard risk factors. They note that "one would increase the probabilities shown [in the Table] by 20 percent for a Type A individual, and decrease them by 20 percent for a Type B" (Levy & Feinleib, 1980, p. 1265). Jenkins presents another affirmative view of the contribution of Type A in his estimate that Type A behavior pattern "has about the same strength of association with coronary artery disease prevalence and incidence as do other standard risk factors" (Jenkins, 1978).

A number of other studies offer conflicting results regarding the relationship between pre-infarction psychological factors and coronary mortality and morbidity. These all may be measuring differing phenomena, given the variety of instruments, methods, research designs, and study populations. As noted, most of the work on psychosocial factors has been carried out primarily in connection with tracing etiology of the disease, and the specific role of the factors remains a matter of controversy (Hackett & Rosenbaum, 1980).

Nevertheless, the relevance of such research for the post-infarction period is obvious. If the same factors of psychological predisposition and response continue to operate, they may constitute important influences upon recurrence of heart attacks. As clinicians and researchers point out, however, the factors which determine development of the disease may not be the same as those which determine its course after the acute phase. Important empirical questions on this whole issue remain for resolution.

Psychological Status and Psychosocial Adaptation

The discussion thus far has centered on morbidity and mortality in the post-infarction patient population. The possible relationships between psychological factors and long-term *non-physical* outcomes seems less well-defined, judging by research thus far. Numerous reports point up the prevalence of anxiety and depression in the period immediately following myocardial infarction, and while rates vary among studies, the prominence of these problems is evident (Cassem & Hackett, 1971; Gentry & Haney, 1975; Stern, Pascale & McLoone, 1976; Wishnie, Hackett, & Cassem, 1971; Wynn, 1967). Associations have been found between psychological state early in the illness and the later appearance of such characteristics many months later, particularly in regard to anxiety and depression. Thus, it would appear that the patient with early emotional stability, able to manage anxiety and depression effectively, might be less likely to have these problems later in his illness career (Gulledge, 1979; Stern, Pascale & Ackerman, 1977). Other studies centering on more general notions of morale and well-being also showed association between these "favorable" responses and later measures of positive adjustment to the illness.

Other elements of the psychological state involving depression and anxiety may also serve to complicate the course of long-term recovery and adjustment

(Garrity & Klein, 1971; Kavanagh, Shephard & Tuck, 1975; Naismith, Robinson, Shaw, & MacIntyre, 1979; Obier, MacPherson, & Haywood, 1977). For example, hypochondriasis, anxiety over sexual activity, loss of self-esteem, and a tendency toward retreatism and dependency are among some of the conditions which have been described in clinical reports. Much of the research in this area is descriptive, reviewing the nature of the problems and their possible relevance to cardiac rehabilitation and recovery. In general, however, the linkages between psychological state early in the illness and long-term outcomes remain to be clearly established. Few systematic attempts have been made to track the changing relationships between emotional state and the physical and non-physical outcomes of the disease in large populations of coronary patients.

In studies of the relationship between psychological state or emotional factors and long-term adjustment, a particular complicating issue has been the problem of measuring the effects of confounding variables, including the physiological and pharmacological influences on mood and behavior. Thus, in some cases scores on personality measures may be a product of states produced as side effects of the drug regimen. Or the "personality scores" may be a consequence of general physiological response to changes and disturbances in the cardiovascular system which have triggering effects on other body systems. In some instances apparent poor psychological and social adjustment to the illness may be symptomatic of the illness itself, a reflection of underlying physiological process, rather than a separate phenomenon of reaction and adaptation to the illness condition.

The distinction may be important from the practical standpoint, as well as from the standpoint of understanding the nature of interrelated factors in recovery and rehabilitation. For example, patients with apparent illness-based, poor psychosocial adjustment may require a different course of support and services, as compared with those patients whose adjustment problems stem from other sources. It seems clear that the general issue remains to be clarified through development of better measures of gradations in physical status, of biological process, psychosocial status, and their interrelations.

Coronary Disease and Pre-Existing Mental Illness

Another element complicating recovery and long-term rehabilitation is the level of emotional illness antecedent to the acute phase of heart disease. Although psychiatric epidemiological surveys present varying estimates, it is apparent that in the general population significant proportions suffer from emotional or psychiatric problems in differing degrees of severity (Dohrenwend, 1975; Weissman, Myers, & Harding, 1978). In fact, a number of these epidemiological estimates rank only a minority segment of the adult populations studied as free of some degree of emotional illness.

Despite the fact that previous mental health may play a role in response to disease, the interaction between pre-existing mental illness and recovery and rehabilitation after myocardial infarction has not been well explicated in the research literature. Some indicators of the parameters are available in a few studies. For example, among 203 patients with a first myocardial infarction, 9 percent were classified by Cay, Vetter, Philip, and Dugard (1972) as having had psychiatric illness and therapy preceding their admission. In a study of 68 patients with myocardial infarction, Stern, Pascale, and Ackerman (1977) report that 22 percent had anxiety or depressive symptomatology in the hospital, and an approximate half of these had sought professional counseling during the year preceding the heart attack.

In general, however, the extent to which the range of emotional disorders in the general population is reflected in heart patient populations remains to be determined. Given the fact of high prevalence of cardiovascular disorders, it seems unlikely that persons with heart disease are exempt in some unique way from the range of emotional illnesses and symptomatology afflicting the population as a whole.

Though few empirical studies of heart patients report on the matter, it seems evident that pre-existing neurotic or psychotic symptoms may considerably complicate coping and adaptation to cardiac disease. Some clinical reports and materials advising physicians duly note that psychiatric problems in varying degrees of severity may constitute one of the dangers to recovery in the acute phase. Typically, such commentaries suggest tranquilizers or other mood-altering drugs as appropriate solutions. Their role in long-term care is generally less well specified.

How emotional problems complicate the stresses of long-term chronic cardiac disease constitutes only one side of the issue. The other side is that physical, psychological, social, and economic stresses of cardiac disease may exacerbate emotional problems and adversely affect mental health. This issue of interacting mental illness and cardiac disease has implications for both patients and for those with whom they live or associate. Spouses and children of patients most often bear persisting burdens of the dual problems of emotional and physical ailments. However, despite their ubiquity, we have little research thus far on manifestations of mental illness which develop in conjunction with continuing stresses associated with heart disease over the years. And the burdens, correlates, predictors, and consequences have not yet been adequately identified within the varying sub-types of patients who comprise the populations of heart patients in the chronic phase. In general, it appears cardiology, psychiatry, and epidemiology have given little attention to this matter. Medical School curricula as well typically offer little training to new physicians concerning the emotional consequences of chronic illness, such as heart disease. This issue is one which deserves to be addressed more thoroughly in the future.

Ego Structure, Coping, and Defense Mechanisms

One integral feature of the adaptive process in illness is that the individual passes through phases or stages of reinterpreting and integrating the experience. Some attempts have been made to specify models by which these processes occur, based on small series of heart patients and on observations drawn from clinical practice. Phases of initial denial, readjustment, reformulation, changes in self-image, and alterations of goals have been described, with most centering on the phases immediately following an acute event (Idelson, Croog, & Levine, 1974; Josten, 1970; Moos & Tsu, 1977). In what ways are processes of coping and stages of adjustment, for example, generally characteristic for all heart patients and which styles or variations in adaptive processes deserve specification? Thus far, there has been little empirical testing of the models, and research on possible alternate models for sub-segments within the heart patient population has received little attention.

According to prominent theories of personality, important components of adaptive processes are the mechanisms of defense by which the ego maintains its integrity and balance. In empirical studies of heart patients the full range of these mechanisms of defense and their functions in the adaptive process have generally been overlooked. Instead, major focus has been devoted virtually solely to the mechanism of denial. The importance of denial in the long-term illness process has been shown first in the pre-illness stage, influencing the time and occurrence of seeking medical care (Hackett & Cassem, 1969). In some work with patients in the immediate post-infarction period, studies have pointed out positive functions of initial denial, linking it with reduction of anxiety (Hackett & Rosenbaum, 1980).

However, the long term functions and implications of denial are less clear. Some studies have pointed up positive effects of initial denial in noting low mortality rates among deniers in periods immediately following heart attacks and in later rehabilitation outcomes (Stern, Pascale, McLoone, 1976; Stern et al. 1977).

Over the long-term, what happens to heart patients who deny their illness? Even in the case of this comparatively well researched area we have few data on subsequent adjustment and survival. Do the initially strong deniers remain so over the years? If they disregard their health, do they die in higher proportions than non-deniers? Are there degrees of denial or gradations which can be identified as salutary for specified populations?

The conditions and time periods in which denial constitutes a constructive response remain unclear. Over many months and years the patient denying his or her own heart disease may undertake behavior apparently inimical to health, such as extreme exertion, overwork, disregard to medications and dietary instructions from the physicians. If the quality of their lives is improved, if they can thereby gain satisfaction and function as "normal" individuals, is the denial maladaptive? Or is it beneficial in the sense that a short life of satisfaction can be preferable to a longer one of restrictions and invalidism? The questions illustrate some general problems associated with the lack of empirical data on which generalizations can be based.

Much of this research on denial is based on studies of small numbers of patients, and considerations of variation in definition, validity of measures, sampling, and lack of standardized instruments suggest need for caution in interpretation. Nonetheless, these suggestive findings help promise continued constructive controversy about the role of psychological coping mechanisms in affecting later physiological state, mortality and rehabilitation.

These problems relating to the denial mechanism in heart disease are one aspect of larger issues of relationships between post-hospital outcome variables and components of personality organization, coping process, and the defense mechanisms. Many of the theoretical approaches and findings in this area have been developed in studies of patients with mental illness. The nature of their possible application to persons with cardiac disease and other chronic illness remains as a challenge for empirical testing and validation.

Psychological Factors, Risk Factor Reduction, and Rehabilitation

Another type of influence of the psychological component upon outcomes concerns preventive behavior and the coronary risk factors. Smoking, hypertension, diet, and exercise level are all potentially modifiable insofar as they involve personal action such as following a regimen of hypertensive medications, adherence to dietary restrictions, exercising, and elimination of smoking (Dawber, 1980; Heiss, Haskell, Mowery, Criqui, Brockway, & Tyroler, 1980; Levy & Feinleib, 1980; Orleans, 1979). The psychological state of the patient may play an important part in determining preventive action to reduce risk factors.

One complication here is that the beneficial effects or risk factor reduction are less well established for persons with chronic coronary disease than for randomly selected populations. If psychological state makes a difference in risk factor reduction, does it thus empirically affect the course of coronary disease in patients who have had heart attacks? The matter may be particularly difficult to resolve, given problems of measurement of risk factor reduction, psychological factors, and physical and psychosocial outcomes in study populations.

Aside from the issue of mortality and morbidity, however, there are important questions about the effect of risk factor reduction upon emotional state and adjustment to the illness. For example, while exercise may or may not have a beneficial effect in prolonging life, its adherents maintain that it has merit in increasing psychological well-being (Hackett & Cassem, 1973; Heinzelmann, 1973; NHLBI, 1979). Hence the psychological resiliency and drive which leads patients to exercise as part of risk reduction may lead to other beneficial effects in adjustment and quality of life.

GAPS AND NEEDS IN THE RESEARCH LITERATURE: PSYCHOSOCIAL FACTORS IN RECOVERY AND REHABILITATION

In many ways our potential for developing generalizations about long-term recovery is limited by the nature of reports in the research literature, their strengths, their differing emphases, and their gaps and flaws. Hence, in considering directions of research on psychosocial aspects of recovery and rehabilitation, it is useful to note briefly some of the principal parameters which shape them. These include issues involving (a) conceptualization, (b) methods, and (c) the availability and form of documentation and empirical data.

1. Conceptual Issues

A core problem for characterization of psychosocial factors in recovery and rehabilitation lies in the nature of conceptualization of the dependent variable. What constitutes recovery and rehabilitation—in terms of the psychosocial areas—remains poorly defined. The scientific literature on heart disease reflects limited conceptualization and lack of agreement concerning criteria applicable to the broad range of heart patients with heterogeneous social, psychological, and economic characteristics. Most frequently the criteria employed consist of relatively simple measures in such areas as work return and functional capacity.

Moreover, in studies of long-term careers of heart patients, few models sufficiently take into account such issues as the following:

(a) The recovery process is an ongoing one, changing and shifting over time as new experiences are incorporated, integrated, and as the individual, both consciously and unconsciously, re-evaluates the initial acute experience and the current condition of chronic illness.

(b) In the post-hospital phase, adjustments to the illness are comprised of a series of adaptations in various spheres of the life of the individual, including the physical, the emotional, family and social relationships, work, financial expenditures, and sexual behavior, among others. These areas are not only interrelated in complex ways, but they have a dynamic aspect as well, with the relationships constantly changing over time.

(c) Degree of adaptation to the illness in each principal life area is not uniform at any particular point in time. Thus, the patient may have a favorable self-image, anxieties about the illness in the work situation, objectively competent work performance, and disturbance in role relationships with family members as a consequence of the heart disease. Presently, we have only limited means of deriving an additive measure of the total *gestalt* of the patient at a particular time. Since there is ongoing change in both external events and internal processes, conditions in each of the life areas are in constant flux. There may be, for example, less anxiety about heart disease at work, but there may be persisting stress and exertion on the job of a type objectively dangerous to health. Judging by the current theoretical literature, it still remains unclear how such phenomena can be best conceptualized and accurately measured in empirical research.

(d) The norms, values, and standards which shape the changing response and "adjustment" over the years of chronic disease experience vary among subgroups of heart patients in the population, differing by age, sex, occupational group, ethnic origin, and religious affiliation. How these operate within such sub-groups is not clear.

(e) How physiological process and behavioral patterns interact over time is also rarely approached in consideration of the long-term psychosocial factors in recovery and rehabilitation. Behavioral changes and life decisions may be stimulated by perceived symptoms, but it is likely that they are also affected in subtle ways by physiological processes, such as endocrine changes, effects on the nervous system induced by medications, and the responses of other major body systems to physiological change and functional limitation in the cardiovascular system.

2. Some Methodological Issues

A second principal parameter lies in the nature of the research reports themselves and the character of conclusions which may be drawn from empirical studies. Potential for generalization is hampered by such factors as the following: (1) a lack of systematic research in many principal areas pertaining to recovery and rehabilitation, particularly those concerned with sociological and anthropological variables; (2) relative inattention to variability within sub-groups, differing by age, sex, cardiovascular status, social class, ethnic origin, and personal ideology and values; (3) minimal use of control groups; and (4) few standardized instruments for measurement.

Where standardized measures have been employed, such as in regard to psychological characteristics or physical disability, their application in some studies may be questionable. For example, measures developed for use with mental patients may have acceptable validity levels with these specific populations, but may not be equally appropriate for other populations without psychopathology. Some critics question the utility of psychometric as opposed to behavioral measures in assessing outcomes in the chronic illness phase, maintaining that the record of observed behavior is more useful in evaluation than indicators of what a patient says he thinks or believes at the moment (National Heart, Lung and Blood Institute, 1979; Oberman, Ray, Turner, Barnes, & Grooms, 1975). Such conditions relating to conceptualization and methods are generic, of course, characteristic of many areas of research. Certainly studies of psychosocial factors in long-term recovery and rehabilitation are not unique in regard to such problems. We note them here, however, as they have set the context and frame of reference within which we review principal issues, findings, and directions of research.

3. Availability and Form of Documentation and Empirical Data

One consequence of the shaping of past research is that we can only draw upon limited published data concerning such areas as the following:

(a) The long-term, psychosocial processes of recovery, rehabilitation and adjustment to chronic illness such as heart disease is as yet poorly documented. Though a considerable number of people live for many years with heart disease, their patterns of personal coping, and changes in their adjustments to the illness in various areas of their lives have only infrequently been systematically researched. Main emphasis has been upon the first year or two following an acute cardiac event.

(b) Documentation of change and process within various important subgroups is generally lacking. For example, though cardiovascular disease afflicts females as well as males, virtually no studies are available on the female heart patient and her psychosocial adjustment. Similar comments can be made concerning the aged and the young, as well as persons other than "middle class," middle-aged, white males in American society.

(c) Changes in primary life areas and activities are largely undocumented, insofar as they relate to long-term recovery and living with heart disease. These include the changing influence of the family over the years, religion, work and retirement, sexuality, and the aging process.

(d) Minimal differentiation is made between the patient with one heart attack and those with multiple cardiac events in reports on psychosocial processes of recovery and rehabiliation. Analysis of long-term psychosocial factors rarely systematically controls for level of physical impairment, type of cardiac damage, occluded vessels, etc. Yet we cannot assume that the same psychosocial processes occur in patients with simple myocardial infarction, as compared with those with multiple episodes—or that the problems are somehow a multiplicative or additive function of number of acute cardiac episodes.

CONCLUSION

"What will happen to me? What can I do to prevent another heart attack? What should I be doing now?" These questions are representative of the practical concerns of many patients after a heart attack, and in another way they reflect the research concerns of many professionals in the biomedical and sociomedical communities as well. In this paper concerning lines of research on social and psychological aspects of the recovery of heart patients, we have pointed up areas of progress as well as prominent questions which remain to be answered.

It is well known that most heart patients who leave the hospital apparently do well and become re-engaged in their lives. However, data from the Social Security Administration indicate also great economic and social costs, associated with the fact that persons with cardiac disorders constitute the largest proportion of those receiving disability benefits. Beyond this, millions of heart patients may be living with some degree of outright physical disability—or with more subtle social, psychological and physical impairment associated with their chronic cardiac illness. And it is even more difficult to trace out the nature of the impairments and their costs and consequences for individuals, the community, and society.

Understanding the post-hospital recovery and rehabilitation processes among cardiac patients requires new conceptual approaches and more creative research if we are to proceed. For purposes of this chapter we have organized materials in terms of a multi-dimensional model, referring to principal life areas of patients and to applications of their armory of resources. The approach has pointed up some of the complex ways in which elements in each of the major life areas interweave in helping determine the long-term fate of the heart patient in terms of physical outcomes, quality of life, productive capacity, and social and psychological adjustment. The materials at the same time point up the fact that empirical data are meager in some principal areas—including many of central concern.

Among the various issues on which we need further empirical data for understanding recovery and rehabilitation of coronary patients, certain ones should have particular priority. First is the need for further specification of the nature of adjustment and adaptation to the disease, with particular reference to changes over the succeeding life span of the patient. A second one is the need for basic empirical documentation. In previous research, the phenomena of variation in adaptive processes, problems and use of resources have hardly been touched upon in relation to male-female differences, age groups, social class, ethnic and racial populations, and residents of non-metropolitan area. Even less is known about the social and psychological sequelae of heart disease among non-Western populations, particularly those with other than the Judaeo-Christian tradition.

A series of questions drawn from this review help point to other priority areas. For example, which intervention and support services provide patients the most benefit? What critical elements and processes in the families of heart patients are relevant to the course of their disease and their adjustment to it? In what ways do personality factors make a difference in the disease? What is the relationship between religious faith and belief to the processes of adjustment and adaptation to chronic heart disease? In what ways do the value systems of a community influence health care practices which in turn have some direct impact on the long-term fate of persons living with coronary disease?

Fortunately research in this area can be aided also by transferability of theory, methods, research instruments and findings from other relevant areas of social, psychological and medical research. These include studies in such fields as coping processes, social supports, family response to illness crisis, the role of psychosocial factors in illness, adjustment to problems of aging, factors in utilization and organization of services, relationships between work and physical and mental health.

Exploration of these issues of social and psychological factors in recovery has promise in many ways. It can provide a more systematic basis for planning programs, designating target populations with priority needs, and aiding heart patients in maintaining their lives as constructive members of society. Beyond this, however, such data can help produce generalizations relevant to understanding long-term recovery and rehabilitation in the case of other chronic illnesses as well. By increasing our knowledge of how men and women cope over the years with a life-threatening, often debilitating illness condition, such research may help us in dealing also with more basic existential questions—how men and women in the face of harsh circumstance can cope with the conditions of life and survival in the social context.

REFERENCES

Acker, J. E., Jr. Medical benefits and concerns in cardiac rehabilitation. In M. L. Pollock & D. H. Schmidt (Eds.), *Heart disease and rehabilitation*. Boston: Houghton Mifflin, 1979.

Adsett, C. A., & Bruhn, J. G. Short-term group psychotherapy for post-myocardial infarction patients and their wives. *The Canadian Medical Association Journal*, September 28, 1968, *99*, 577–584.

American Heart Association. *Directory: Cardiac rehabilitation units, 1975–76*. Dallas, Texas: January, 1976.

American Jurisprudence (2nd ed.). Workmen's compensation §300: Rupture, hernia, hemorrhage, stroke. Rochester, N.Y.: Lawyers Cooperative, 1966, *82*, 87–90.

Bakke, E. W. *The unemployed man*. New York: E. P. Dutton & Co., 1934.

Becker, M. H. Psychosocial aspects of health-related behavior. In H. W. Freeman, S. Levine, & L. G. Reeder (Eds.), *Handbook of medical sociology* (3rd ed.). Englewood Cliffs, N.J.: Prentice Hall, 1979.

Bloom, S. W., & Wilson, R. N. Patient-practitioner relationships. In H. W. Freeman, S. Levine, & L. G. Reeder (Eds.), *Handbook of medical sociology* (3rd ed.). Englewood Cliffs, N.J.: Prentice Hall, 1979.

Blumenthal, J. A., Williams, R. B., Kong, Y., Schanberg, S. M. & Thompson, L. W. Type A behavior and coronary atherosclerosis. *Circulation*, 1978, *58*, 634–639.

Bove, A. A. The cardiovascular response to stress. *Psychosomatics*, 1977, *18*, 13–17.

Brush, L. F. Heart injuries: When are they compensable? *New York State Bar Journal*, January, 1981, *53*, 23ff.

Cannon, W. *The wisdom of the body*. New York: W. W. Norton, 1932.

Caplan, G. *The principles of preventive psychiatry*. New York: Basic Books, 1964.

Caplan, G. *Support systems and community mental health*. New York: Behavioral Publications, 1974.

Caplan, G., & Killilea, M. (Eds.). *Support systems and mutual help: Multidisciplinary explorations.* New York: Grune & Stratton, 1976.

Caplan, R. D., Cobb, S., French, J. R. P., Jr., Harrison, R. V., & Pinneau, S. R., Jr. *Job demands and worker health: Main effects and occupational differences.* (U.S. Dept. of Health, Education, and Welfare Publ. No. N1OSH 75-160). Washington, D.C., U.S. Govt, Printing Office, April 1975.

Cassem, N. H., & Hackett, T. P. Psychiatric consultation in a coronary care unit. *Annals of Internal Medicine,* July 1971, *75,* 9–14.

Cay, E. L., Vetter, N., Philip, A. E., & Dugard, P. Psychological status during recovery from an acute heart attack. *Journal of Psychosomatic Research,* 1972, *16,* 425–435.

Chambers, W. N., & Reiser, M. F. Emotional stress and the precipitation of congestive heart failure. *Psychosomatic Medicine,* 1953, *15,* 38–60.

Comstock, G. W., & Partridge, K. B. Church attendance and health. *Journal of Chronic Diseases,* 1972, *25,* 665–672.

Cromwell, R. L., Butterfield, E. C., Brayfield, F. M., & Curry, J. J. *Acute myocardial infarction: Reaction and recovery.* St. Louis: C. V. Mosby Company, 1977.

Croog, S. H. Social aspects of cardiac rehabilitation: A selective review. In N. Wenger & H. Hellerstein (Eds.), *Rehabilitation of the patient after myocardial infarction.* New York: John Wiley and Sons, 1978.

Croog, S. H. The family as a source of stress. In S. Levine & N. A. Scotch (Eds.)., *Social stress.* Chicago: Aldine, 1970.

Croog, S. H., & Fitzgerald, E. F. Subjective stress and serious illness of a spouse: Wives of heart patients. *Journal of Health and Social Behavior,* 1978, *19,* 166–178.

Croog, S. H., & Levine, S. Religious identity and response to serious illness: A report on heart patients. *Social Science and Medicine,* 1972, *6,* 17–32.

Croog, S. H., & Levine, S. *The heart patient recovers: Social and psychological factors.* New York: Human Sciences Press, 1977.

Croog, S. H., & Levine, S. *Life after a heart attack: Social and psychological factors after eight years.* New York: Human Sciences Press, 1982.

Croog, S. H., Levine, S., & Lurie, Z. The heart patient and the recovery process: A review of directions of research on social and psychological factors. *Social Science and Medicine,* 1968, *2,* 111–164.

Croog, S. H., Lipson, A., & Levine, S. Help patterns in severe illness: The role of kin network and non-family resources. *Journal of Marriage and the Family,* 1972, *34,* 32–41.

Davidson, D. M. The family and cardiac rehabilitation. *Journal of Family Practice,* 1979, *8,* 253–261.

Dawber, T. R. *The Framingham study: The epidemiology of atherosclerotic disease.* Cambridge, Massachusetts: Harvard University Press, 1980.

Dawber, T. R. Foreword. In S. H. Croog & S. Levine, *Life after a heart attack: Social and psychological factors after eight years.* New York: Human Sciences Press, 1982.

DeBusk, R. F., Houston, N., Haskell, W., Fry, G., & Parker, M. Exercise training soon after myocardial infarction. *The American Journal of Cardiology,* 1979, *44,* 1223–1229.

Deegan, Fr. J. D. Coping with coronary heart disease: A pastoral care approach. *Minnesota Medicine,* January 1977, *60,* 30A–B.

Doehrman, S. R. Psycho-social aspects of recovery from coronary heart disease. *Social Science and Medicine,* 1977, *11,* 199–218.

Dohrenwend, B. P. Sociocultural and socio-psychological factors in the genesis of mental disorder. *Journal of Health and Social Behavior,* 1975, *16,* 365–392.

Dumont, M. P. Self-help treatment programs. *American Journal of Psychiatry,* 1974, *131,* 631–635.

Dunbar, F. *Mind and body: Psychosomatic medicine.* New York: Random House, 1948.

Dunbar, J. M., & Stunkard, A. J. Adherence to diet and drug regimen. In R. Levy, B. Rifkind, B. Dennis & N. Ernst (Eds.), *Nutrition, lipids, and coronary heart disease.* New York: Raven Press, 1979.

Dyer, Fr. Mark. Some religious aspects of support systems: Neo-pentecostal groups. In G. Caplan & M. Killilea (Eds.), *Support systems and mutual help: Multidisciplinary explorations.* New York: Grune & Stratton, 1976.

Eliot, R. S., & Buell, J. C. *Environmental and behavioral influences in the major cardiovascular disorders.* Paper presented at the First Annual Meeting of the Academy of Behavioral Medicine Research. Snowbird, Utah: June, 1979.

Engel, G. L. Sudden and rapid death during psychological stress. *Annals of Internal Medicine,* 1971, *74,* 771–782.

Finlayson, A., & McEwen, J. *Coronary heart disease and patterns of living.* New York: Prodist, 1977.

Frank, K. A., Heller, S. S., Kornfeld, D. S., Sporn, A. A., & Weiss, M. B. Type A behavior pattern and coronary angiographic findings. *Journal of the American Medical Association,* 1978, *240,* 761–763.

Garrity, T. F. Vocational adjustment after first myocardial infarction: Comparative assessment of several variables suggested in the literature. *Social Science and Medicine,* 1973, *7,* 705–717.

Garrity, T. F. *Behavioral adjustment after myocardial infarction: A selective review of recent descriptive, correlational and intervention research.* Paper presented at the First Annual Meeting of the Academy of Behavioral Medicine Research. Snowbird, Utah: June, 1979.

Garrity, T. F., & Klein, R. F. A behavioral predictor of survival among heart attack patients. In E. Palmore & F. G. Jeffers (Eds.), *Prediction of life span.* Lexington: D. C. Heath and Company, 1971.

Gentry, W. D. Preadmission behavior. In W. D. Gentry & R. B. Williams, *Psychological aspects of myocardial infarction and coronary care* (2nd ed.). St. Louis: C. V. Mosby, 1979.(a)

Gentry, W. D. Psychosocial concerns and benefits in cardiac rehabilitation. In M. L. Pollock & D. H. Schmidt (Eds.), *Heart disease and rehabilitation.* Boston: Houghton Mifflin, 1979.(b)

Gentry, W. D., & Haney, T. Emotional and behavioral reaction to acute myocardial infarction. *Heart and Lung,* 1975, *4,* 738–745.

Gore, S. *The influence of social support in ameliorating the consequences of job loss.* Unpublished dissertation, University of Michigan, 1973.

Gulledge, A. D. Psychological aftermaths of myocardial infarction. In W. D. Gentry & R. B. Williams, Jr. (Eds.). *Psychological aspects of myocardial infarction and coronary care* (2nd ed). St. Louis: C. V. Mosby, 1979.

Hackett, T. P. The use of groups in the rehabilitation of the post-coronary patient. *Advances in Cardiology,* 1978, *24,* 127–135.

Hackett, T. P., & Cassem, N. H. Factors contributing to delay in responding to the signs and symptoms of acute myocardial infarction. *The American Journal of Cardiology,* 1969, *24,* 651–658.

Hackett, T. P., & Cassem, N. H. Psychological adaptation to convalescence in myocardial infarction patients. In J. P. Naughton & H. K. Hellerstein (Eds.), *Exercise testing and exercise training in coronary heart disease.* New York: Academic Press, 1973.

Hackett, T. P., & Cassem, N. H. White collar and blue collar responses to heart attack. *Journal of Psychosomatic Research,* 1976, *20,* 85–95.

Hackett, T. P., & Rosenbaum, J. F. Emotion, psychiatric disorders, and the heart. In E. Braunwald (Ed.), *Heart Disease.* Philadelphia, Pa.: W. B. Saunders, 1980.

Halberstam, M. J., & Lesher, S. *A coronary event.* New York: Popular Library, 1978.

Heinzelmann, F. Social and psychological factors that influence the effectiveness of exercise programs. In J. P. Naughton & H. K. Hellerstein (Eds.), *Exercise testing and exercise training in coronary heart disease.* New York: Academic Press, 1973.

Heiss, G., Haskell, W., Mowery, R., Criqui, M. H., Brockway, M., & Tyroler, H. A. Plasma high-density lipoprotein cholesterol and socioeconomic status. *Circulation*, 1980, *62*, Supplement IV, IV–108–IV–114.

Hellerstein, H. K., & Friedman, E. H. Sexual activity and the post-coronary patient. *Archives of Internal Medicine*, 1970, *125*, 987–999.

Hellmuth, G. A. Is workmen's compensation a barrier to cardiac employment? *Archives of Environmental Health*, 1970, *20*, 404–409.

Hill, J., Hampton, J. R., & Mitchell, J. R. A randomized trial of home-versus-hospital management for patients with suspected myocardial infarction. *Lancet*, 1978, *1*, 837–841.

Hollender, M. H. *The psychology of medical practice*. Philadelphia: W. B. Saunders, 1958.

House, J. S. Occupational stress as a precursor to coronary disease. In W. D. Gentry & R. B. Williams, Jr. (Eds.), *Psychological aspects of myocardial infarction and coronary care*. St. Louis: The C. V. Mosby Co., 1975.

Humphries, J. O. Survival after myocardial infarction. *Modern concepts of cardiovascular disease*, 1977, *46*, 51–56.

Ibrahim, M., Feldman, J. G., Sultz, H. A., Staiman, M. G., Young, L. J., & Dean, D. Management after myocardial infarction: A controlled trial of the effect of group psychotherapy. *International Journal of Psychiatry in Medicine*, 1974, *5*, 253–268.

Idelson, R. K., Croog, S. H., & Levine, S. Changes in self-concept during the year after a first heart attack: A natural history approach. *American Archives of Rehabilitation Therapy*, 1974, *22*, 10–21, 25–31.

Jenkins, C. D. Psychologic and social precursors of coronary disease. *New England Journal of Medicine*, 1971, *284*, 244–255, 307–317.

Jenkins, C. D. Recent evidence supporting psychologic and social risk factors for coronary disease. *New England Journal of Medicine*, 1976, *294*, 987–994, 1033–1038.

Jenkins, C. D. Behavioral risk factors in coronary artery disease. *Annual Review of Medicine*, 1978, *29*, 543–562.

Jenkins, C. D. The coronary-prone personality. In W. D. Gentry & R. B. Williams, Jr. (Eds.), *Psychological aspects of myocardial infarction and coronary care* (2nd ed.). St. Louis: C. V. Mosby, 1979.

Jenkins, C. D., Zyzanski, S. J., & Rosenman, R. H. Risk of new myocardial infarction in middle-aged men with manifest coronary heart disease. *Circulation*, 1976, *53*, 342–347.

Johnson, L. B. *The vantage point: Perspectives of the presidency, 1963–1969*. New York: Holt, Rinehart & Winston, 1971.

Josten, J. Emotional adaptation of cardiac patients. *Scandinavian Journal of Rehabilitative Medicine*, 1970, *2–3*, 49–52.

Kannel, W. B., Sorlie, P., & McNamara, P. M. Prognosis after initial myocardial infarction: The Framingham Study. *American Journal of Cardiology*. 1979, *44*, 53–59.

Kaplan, B. H., Cassel, J. C., & Gore, S. Social support and health. *Medical Care*, May 1977, 15 (Supplement), 47–58.

Kavanagh, T., Shephard, R. J., & Tuck, J. A. Depression after myocardial infarction. *The Canadian Medical Association Journal*, 1975, *113*, 23–27.

Klein, R. F., Garrity, T. F., & Gelein, J. Emotional adjustment and catecholamine excretion during early recovery from myocardial infarction. *Journal of Psychosomatic Research*, 1974, *18*, 425–435.

Krantz, D. S. Cognitive processes and recovery from heart attack: A review and theoretical analysis. *Journal of Human Stress*, 1980, *6*, 27–38.

Krantz, D. S., Baum, A., & Wideman, M. V. Assessment of preferences for self-treatment and information in health care. *Journal of Personality and Social Psychology*, 1980, *39*, 977–990.

Kuller, L. H. Natural history of coronary heart disease. In M. L. Pollock & D. H. Schmidt (Eds.), *Heart disease and rehabilitation*. Boston: Houghton Mifflin, 1979.

Lear, M. *Heartsounds*. New York: Simon & Schuster, 1980.

Leighton, A. H. *My name is legion*. New York: Basic Books, 1959.

Lesher, S. After a heart attack, there comes a will to live—well. *The New York Times Magazine,* January 27, 1974, *1,* 9–32.

Levin, L. S., Katz, A. H., & Holst, E. *Self-care: Lay initiatives in health*. (2nd ed.). New York: Prodist, 1979.

Levine, S., White, P. E., & Paul, B. D. Community interorganizational problems in providing medical care and social services. *American Journal of Public Health, 1963, 53,* 1183–1195.

Levy, R. I., & Feinleib, M. Risk factors for coronary artery disease and their management. In E. Braunwald (Ed.), *Heart disease*. Philadelphia: W. B. Saunders, 1980.

Litman, T. J. The family as a basic unit in health and medical care: A social-behavioral overview. *Social Science and Medicine, 1974, 8,* 495–519.

Lown, B., Verrier, R. L., & Rabinowitz, S. H. Neural and psychologic mechanisms and the problem on sudden cardiac death. *American Journal of Cardiology. 1977, 39,* 890–902.

Maccoby, N., Farquhar, J. W., Wood, P. D., & Alexander, J. Reducing the risk of CV disease: Effects of a community-based campaign on knowledge and behavior. *Journal of Community Health, 1977, 3,* 100–114.

Marston, M. Compliance with medical regimens: A review of the literature. *Nursing Research,* 1970, *19,* 312–323.

Mather, H., et al. Acute myocardial infarction: Home and hospital treatment. *British Medical Journal, 1971, 3,* 334–338.

Mather, H. G., et al. Myocardial infarction: A comparison between home and hospital care for patients. *British Medical Journal, 1976, 1,* 925–929.

Mayou, R., Foster, A., & Williamson, B. Psychological and social effects of myocardial infarction on wives. *British Medical Journal, 1978, 1,* 699–701.

McLane, M., Krop, H., & Mehta, J. Psychosexual adjustment and counseling after myocardial infarction. *Annals of Internal Medicine,* 1980, *92,* 514–519.

Moos, R. H., & Tsu, V. D. The crisis of physical illness: An overview. In R. H. Moos (Ed.), *Coping with physical illness*. New York: Plenum, 1977.

The multiple risk factor intervention trial (MRFIT). A national study of primary prevention of coronary heart disease. *Journal of the American Medical Association, 1976, 235,* 825–828.

Nagle, R., Gangola, R., & Picton-Robinson, I. Factors influencing return to work after myocardial infarction. *Lancet, 1971, 2,* 454–456.

Naismith, L. D., Robinson, J. F., Shaw, G. B., & MacIntyre, M. M. J. Psychological rehabilitation after myocardial infarction. *British Medical Journal, 1979, 1,* 439–442.

National Commission on State Workmen's Compensation Laws. *Compendium on workmen's compensation*. Washington, D.C.: U.S. Government Printing Office, 1973.

National Heart, Lung and Blood Institute. *Proceedings of the Workshop on Physical Conditioning and Training,* National Institutes of Health, Bethesda, Maryland, May 16–17, 1979.

Naughton, J. Vocational aspects of rehabilitation after myocardial infarction. In N. K. Wenger & H. K. Hellerstein (Eds.), *Rehabilitation of the coronary patient*. New York: John Wiley and Sons, 1978, pp. 283–294.

Naughton, J., & Hellerstein, H. K. (Eds.). *Exercise testing and exercise training in coronary heart disease*. New York: Academic Press, 1973.

Ness, R. C. The impact of indigenous healing activity: An empirical study of two fundamentalist churches. *Social Science and Medicine,* 1980, *14B,* 167–180.

Nuckolls, K. B., Cassel, J. C., & Kaplan, B. H. Psychosocial assets, life crisis and the prognosis of pregnancy. *American Journal of Epidemiology, 1972, 95,* 431–441.

Oberman, A., Ray, M., Turner, M. E., Barnes, G., & Grooms, C. Sudden death in patients evaluated for ischemic heart disease. *Circulation, 1975, 52* (Supplement III), 170–175.

Obier, K., MacPherson, M., & Haywood, J. L. Predictive value of psychosocial profiles following acute myocardial infarction. *Journal of the National Medical Association,* 1977, *69,* 59–61.

Orleans, C. S. Behavioral approaches to risk reduction in coronary patients. In W. D. Gentry & R. B. Williams, Jr. (Eds.), *Psychological aspects of myocardial infarction and coronary care* (2nd ed.). St. Louis: C. V. Mosby, 1979.

Paffenbarger, R. S., Laughlin, M. E., Gima, A. S., & Black, R. A. Work activity of longshoremen as related to death from coronary heart disease and stroke. *The New England Journal of Medicine,* 1970, *282,* 1109–1114.

Pattison, E. M., Lapins, N. A., & Doerr, H. A. Faith healing: A study of personality and function. *Journal of Nervous and Mental Disorders,* 1973, *157,* 397–409.

Pratt, L. *Family structure and effective health behavior: The energized family.* Boston: Houghton Mifflin, 1976.

Proudfit, W. L., Bruschke, A. V. G., & Sones, F. M., Jr. Natural history of obstructive coronary artery disease: Ten year study of 601 non-surgical cases. *Progress in Cardiovascular Diseases,* 1978, *21,* 53–78.

Radcliffe-Brown, A. R. Taboo. In *Structure and function in primitive society.* London: Cohen and West, 1952.

Rahe, R. H., Ward, H. W., & Hayes, V. Brief group therapy in myocardial infarction rehabilitation: Three to four-year follow-up of a controlled trial. *Psychosomatic Medicine,* 1979, *41,* 229–242.

Roskies, E., Spevack, M., Surkis, A., Cohen, C., & Gilman, S. Changing the coronary prone (Type A) behavior pattern in a non-clinical population. *Journal of Behavioral Medicine,* 1978, *1,* 201–216.

Ruskin, H. D., Stein, L. L., Shelsky, I. M., & Bailey, M. A. MMPI: Comparison between patients with coronary heart disease and their spouses together with other demographic data. *Scandinavian Journal of Rehabilitative Medicine.* 1970, *2–3,* 99–104.

Sackett, D., & Haynes, R. B. (Eds.). *Compliance with therapeutic regimens.* Baltimore: Johns Hopkins University Press, 1976.

Scalzi, C. C., & Dracup, K. Sexual counseling of coronary patients. In W. D. Gentry & R. B. Williams, Jr. (Eds.), *Psychological aspects of myocardial infarction and coronary care* (2nd ed.). St. Louis: C. V. Mosby, 1979.

Shapiro, S., Weinblatt, E., & Frank, C. W. Return to work after first myocardial infarction. *Archives of Environmental Health,* January 1972, *24,* 17–26.

Skelton, M., & Dominian, J. Psychological stress in wives of patients with myocardial infarction. *British Medical Journal,* 1973, *2,* 101–103.

Smith, R. T. Rehabilitation of the disabled: The role of social networks in the recovery process. *International Rehabilitative Medicine,* 1979, *1,* 63–72.

Smith, R. T. Role of social resources in cardiovascular rehabilitation. *Proceedings of the Workshop on Physical Conditioning and Rehabilitation,* National Heart, Lung and Blood Institute, May 16–17, 1979.

Stern, M. J., & Pascale, L. Psychosocial adaptation post-myocardial infarction: The spouse's dilemma. *Journal of Psychosomatic Research,* 1979, *23,* 83–87.

Stern, M. J., Pascale, L., & Ackerman, A. Life adjustment post-myocardial infarction: Determining predictive variables. *Archives of Internal Medicine,* 1977, *137,* 1680–1685.

Stern, M. J., Pascale, L., & McLoone, J. B. Psychosocial adaptation following an acute myocardial infarction. *Journal of Chronic Diseases,* 1976, *29,* 513–526.

Surwillo, W. W., & Hobson, D. P. Brain electrical activity during prayer. *Psychological Reports,* 1978, *43,* 135–143.

Syme, S. L. Life style intervention in clinic-based trials. *American Journal of Epidemiology,* 1978, *108,* 87–91.

Szasz, T. S., & Hollender, M. H. A contribution to the philosophy of medicine: The basic models of the doctor-patient relationship. *A.M.A. Archives of Internal Medicine,* 1956, *97,* 585–592.

Treitel, R. *Rehabilitation of disabled adults, 1972.* Social Security Survey of the Disabled: 1972. Disabled and non-disabled adults. Social Security Administration, Office of Research and Statistics. Report No. 3, 1977. DHEW Publication No. (SSA) 77–11717.

U.S. Department of Health, Education and Welfare, Public Health Service, Office of the Assistant Secretary for Health. *Health-United States: 1978.* (DHEW Pub. No. PHS 78–1232) Washington, D.C.: U.S. Government Printing Office, December 1978.

Vaux, K. Religion and health. *Preventive Medicine,* 1976, *5,* 522–536.

Weissman, M. M., Myers, J. K., & Harding, P. S. Psychiatric disorders in a U.S. urban community: 1975–1976. *American Journal of Psychiatry,* 1978, *135,* 459–462.

Wenger, N. K. Patient and family education after myocardial infarction. *Postgraduate Medicine,* 1975, *57,* 129–134.

Wishnie, H. A., Hackett, T. P., & Cassem, N. H. Psychological hazards of convalescence following myocardial infarction. *Journal of the American Medical Association,* February 22, 1971, *215,* 1292–1296.

Wynn, A. Unwarranted emotional distress in men with ischaemic heart disease (IHD). *The Medical Journal of Australia,* November 4, 1967, 847–851.

Author Index

Numbers in *italics* refer to the pages on which the complete references are listed.

Subject Index